NEW APPROACHES TO THE STUDY OF BENIGN PROSTATIC HYPERPLASIA

Workshop Organizing Committee

Allen E. Buhl, PhD
Donald B. Carter, PhD
Frances A. Kimball, PhD

Workshop Host

The Upjohn Company

PROGRESS IN CLINICAL AND BIOLOGICAL RESEARCH

RECENT TITLES

Vol 115: **Prevention of Hereditary Large Bowel Cancer,** John R.F. Ingall, Anthony J. Mastromarino, *Editors*

Vol 116: **New Concepts in Thyroid Disease,** Roberto J. Soto, Gerardo Sartorio, Ismael de Forteza, *Editors*

Vol 117: **Reproductive Toxicology,** Donald R. Mattison, *Editor*

Vol 118: **Growth and Trophic Factors,** J. Regino Perez-Polo, Jean de Vellis, Bernard Haber, *Editors*

Vol 119: **Oncogenes and Retroviruses: Evaluation of Basic Findings and Clinical Potential,** Timothy E. O'Connor, Frank J. Rauscher, Jr., *Editors*

Vol 120: **Advances in Cancer Control: Research and Development,** Paul F. Engstrom, Paul N. Anderson, Lee E. Mortenson, *Editors*

Vol 121: **Progress in Cancer Control III: A Regional Approach,** Curtis Mettlin, Gerald P. Murphy, *Editors*

Vol 122: **Advances in Blood Substitute Research,** Robert B. Bolin, Robert P. Geyer, George J. Nemo, *Editors*

Vol 123: **California Serogroup Viruses,** Charles H. Calisher, Wayne H. Thompson, *Editors*

Vol 124: **Epilepsy: An Update on Research and Therapy,** Giuseppe Nisticò, Raoul Di Perri, H. Meinardi, *Editors*

Vol 125: **Sulfur Amino Acids: Biochemical and Clinical Aspects,** Kinya Kuriyama, Ryan J. Huxtable, Heitaroh Iwata, *Editors*

Vol 126: **Membrane Biophysics II: Physical Methods in the Study of Epithelia,** Mumtaz A. Dinno, Arthur B. Callahan, Thomas C. Rozzell, *Editors*

Vol 127: **Orphan Drugs and Orphan Diseases: Clinical Realities and Public Policy,** George J. Brewer, *Editor*

Vol 128: **Research Ethics,** Kåre Berg, Knut Erik Tranøy, *Editors*

Vol 129: **Zinc Deficiency in Human Subjects,** Ananda S. Prasad, Ayhan O. Çavdar, George J. Brewer, Peter J. Aggett, *Editors*

Vol 130: **Progress in Cancer Control IV: Research in the Cancer Center,** Curtis Mettlin, Gerald P. Murphy, *Editors*

Vol 131: **Ethopharmacology: Primate Models of Neuropsychiatric Disorders,** Klaus A. Miczek, *Editor*

Vol 132: **13th International Cancer Congress,** Edwin A. Mirand, William B. Hutchinson, Enrico Mihich, *Editors.* Published in 5 Volumes: Part A: **Current Perspectives in Cancer.** Part B: **Biology of Cancer (1).** Part C: **Biology of Cancer (2).** Part D: **Research and Treatment.** Part E: **Cancer Management**

Vol 133: **Non-HLA Antigens in Health, Aging, and Malignancy,** Elias Cohen, Dharam P. Singal, *Editors*

Vol 134: **Globin Gene Expression and Hematopoietic Differentiation,** George Stamatoyannopoulos, Arthur W. Nienhuis, *Editors*

Vol 135: **Developmental Pharmacology,** Stuart M. MacLeod, Allan B. Okey, Stephen P. Spielberg, *Editors*

Vol 136: **Hypoxia, Exercise, and Altitude: Proceedings of the Third Banff International Hypoxia Symposium,** John R. Sutton, Charles S. Houston, Norman L. Jones, *Editors*

Vol 137: **PCB Poisoning in Japan and Taiwan,** Masanori Kuratsune, Raymond E. Shapiro, *Editors*

Vol 138: **Chemical Taxonomy, Molecular Biology, and Function of Plant Lectins,** Irwin J. Goldstein, Marilynn E. Etzler, *Editors*

Vol 139: **Difficult Decisions in Medical Ethics: The Fourth Volume in a Series on Ethics, Humanism, and Medicine,** Doreen Ganos, Rachel E. Lipson, Gwynedd Warren, Barbara J. Weil, *Editors*

Vol 140: **Abnormal Functional Development of the Heart, Lungs, and Kidneys: Approaches to Functional Teratology,** Casimer T. Grabowski and Robert J. Kavlock, *Editors*

Vol 141: **Industrial Hazards of Plastics and Synthetic Elastomers,** Jorma Järvisalo, Pirkko Pfäffli, Harri Vainio, *Editors*

Vol 142: **Hormones and Cancer,** Erlio Gurpide, Ricardo Calandra, Carlos Levy, Roberto J. Soto, *Editors*

Vol 143: **Viral Hepatitis and Delta Infection,** Giorgio Verme, Ferruccio Bonino, Mario Rizzetto, *Editors*

Vol 144: **Chemical and Biological Aspects of Vitamin B_6 Catalysis,** A.E. Evangelopoulos, *Editor.* Published in 2 volumes. Part A: **Metabolism, Structure, and Function of Phosphorylases, Decarboxylases, and Other Enzymes.** Part B: **Metabolism, Structure, and Function of Transaminases.**

Vol 145: **New Approaches to the Study of Benign Prostatic Hyperplasia,** Frances A. Kimball, Allen E. Buhl, and Donald B. Carter, *Editors*

See pages following the index for previous titles in this series.

NEW APPROACHES TO THE STUDY OF BENIGN PROSTATIC HYPERPLASIA

Proceedings of the Ninth Brook Lodge Workshop on Problems in Reproductive Physiology, held in Augusta, Michigan, September 26–27, 1983

Editors

FRANCES A. KIMBALL, PhD
Fertility Research
The Upjohn Company
Kalamazoo, Michigan

ALLEN E. BUHL, PhD
Fertility Research
The Upjohn Company
Kalamazoo, Michigan

DONALD B. CARTER, PhD
Molecular Biology Research
The Upjohn Company
Kalamazoo, Michigan

ALAN R. LISS, INC. • NEW YORK

Address all Inquiries to the Publisher
Alan R. Liss, Inc., 150 Fifth Avenue, New York, NY 10011

Printed in the United States of America.

Library of Congress Cataloging in Publication Data

Brook Lodge Workshop on Problems in Reproductive
Physiology (9th: 1983: Augusta, Mich.)
New approaches to the study of benign prostatic
hyperplasia.

(Progress in clinical and biological research; v. 145)
"Host, the Upjohn Company."
Includes index.
1. Prostate gland—Hypertrophy—Congresses.
2. Prostate gland—Hypertrophy—Animal models—Congresses. 1. Buhl, Allen E. II. Carter, Donald B.
III. Kimball, Frances A. IV. Upjohn Company. V. Title.
VI. Series.
RC 899.B76 1983 616.6′5 83-26833
ISBN 0-8451-0145-5

Contents

Contributors and Participants

***Edward P. Ajemian,** Bronson Medical Center, Kalamazoo, MI 49001

***Georg Bartsch,** Department of Urology, University of Innsbruck, Innsbruck, Austria **[159]**

***John A. Belis,** Department of Urology, West Virginia University School of Medicine, Morgantown, WV 26506 **[345]**

***Bijoy K. Bhuyan,** The Upjohn Company, Kalamazoo, MI 49001

A. Brüngger, Department of Pathology, University of Basel, Basel, Switzerland **[159]**

***Allen E. Buhl,** Fertility Research, The Upjohn Company, Kalamazoo, MI 49001 **[xiii]**

***J. Allan Campbell,** The Upjohn Company, Kalamazoo, MI 49001

***Donald B. Carter,** Molecular Biology Research, The Upjohn Company, Kalamazoo, MI 49001 **[xiii]**

***Leland W.K. Chung,** Department of Pharmacology, School of Pharmacy, University of Colorado, Boulder, CO 80309 **[291]**

***Gerald R. Cunha,** Department of Anatomy, University of California Medical School, San Francisco, CA 94143 **[67,81]**

***Roger S. Cunningham,** The Upjohn Company, Kalamazoo, MI 49001

G. Daxenbichler, Department of Gynecology, University of Innsbruck, Innsbruck, Austria **[159]**

***Raymond M. DeHaan,** The Upjohn Company, Kalamazoo, MI 49001

William R. Fair, Department of Surgery/Division of Urology, Washington University School of Medicine, St. Louis, MO 63110 **[181]**

***Richard Frederickson,** Department of Anatomy, West Virginia University Medical Center, Morgantown, WV 26506 **[143]**

***Earl S. Gerard,** The Upjohn Company, Kalamazoo, MI 49001

***Ernest A. Gilling,** The Upjohn Company, Kalamazoo, MI 49001

***Denis J. Gospodarowicz,** Cancer Research Institute, University of California Medical Center, San Francisco, CA 94143 **[103]**

Warren D.W. Heston, Department of Surgery/Division of Urology, Washington University School of Medicine, St. Louis, MO 63110 **[181]**

H. Hintner, Department of Dermatology, University of Innsbruck, Innsbruck, Austria **[159]**

***John T. Isaacs,** Department of Urology and Oncology, Johns Hopkins University School of Medicine, Baltimore, MD 21205 **[217]**

***William B. Isaacs,** Department of Urology and Pharmacology, Johns Hopkins University School of Medicine, Baltimore, MD 21205 **[307]**

Stephen C. Jacobs, Department of Urology, Medical College of Wisconsin, Milwaukee, WI 53226 **[197]**

***Fred Kagan,** The Upjohn Company, Kalamazoo, MI 49001

*Indicates participant of Workshop on Problems in Reproductive Physiology.

The boldface number in brackets indicates the opening page number of a contributor's article.

***James P. Karr**, Department of Experimental Surgery, Roswell Park Memorial Institute, Buffalo, NY 14263 **[257]**

***Benita S. Katzenellenbogen**, Department of Physiology and Biophysics, University of Illinois, Urbana, IL 61801

***L.H. Li**, The Upjohn Company, Kalamazoo, MI 49001

Eli F. Lizza, Department of Urology, West Virginia University School of Medicine, Morgantown, WV 26506 **[345]**

***Mark A. Lucas**, Bronson Medical Center, Kalamazoo, MI 49001

***Thomas A. Marks**, The Upjohn Company, Kalamazoo, MI 49001

Ch. Marth, Department of Gynecology, University of Innsbruck, Innsbruck, Austria **[159]**

***Patricia L. Kemp**, The Upjohn Company, Kalamazoo, MI 49001

Untae Kim, Department of Pathology, Roswell Park Memorial Institute, Buffalo, NY 14263 **[257]**

***Frances A. Kimball**, Fertility Research, The Upjohn Company, Kalamazoo, MI 49001 **[xiii]**

***Kenneth T. Kirton**, The Upjohn Company, Kalamazoo, MI 49001

***James W. Lauderdale**, The Upjohn Company, Kalamazoo, MI 49001

W. Dwayne Lawrence, Department of Pathology, Massachusetts General Hospital, Boston MA 02114 **[67]**

Russell K. Lawson, Department of Urology, Medical College of Wisconsin, Milwaukee, WI 53226 **[197]**

Karl H. Leissner, Department of Surgery, Mölndal's Hospital, Mölndal, Sweden 431 80 **[333]**

***Robert A. Lepley**, The Upjohn Company, Kalamazoo, MI 49001

***Ronald W. Lewis**, Department of Urology, Tulane University Delta Regional Primate Research Center, Covington, LA 70433 **[235]**

Lucinda Mata, Department of Cell Biology, Glubenkian Institute of Science, Oeiras, Portugal **[143]**

James Matsuura, Department of Pharmacology, School of Pharmacy, University of Colorado, Boulder, CO 80309 **[291]**

***Michael G. Mawhinney**, Departments of Urology and Pharmacology/Toxicology, West Virginia University School of Medicine, Morgantown, WV 26506 **[143]**

***John E. McNeal**, Division of Urology, Stanford University Medical Center, Stanford, CA 94305 **[27]**

Gary J. Miller, Department of Pathology, University of Colorado Health Sciences Center, Denver, CO 80262 **[291]**

***William L. Miller, Jr.**, The Upjohn Company, Kalamazoo, MI 49001

Gerald P. Murphy, Department of Experimental Surgery, Roswell Park Memorial Institute, Buffalo, NY 14263 **[257]**

***Gary L. Neil**, The Upjohn Company, Kalamazoo, MI 49001

***Melvin L. Noah**, The Upjohn Company, Kalamazoo, MI 49001

***Peter Ofner**, Department of Urology, Tufts University School of Medicine, Boston, MA 02111 **[363]**

***Richard F. Parrish**, Department of Surgery/Division of Urology, Washington University School of Medicine, St. Louis, MO 63110 **[181]**

***L. Susan Pletscher**, Department of Surgery/Division of Urology, Washington University School of Medicine, St. Louis, MO 63110 **[181]**

***Martin I. Resnick**, Department of Urology, Case Western Reserve, Cleveland, OH 44106

***Stanley J. Robboy**, Department of Pathology, Massachusetts General Hospital, Boston, MA 02114 **[67]**

Audrey K. Rocco, Department of Pharmacology, School of Pharmacy, University of Colorado, Boulder, CO 80309 **[291]**

***Keith Roe,** The Upjohn Company, Kalamazoo, MI 49001

H.P. Rohr, Department of Pathology, University of Basel, Basel, Switzerland **[159]**

Meredith N. Runner, Department of Molecular, Cellular, and Developmental Biology, University of Colorado, Boulder, CO 80309 **[291]**

Håkan Salander, Department of Surgery, Vänerborg's Hospital, Vänerborg, Sweden 46201 **[55]**

Avery A. Sandberg, Department of Genetics and Endocrinology, Roswell Park Memorial Institute, Buffalo, NY 14263 **[257]**

***Francis J. Schwende,** The Upjohn Company, Kalamazoo, MI 49001

U. Schweikert, Department of Internal Medicine, University of Bonn, Bonn, Federal Republic of Germany **[159]**

***Thomas C. Smith,** The Upjohn Company, Kalamazoo, MI 49001

***Charles H. Spilman,** The Upjohn Company, Kalamazoo, MI 49001

U. Stanzl, Department of Dermatology, University of Innsbruck, Innsbruck, Austria **[159]**

***Michael T. Story,** Department of Urology, Medical College of Wisconsin, Milwaukee, WI 53226 **[197]**

Russell Tackett, Department of Surgery/Division of Urology, Washington University School of Medicine, St. Louis, MO 63110 **[181]**

William F. Tarry, Department of Urology, West Virginia University School of Medicine, Morgantown, WV 26506 **[345]**

Louis Terracio, Department of Anatomy, University of South Carolina School of Medicine, Columbia, SC 29208 **[363]**

Timothy C. Thompson, Department of Pharmacology, School of Pharmacy, University of Colorado, Boulder, CO 80309 **[291]**

Mark O. Thornton, Departments of Urology and Pharmacology/Toxicology, West Virginia University Medical Center, Morgantown, WV 26506 **[143]**

***Lars-Eric Tisell,** Department of Surgery I, University of Göteborg, Sahlgren's Hospital, Göteborg, Sweden 413 45 **[55, 333]**

***Paul L. Van Den Brink,** Bronson Medical Center, Kalamazoo, MI 49001

Richard L. Vena, Department of Urology, Tufts University School of Medicine, Boston, MA 02111 **[363]**

***Patrick C. Walsh,** Department of Urology, Johns Hopkins Hospital, Baltimore, MD 21205 **[1]**

***Max S. Wicha,** Department of Internal Medicine, University of Michigan Simpson Memorial Research Institute, Ann Arbor, MI 48109 **[129]**

***John W. Wilks,** The Upjohn Company, Kalamazoo, MI 49001

***Yang-Dar Yuan,** The Upjohn Company, Kalamazoo, MI 49001

***Robert G. Zimbelman,** The Upjohn Company, Kalamazoo, MI 49001

Preface

This, the Ninth Brook Lodge Conference on Problems of Reproductive Physiology, is the latest in a series of small meetings held over 22 years. The topics for these meetings reflect the changing state of knowledge on various topics and interests of the organizers. The rapid increase in information on human benign prostatic hyperplasia and the search for a medical method to intervene in this process stimulated the organizers to focus the 1983 workshop on this topic. The first four speakers provide histological and morphological background for the molecular and biochemical studies described subsequently. The interactions of biochemist, physiologist, pathologist, and physician as they focus their thoughts and talents on this area are apparent in the discussions of presentations. This workshop was planned to provide insight and a sense of synthesis for the participants. For the reader, the record of the proceedings should serve as a useful record to the state of the art in this research area.

Benign prostatic hyperplasia, a commonly occurring condition in older men, is currently treated at the onset of urethral blockage with mechanical or surgical manipulation. Examination of the physical relationship, biochemical interactions, and hormonal influences in this complex tissue could further advance the understanding of this disease. A more complete understanding of the prostate physiology should be reflected in our ability to better control this organ and to treat its dysfunction.

The efforts of many individuals made these Proceedings possible. Members of the research community at The Upjohn Company planned and organized the program. This meeting was a success because of the contributions of the workshop participants who prepared manuscripts and participated in the discussions. We also wish to thank Drs. Georg Bartsch, Gerald R. Cunha, John E. McNeal, and Michael G. Mawhinney for serving as session chairpersons. The hospitality provided by the staff at Brook Lodge was an important feature in providing the atmosphere for this workshop. The skillful efforts of Marcia Campbell and Edna Rose in preparation of the discussions are appreciated.

Frances A. Kimball, PhD
Allen E. Buhl, PhD
Donald B. Carter, PhD

New Approaches to the Study
of Benign Prostatic Hyperplasia, pages 1–25

HUMAN BENIGN PROSTATIC HYPERPLASIA: ETIOLOGICAL CONSIDERATIONS

Patrick C. Walsh, M.D.

Director, The James Buchanan Brady Urological
Institute of the Johns Hopkins Hospital
Baltimore, Maryland 21205

Benign prostatic hyperplasia (BPH) is probably the most common neoplastic growth that occurs in men. Beginning with the early observations of Morgagni (1760) it was recognized that BPH arose from the inner periurethral glands of the prostate; a century later surgical techniques were developed for the removal of this tissue. Although over the ensuing years these advances have provided a logical and satisfactory form of treatment for this disorder, much remains to be learned about the causes, pathogenesis, and possible medical management of prostatic hyperplasia. It is estimated that 75% of males over 50 years of age have symptoms arising from BPH and that over 290,000 surgical procedures are performed each year to relieve this condition. This makes BPH the second leading cause of surgery in men with an overall medical cost that well exceeds $1 billion per year in the United States. These facts emphasize the need for further investigation to uncover the etiology of this disorder and to provide alternative forms of treatment.

NATURAL HISTORY

As demonstrated by Swyer many years ago (1944), there is a very slow increase in the size of the prostate from the time of birth until puberty. At that time a rapid increase in size occurs that continues until after the third decade is reached. The size of the prostate then remains constant until about the age of 45. Thereafter there is a gradual increase in prostatic weight.

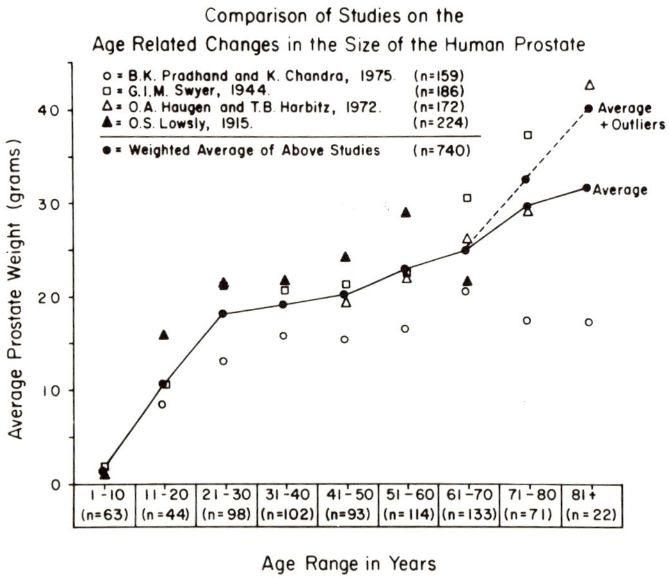

Fig. 1. Age-related changes in the size of the human prostate. Data summarized from 4 published autopsy series from a total of 740 human subjects. (Published with permission of Stephen Berry).

The data in Fig. 1 have been compiled by Stephen Berry from 4 major autopsy series comprising a total of 740 human specimens in which the size of the human prostate has been correlated with age (Lowsley 1915; Swyer 1944; Haugen Harbitz 1972; Pradhan, Chandra 1975). The solid line connecting the dark circles denotes the weighted average obtained from the 4 studies. Two of the 4 studies contained a few specimens that were extremely large and could be shown to be outliers from the general average and when they are included they raise the overall average as shown by the broken line.

In other autopsy series, histologic criteria have been utilized to define the presence of BPH at various ages. Fig. 2 summarizes data from 5 autopsy series based upon a total of 1,067 human subjects (Moore 1943; Swyer 1944; Franks 1954; Haugen, Harbitz 1972; Pradhan, Chandra 1975). Histologically BPH is rarely identified in men under the age of 40 years. However, beginning in the forties the incidence of BPH increases from an average of 23% to 88% by the 9th decade. Although this reflects the incidence of BPH as determined in histological sections by the pathologist, it does not indicate the sizes of the prostates associated with this disease. On Fig. 2 we have reproduced the data on

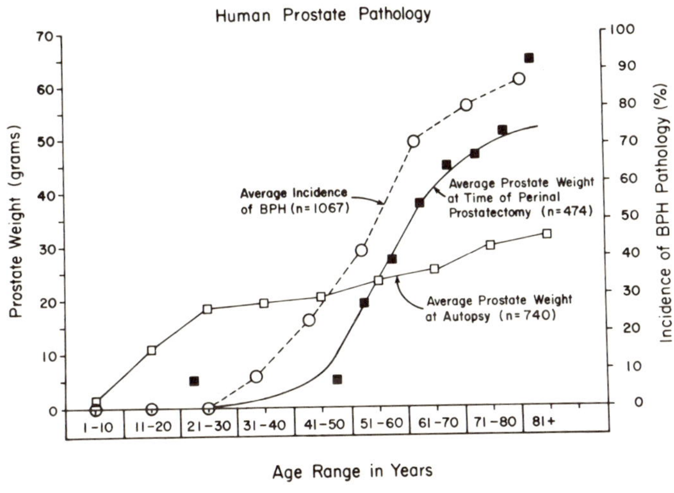

Fig. 2. Age-related alterations in human prostatic pathology: incidence of BPH at autopsy in 1,067 men based on histological criteria (open circles); average prostatic weight at autopsy in 740 men (open boxes); average prostatic weight at time of simple perineal prostatectomy for BPH in 474 men (closed boxes). (Reproduced with permission of Stephen Berry).

average prostatic weight at autopsy from 740 patients and have also included the average prostatic weight at the time of simple perineal prostatectomy performed for BPH in the early part of the century at the Brady Urological Institute (Gover, 1923).

These data indicate that with age there is a gradual increase in average prostatic weight beginning at approximately the fifth decade; this finding is accompanied by an increase in the incidence of BPH identified histologically by the pathologist. In addition, the amount of tissue removed at the time of simple prostatectomy appears to increase as well with advancing age. These data support the progressive nature of this disease in the aging male.

Although most patients over the age of 50 will have histological evidence of benign prostatic hyperplasia and many patients will suffer symptoms resulting from urethral compression, not all patients require a prostatectomy for relief of these symptoms. In 1967 Lytton et al suggested that the probability of a 40-year old man requiring an operation for BPH, if he lives to 80 years of age, is approximately 10%. Recently, Birkhoff (1983) suggested that because the rate of prostatectomy has doubled since that study was performed the chance now of a 50-year old man requiring a prostatectomy during his lifetime is 20-25%.

ETIOLOGY

Although in aging men the development of BPH is almost a universal phenomenon, the cause and pathogenesis of this disorder are poorly understood. Attempts at identifying risk factors based on epidemiological studies have not been very helpful. Recently Rotkin (1983) summarized these data and suggested that " there are no confirmable data to suggest relationships of sociocultural variables, celibacy, specific blood groups, use of tobacco and/or alcohol, gerontologic conditions, such as coronary heart disease, cerebral vascular disease, hypertension, diabetes mellitus, and cirrhosis of the liver, to the onset of BPH". Furthermore, he concluded that there was no further information to support the claimed association of BPH as a precursor developing into prostatic cancer.

Based upon all available information, it appears clear that the two major factors necessary for the onset of BPH in men are the presence of the testes and aging. Consequently, much research has been directed at identifying a hormonal cause for BPH. Although there is conflicting information, there are several factors that strongly support the possibility that BPH in men is under endocrine control: 1) BPH does not occur in men who are castrated prior to puberty; 2) regression of established BPH has been reported to occur following castration; and 3) in an animal model BPH can be reproduced by hormones. What is the nature of these hormonal influences?

Over the past decade the factors that interact to cause the development of BPH have come under intense scrutiny. The various theories and approaches to this problem can be distilled down to 3 possibilities (Grayhack 1983): 1) BPH reflects merely a reaction of normal prostatic cells to an abnormal endocrine environment; 2) BPH reflects a stimulated growth of substantially altered prostatic cells by a minimally altered hormonal environment; or 3) BPH reflects a variable mixture of these factors. The remainder of this manuscript will be directed at a detailed discussion of various etiological factors that have been considered to be important in the pathogenesis of BPH.

Role of the Testis in the Pathogenesis of BPH

It is generally believed that BPH does not occur in patients who are castrated prior to puberty and is rare in males who are castrated prior to the age of 40. Only one documented exception has been reported by Scott (1953) who performed a prostatectomy on a 60-year old man with urinary retention who had been castrated at the age of 28 years. Whether the testes play a permissive or active role in the development of BPH is uncertain. Theoretically, the most convincing way to demonstrate a direct effect of the testes on BPH would be the demonstration of regression following castration of patients with established BPH. As stated by Huggins and Stevens in 1940, "Whether benign hypertrophy of the prostate is under endocrine control or not is a problem of immediate interest since not all workers are agreed on this point. Determination of the effect of castration on this disease is one of the most critical ways to settle this problem, but contradiction of opinion exists at the present time as to the effect of removal of the gonads on enlargement of the prostate." Unfortunately, this statement is as true today as it was in 1940. In a classic study by White in 1895, 111 men were castrated for the treatment of bladder outlet obstruction with approximately 87% showing rapid atrophy of the prostatic enlargement after orchiectomy. The following year Cabot presented a longer followup of 61 cases with substantial improvement demonstrated in 84% of men undergoing orchiectomy for BPH. These reports were followed quickly by other publications reporting failure of relief of prostatic enlargement following castration, and 30 to 40 years elapsed before Deming and associates revived the subject. They reported no effect of castration on prostatic enlargement in 1 patient whom they followed for 3 months. In 1940, Huggins and Stevens castrated 3 men for treatment of BPH and reported that atrophy was not present 29 days after castration in 1 patient but appeared in the other 2 at 86 and 91 days after the operation, respectively. They concluded that "the prostatic epithelium, at least, is under the control of the testes."

Believing that more data were necessary to prove a relationship between established BPH and the testes, and recognizing that purposeful castration of a large number of men with the condition is not feasible, Wendel et al (1972) compared the histological findings of BPH in patients with prostatic carcinoma who had been treated with castration and estrogen therapy with the histological findings in patients with prostatic cancer who were not treated. They concluded that the BPH present in patients with carcinoma of the prostate treated with orchiectomy and estrogen is a lower grade than that found in those patients not receiving this treatment. Infolding of the acinar epithelium and the secretory phase were virtually absent in the group receiving orchiectomy and estrogen, as compared with their presence in patients not having this treatment. This finding in patients with occult or untreated prostatic cancer suggests that the differences are correlated with orchiectomy and estrogen and not with the presence of carcinoma itself. They believe that their observations support the theory that the cells of BPH are subject to continuing stimulation by the testes. Summarizing all of these findings, one returns to the conclusion of Huggins and Stevens (1940) that "the prostatic epithelium, at least, is under the control of the testes."

In all of these studies, there has been no accurate quantitation of the stromal component of the disease. It is well recognized that in experimental animals following castration there is more rapid and complete regression of epithelial components than their stromal counterparts (Neubauer et al 1981). Consequently, it is possible that castration may have its most powerful influence in those cases of BPH characterized by epithelial overgrowth and the least influence in those cases in which the disease is mainly stromal. In the future, further attempts should be made to clarify the influence of the testes on BPH. By using potent LHRH agonists or through the use of inhibitors of steroidogenesis, one should be able to reversibly suppress testicular function in men with established BPH in an attempt to clarify the influence of testicular secretions on growth. In designing such experiments, it will be important to determine the pretreatment histology of the prostate and to evaluate response utilizing quantitative measurements of prostatic size (obtained by computerized tomography or sonography) and by independent urodynamic evaluations. In this way, it should be possible to identify whether or not the testes influence growth of BPH. If so, further attempts will be necessary to determine whether the role of the testes is merely permissive or whether they exert an active influence in the induction of the disease.

The "Dihydrotestosterone Thesis" in the Pathogenesis of BPH

It is well recognized that dihydrotestosterone (DHT) is the major intracellular androgenic metabolite within the prostate (Bruchovsky, Wilson 1968; Anderson, Liao 1968). Recognizing the central regulatory role of DHT in growth of the prostate, Wilson and coworkers first suggested that DHT accumulation might be implicated in the etiology of BPH. This suggestion was based initially on an investigation of several different animal species to determine whether the capacity of the prostate to form DHT could be correlated with prostatic growth (Wilson, Gloyna 1970). Their study demonstrated that in most animals the prostate loses its ability to form DHT with age. However, in 2 animal species, the dog and man, high rates of DHT formation persist throughout life. Because these are the two animal species that spontaneously develop prostatic hyperplasia, they proposed that BPH might be the result of the unregulated production of DHT over many years. To explore this possibility further, Siiteri and Wilson (1970) measured the androgen content in normal and hyperplastic human prostates. Although they found no significant difference in the content of testosterone in the 2 types of tissue, the content of DHT was 3-4 fold greater in hyperplastic tissue than in normal glands. Subsequently, this observation has been confirmed by other investigators and for the past dozen years research into the etiology of BPH has focussed on factors that may be responsible for the accumulation of supranormal levels of DHT and the mechanism by which this induces prostatic hyperplasia (Geller, et al 1976; Hammond 1978; Meikle et al 1978; Krieg et al 1979).

Recently, while investigating the value of using measurements of DHT content as a marker for the hormonal responsiveness of prostatic cancer, our laboratory noted that the content of DHT in normal and benign hyperplastic tissues obtained at open surgical procedures was similar (Walsh et al, 1983). We measured DHT content in normal peripheral and benign hyperplastic prostatic tissue obtained at open surgical procedures on 29 men ages 36 to 82 years. The DHT content in normal prostates (mean $\pm$ SE, 5.1 $\pm$ 0.4 ng/g tissue) and in BPH (5.0 $\pm$ 0.4) was similar. In 11 patients in whom both normal and hyperplastic prostatic tissue was harvested simultaneously at the same operation, there was no significant difference in the content of DHT in the 2 types of tissue. These findings failed to confirm the widespread belief that DHT content is elevated in BPH. Our data differ from the reported literature in one major respect: the DHT content of normal peripheral prostate in this study is 3-4 times higher than previously reported (Table 1). In reviewing the literature to determine why we were unable to confirm the findings of others, we learned that the "elevated" levels of DHT in BPH reported by others were based upon measurements performed on surgically removed specimens whereas the "low levels" of DHT in normal tissue were based upon measurements performed on tissues obtained at autopsy. This observation suggested that the conditions of tissue harvesting may have significantly influenced the endogenous levels of androgen within the prostate. To explore this possibility further DHT content was measured in 7 cadavers ranging in age from 19 to 82 years of age. The results of this experiment suggested that the DHT content of

Table 1. Summary of published data on DHT content in normal and hyperplastic prostatic tissue.

Authors	Source of tissue		DHT ng/g tissue + SE	
	Normal	BPH	Normal	BPH
Siiteri & Wilson	Autopsy	Surgery	1.3±0.5	6.0±1.0
Geller, et al	Autopsy	Surgery	2.1±0.3	5.6±0.9
Hammond	Autopsy	Surgery	1.3±0.3	5.5±0.5
Meikle, et al	Autopsy	Surgery	1.3±0.6	4.0±1.9
Krieg, et al	Autopsy	Surgery	1.6±1.0	4.5±1.4
Walsh et al (in press)	Surgery	Surgery	5.1±0.4	5.0±0.4
	Autopsy	Autopsy	0.7±0.1	1.0±0.2

prostatic tissue removed at autopsy is facticiously low (0.7-1.0 ng/g tissue) (Table 1). Several investigators have justified the use of prostatic tissue procured at autopsy for the measurement of DHT content by demonstrating that when prostatic tissue was incubated at 20°C there was no fall in DHT content. However, the unclothed body of an adult in an environmental temperature of 60° F only cools at 1° F per hour during the first 3 hours after death and then 2° F per hour during the next 3 hours. If the body is clothed, the rate of cooling is 66% slower (Marshall, Hohre, 1962). These facts encouraged us to determine the influence of incubations performed at 37° C on DHT content. When *in vitro* incubations of fresh prostatic tissue were performed at 37° C, DHT content was reduced to low levels within 2 hours.

The findings in this study that DHT content in BPH is identical to levels in normal tissue question the role of DHT accumulation as a causative factor in the etiology of

BPH. The speculative role of DHT as a causative factor in BPH has been supported experimentally by studies in the dog which demonstrated: 1) canine BPH is characterized by increased prostatic dihydrotestosterone concentration (Gloyna et al 1970); and 2) steroid treatment regimens that increase prostatic growth in the dog increase prostatic DHT concentrations (Moore et al 1979). However, recent studies from our laboratories have questioned these findings. In age-matched dogs, we could demonstrate no difference in DHT content between dogs with histologically normal prostates and those with spontaneous BPH (Ewing et al). Secondly, although a positive correlation was observed between prostatic weight and DHT content in castrated or intact beagles treated with 11 of 15 different steroid regimens, there were 4 additional treatment regimens (intact or castrated beagles treated with either DHT or 3α- androstanediol alone) which resulted in high concentrations of prostatic DHT but which failed to evoke equivalent increases in prostatic weight (Ewing et al). Finally there was a dramatic biphasic change in prostatic DHT concentrations with advancing age in the beagle. After age 4 years, although DHT content in the prostate fell, the incidence of BPH continued to increase (Ewing et al). In another study, we observed that the prostatic secretory function in the beagle peaks at approximately 4 years of age and then declines dramatically (Brendler et al 1983). However, as the secretory capacity of the prostate diminishes the gland continues to grow and histological changes of BPH become more evident. These data suggest that the factors regulating growth of the canine prostate and at least one differentiated function (i.e. secretion) may be controlled separately and the fact that abnormal growth continues in the face of declining DHT levels suggests that regulatory factors other than DHT may be involved in the etiology of the hyperplastic growth of the dog prostate. Recognizing that human BPH occurs in the presence of normal tissue levels of dihydrotestosterone should focus research efforts to identify other factors that may sensitize this tissue and accelerate growth. Indeed, at the present time this appears to be one of the most fruitful immediate areas for research efforts.

The Role of Estrogen/Androgen Synergism in the Pathogenesis of BPH

The role of estrogens in the physiological regulation of prostatic growth in man is one of great speculation. For years it has been assumed that estrogen may be responsible in some way for the spontaneous development of prostatic hyperplasia in man. This speculation was strengthened by the observation that in the dog, estrogen acts synergistically with androgen in the experimental induction of BPH. Wilson and co-workers (1975) using the dog as a model demonstrated previously that young castrated dogs that were treated for 2 years with either testosterone or DHT failed to develop BPH whereas intact control dogs over a similar interval spontaneously developed the disease. Based upon this observation they speculated that one or more testicular hormones, other than testosterone or DHT, were required for the development of prostatic hyperplasia. Based on these findings Walsh and Wilson (1976) subsequently examined the possible role of estradiol and androstanediol in this process. In this series of experiments, dogs received treatment with androstanediol or DHT with or without estradiol. In the animals treated with androstanediol, the average weight of the prostate increased 10 grams in 1 year and 2 of the 5 animals developed BPH. Even more striking results were produced by the combination of androstanediol plus estradiol - the average increase in gland size was 31.2 grams and all 5 animals had massively enlarged prostates. These results were in striking contrast to previous studies in which prostatic weights of similar animals treated with identical doses of testosterone and DHT averaged only 3.6 and 6.0 grams respectively. Thus, for the first time enlargement of the prostate comparable to that seen in prostatic hyperplasia was produced by hormonal treatment subsequent to early castration in the dog. These results have been confirmed by others subsequently. In addition it has been demonstrated also that when DHT is administered in combination with estradiol prostatic hyperplasia is induced (DeKlerk et al 1979).

To gain insight into the mechanism by which estrogen produces this synergistic effect, the androgen and estrogen receptors in the canine prostate have been characterized. The canine prostate contains high concentrations of an estrogen receptor (Chaisiri et al 1978; Trachtenberg et al 1980, Hawkins et al 1980). Furthermore, when castrated dogs are treated with estradiol, there is a two-fold increase in cytosolic androgen receptor (Moore et al 1979). This observation led Wilson and co-workers to propose that the mechanism of estrogen/androgen synergism in the experimental induction of canine BPH may be explained by estradiol mediated increases in the androgen receptor. Our laboratory subsequently demonstrated that spontaneously arising canine hyperplasia in young dogs was characterized by increases in nuclear androgen receptor content and that the administration of estradiol plus androstanediol to castrate dogs significantly increased the prostatic nuclear androgen receptor content over that found in dogs treated with androstanediol alone (Trachtenberg et al 1980). From this observation we concluded that an increase in nuclear androgen receptor content appeared to be an important event in the development of spontaneously arising and experimentally induced canine prostatic hyperplasia and that the mechanism of androgen/estrogen synergism in the experimental induction of canine BPH may be explained by estradiol-mediated increases in nuclear androgen receptor content (Trachtenberg et al 1980). Although this is an attractive hypothesis to explain the experimental induction of canine prostatic hyperplasia, it is not known yet whether or not estrogen synergism is responsible as well for spontaneous BPH in the dog.

In man, a number of investigators have explored the possibility of estrogen/androgen synergism by measuring steroid hormone levels in the plasma of men as they age. Although some investigators have suggested that there is no alteration in plasma testosterone levels with aging (Harman, Tsitouras 1980), most laboratories agree that with aging there is a gradual fall in plasma testosterone levels. Recently, the reason for the disagreement on this important subject has been explained by the observation that in old age there is attenuation of the early morning rise in testosterone levels that are characteristic of young men (Bremner et al 1983). To correct for this, Zumoff et al (1982) measured 24-hour mean plasma concentrations of androgens and estrogens in healthy men over a wide range of ages. They found that plasma testosterone concentrations showed a slow continuous decline with age, decreasing about 35% between 21 and 85 years of age. However, there was no alteration with age in plasma estrone or estradiol. These findings are in agreement with those of Harman and Tsitouras (1980) but are in contrast to the findings of others which demonstrated an increase in plasma estradiol with age (Rubens et al 1974; Pirke, Doerr 1975). Regardless, whether estradiol concentrations increase or remain stable with aging, because plasma testosterone levels fall there is an alteration in the estrogen to androgen ratio. As emphasized by Wilson (1980), because these endocrine changes probably do not commence until after the initiation of the pathological process it is unlikely that these alterations in plasma hormones are causally linked to the initiation of the hyperplasia. However, it is clear that the continued growth of the hyperplastic process during the fifth and sixth decades takes place on the background of decreased levels of plasma androgen relative to normal or increased levels of plasma estrogen. This is the major evidence that suggests a possible pathogenic role for estrogen in the induction of BPH.

Recognizing that the characterization of steroid hormones in the canine prostate has helped to clarify the estrogen/androgen synergism responsible for the experimental induction of BPH in the dog, similar studies have been carried out in man. The canine prostate contains abundant quantities of a high affinity estrogen receptor. However, reports on estrogen binding in the human prostate have been conflicting (for review see Ekman et al 1983). The percentage of specimens classified as estrogen receptor positive from numerous laboratories is highly variable and the estrogen receptor content differs from one report to another and within the same studies. To explore this subject further we have recently characterized the estrogen receptor in the human prostate and have determined that the human prostate contains multiple sites for estrogen binding in cytosol as well as nuclear preparations (Ekman et al 1983). One class of binding sites (Type I) corresponds to the classical, high affinity estrogen receptor (K_d for {^{3}H} estradiol 0.10 nM). The second class of binding sites (Type II) appears to have a much lower K_d (5-10 nM) and is present in concentrations that interfere with measurement of the classical receptor. The Type I estrogen receptor has been characterized in normal and BPH tissues (Table 2).

In both the cytosol, nuclear salt extractable, and nuclear salt-resistant compartments, the level of the classical estrogen receptor in BPH is significantly lower than in normal tissue. In addition to the estrogen receptor, the progesterone and androgen receptors have also been characterized. Recognizing that estrogens are known to induce the progesterone receptor in breast and uterine target tissues, the existence of a progesterone receptor in human BPH suggests the possibility that this tissue may be under estrogenic stimulation. To

Table 2. Steroid Receptor Content* In Human Prostatic Tissue

Tissue	Receptor	Compartment Cytosol	Nuclear Salt Ext.	Nuclear Salt Res.
Normal	Estrogen-Type I	149±120	30±16	36±24
BPH	Estrogen-Type I	35± 24	5± 7	2± 4
Normal vs BPH	Estrogen-Type I	p<0.01	p<0.01	p<0.02
Normal	Progesterone	408±138	--	--
BPH	Progesterone	452± 57	--	--
Normal vs BPH	Progesterone	N.S.		
Normal	Androgen	387±26	157±17	170±28
BPH	Androgen	428±35	241±12	240±11
%increase BPH	Androgen	10%	54%	41%
p value	Androgen	N.S.	<0.01	<0.01

*fmol/mg DNA

investigate this possibility progesterone receptor content was measured in normal and hyperplastic tissues (Ekman et al 1982). Cytosolic progesterone receptor content in normal and BPH tissue were similar; nuclear salt-extractable and salt-resistant receptors were undetectable (Table 2). These findings failed to provide evidence for preferential estrogenic stimulation of human BPH. When androgen receptor content was measured in the three subcellular compartments, elevated levels of receptor were identified in both the nuclear salt-extractable and salt-resistant compartments in BPH tissue (54% and 41% respectively) (Barrack et al 1983).

In summary, studies on the role of estrogen in the pathogenesis of BPH have been reviewed. Evidence in favor of a role for estrogen includes: 1) experimental induction of BPH in the dog in which estrogen synergizes with 5α-reduced androgens; 2) estrogen induction of the androgen receptor in the canine prostate, a proposed mechanism for estrogen/androgen synergism; 3) alteration in estrogen/androgen production with aging in man favoring a possible role for estrogen in the maintenance, but not induction of BPH; 4) the presence of the classical estrogen receptor in human BPH; and 5) increased nuclear androgen receptor levels in human BPH, similar to findings in spontaneous and experimentally induced canine BPH (Barrack et al 1983). On the other hand, there are also factors that fail to support a role for estrogen in the pathogenesis of BPH: 1) the alterations in estrogen/androgen production which occur with aging appear rather minor and occur after the apparent onset of the disease; 2) cytoplasmic and nuclear estrogen receptor levels in human BPH are significantly lower than in the normal prostate and are considerably lower than estrogen receptor content in the canine prostate; and 3) similar levels of cytosolic progesterone receptor content in normal and BPH tissues, findings that fail to provide evidence for preferential estrogenic stimulation of human BPH (Ekman et al 1982). Thus, although estrogen synergism is an attractive hypothesis as a mechanism for the induction of BPH, further evidence is necessary before this thesis can be accepted. Documentation of definite increases in estrogen stimulation with age are necessary. Furthermore, more information is necessary to document the fact that human BPH is actually a target organ for estrogenic stimulation. In many species, treatment of castrate animals with estrogen produces a marked change in the morphological organization of the prostate from a predominantly atrophic epithelium to one characterized by squamous metaplasia and fibromuscular stroma. In man, when estrogen is administered although squamous metaplasia occurs in the urethra and ducts of the prostate, the acini are rarely involved (Moore, McLellan 1938; Mostofi 1970). This is further evidence against a primary role for estrogens in the stimulation of BPH.

The Role of Stromal-Epithelial Interactions in the Induction of BPH.

Reawakening of the inductive potential of the prostatic stroma during adulthood is a rather recent and particularly attractive hypothesis in the unending search for an answer to the etiology of BPH (McNeal 1978). In the embryo, androgenic hormone is the inducer that triggers the budding of the prostatic ducts from the urethral lining into the adjacent stroma. Cunha (1980) has shown that the mesenchyme is the actual target organ for androgenic steroids that mediates the morphogenetic effects of hormones upon the epithelium. The mesenchyme induces the urogenital epithelium to express its normal program of morphogenesis and cytodifferentiation. McNeal has made the observation that in BPH, gland budding and branching toward a central focus is seen most often as a primary event. He cites the formation of new ductal and acinar architecture, which he states is a forbidden process in adult organs, as evidence for embryonic capacity for this tissue. He feels that some humoral inducing agent from the stroma may be the inciting agent for gland proliferation. He has noted that the earliest changes of BPH occur in a very small area of the prostate which he has termed the transition zone. He feels that the early formation of nodules may represent an entirely local event having no endocrine determinants. In contrast, the growth of nodules, which he finds occurs in men older than age 70, appears synchronized and occurs simultaneously in many nodules of the same gland. This could well represent an endocrine change. Thus, the induction of BPH could be viewed as a multi-factorial event.

At present, there is no solid evidence that "embryonic reawakening" occurs in adult tissues. However, the hypothesis as set forth by McNeal is most attractive and deserves serious consideration and investigation.

SUMMARY - FUTURE DIRECTIONS

The etiology of benign prostatic hyperplasia has been examined and various hypotheses have been reviewed. There is still much to be learned. It remains to be determined whether or not human BPH is under the regulation of the testes. It should be possible to evaluate the role of the testes using various pharmacological manipulations that selectively and reversibly block testicular secretions, e.g. LHRH agonists, antiestrogens, antiandrogens, inhibitors of steroidogenesis. If indeed one can demonstrate an effect of testicular secretions on the growth of BPH, it will remain to be determined whether or not this effect is direct or merely permissive.

Based upon experimental studies in the dog, it appears that the factors regulating growth of the prostate and at least one differentiated function (i.e. secretion) may be controlled separately and furthermore that abnormal growth continues in the face of declining levels of serum testosterone and tissue DHT. These data suggest that regulatory factors other than serum testosterone and tissue levels of DHT may be involved in the etiology of the hyperplastic growth of the dog prostate. Recognizing that human BPH occurs in the presence of normal tissue levels of DHT should focus research efforts to identify other factors that may sensitize this tissue and accelerate growth. In the dog, estrogen serves this function in the experimental induction of the disease. However, it remains to be determined whether estrogenic synergism plays a role in the induction of BPH in man. Additional studies are necessary to determine the relationship between estrogen secretion, aging, and the development of BPH in man. In addition, further evidence needs to be accumulated to document the fact that human BPH is indeed a target organ for estrogenic stimulation.

A recent and attractive area for research involves epithelial-stromal interactions and "embryonic reawakening" in the pathogenesis of BPH. This appears to be an ideal mechanism to explain the early induction of the disease relegating an abnormal endocrine environment to a secondary role involved in the maintenance and proliferation of the disease once it has been induced. This attractive hypothesis needs further work.

ACKNOWLEDGEMENT - This study was supported by the National Institutes of Health Grant AM 19300 of the Department of Health and Human Services. The author wishes to thank his colleagues at the Johns Hopkins University who were involved in the comprehensive study of benign prostatic hyperplasia: Dr. Donald S. Coffey, Dr. Larry L. Ewing, Dr. William W. Scott, Dr. Evelyn Barrack, Dr. Peter Ekman, Dr. John Trachtenberg, Dr. John D. Strandberg, Dr. Barry R. Zirkin, and Stephen J. Berry.

References

Anderson KM, Liao S (1968) Selective retention of dihydrotestosterone by prostatic nuclei. Nature 219:277.

Barrack ER, Bujnovszky P, Walsh PC (1983). Subcellular distribution of androgen receptors in human normal, benign hyperplastic, and malignant prostatic tissues: Characterization of nuclear salt-resistant receptors. Cancer Res 43:1107.

Berry, Stephen (1983). Personal communication.

Birkhoff JD (1983). Natural history of benign prostatic hypertrophy. In Hinman F (ed): "Benign Prostatic Hypertrophy", New York: Springer-Verlag, p 5.

Bremner WJ, Vitiello MV, Prinz PN (1983). Loss of circadian rhythmicity in blood testosterone levels with aging in normal men. J Clin Endocrinol Metab 56:1278.

Brendler CB, Berry SJ, Ewing LL, McCullough AR, Cochran RC, Strandberg JD, Zirkin BR, Coffey DS, Wheaton LG, Hiler ML, Bordy MC, Scott WW, Walsh PC (1983) Spontaneous benign prostatic hyperplasia in the beagle: Age-associated changes in serum hormone levels and the morphology and secretory function of the canine prostate. J Clin Invest 71:1114.

Bruchovsky N, Wilson JD (1968). The conversion of testosterone to 5α-androstane-17ß-ol-one by rat prostate in vivo and in vitro. J Biol Chem 243:2012.

Cabot AT (1896). The question of castration for enlarged prostate. Ann Surg 24:265.

Chaisiri N, Volataire Y, Evans BAJ, Pierrepoint CG (1978). Demonstration of a cytoplasmic receptor protein for estrogen in the canine prostate gland. J Endocrinol 78:131.

Cunha GR, Chung LWK, Shannon JM, Reese BA (1980). Stromal-epithelial interactions in sex differentiation. Biol Reprod 22:19.

DeKlerk DP, Coffey DS, Ewing LL, McDermott IR, Reiner WG, Robinson CH, Scott WW, Strandberg JD, Talalay P, Walsh PC, Wheaton LG, Zirkin BR (1979). Comparison of spontaneous and experimentally induced canine prostatic hyperplasia. J Clin Invest 64:842.

Deming CL (1935). The effect of castration on benign hypertrophy of the prostate in man. J Urol 33:388.

Ekman P, Barrack ER, Greene GL, Jensen EV, Walsh PC (1983). Estrogen receptors in human prostate. Evidence for multiple binding sites. J Clin Endocrinol Metab 57:166.

Ekman P, Barrack ER, Walsh PC (1982) Simultaneous measurement of progesterone and androgen receptors in human prostate: A microassay. J Clin Endocrinol Metab 55:1089.

Ewing LL, Berry SJ, Higginbottom EG. Dihydrotestosterone content of beagle prostatic tissue: Effect of age and hyperplasia. Endocrinology: in press.

Geller J, Albert J, Lopez D, Geller A, Niwayama, G (1976). Comparison of androgen metabolites in benign prostatic hypertrophy (BPH) and normal prostate. J Clin Endocrinol 43:686.

Franks LM (1954). Benign nodular hyperplasia of the prostate: A review. Ann R Coll Surg: 14:92.

Gloyna RE, Siiteri PK, Wilson JD (1970). Dihydrotestosterone in prostatic hypertrophy. II. The formation and content of dihydrotestosterone in the hypertrophic canine prostate and the effect of dihydrotestosterone on prostatic growth in the dog. J Clin Invest 49:1746.

Gover M (1923). A statistical study of the etiology of benign hypertrophy of the prostate gland. Johns Hopkins Hospital Rep 21:231.

Grayhack JT (1983). Directions for future research. In Hinman F (ed): "Benign Prostatic Hypertrophy", New York: Springer-Verlag, p. 313.

Hammond GL (1978). Endogenous steroid levels in the human prostate from birth to old age: A comparison of normal and diseased states. J Endocrinol 78:7.

Harman SM, Tsitouras PD (1980). Reproductive hormones in aging men. I. Measurement of sex steroids, basal luteinizing hormone, and Leydig cell responses to human chorionic gonadotropin. J Clin Endocrinol Metab 51:35.

Haugen OA, Harbitz TB (1972). Prostatic weight in elderly men. Acta Path Microbiol Scand Section A 80:769

Hawkins EF, Trachtenberg J, Hicks LL, Walsh PC (1980). Androgen and estrogen receptors in the canine prostate. J Andrology 1:234.

Huggins C, Stevens R (1940). The effect of castration on benign hypertrophy of the prostate in man. J Urol 43:705.

Krieg M, Bartsch W, Janssen W, Voigt KD (1979). A comparative study of binding metabolism and endogenous levels of androgens in normal, hyperplastic, and carcinomatous human prostate. J Steroid Biochem 11:615.

Lowsley OS (1915). The prostate in old age. Ann Surg 62:716.

Lytton B, Emery JM, Harvard BM (1968). The incidence of benign prostatic hypertrophy. J Urol 99:639.

Marshall TK, Hoare FE (1962). The rectal cooling after death and its mathematical expression. J Forensic Sci 7:56.

McNeal JE (1978). Origin and evolution of benign prostatic enlargement. Invest Urol 15:340.

Meikle AW, Stringham JD, Olsen DC (1978). Subnormal tissue 3α-androstanediol and androsterone in prostatic hyperplasia. J Clin Endocrinol 47:909.

Moore RA (1943). Benign hypertrophy of the prostate. J Urol 50:680.

Moore RA, McLellan AM (1938). A histological study of the effect of the sex hormones on the human prostate. J Urol 40:641.

Moore RJ, Gazak JM, Quebbeman JF, Wilson JD (1979). Concentration of dihydrotestosterone and 3α-androstanediol in naturally occurring and androgen induced prostatic hyperplasia in the dog. J Clin Invest 64:1003.

Moore RJ, Gazak JM, Wilson JD (1979). Regulation of cytoplasmic dihydrotestosterone binding in dog prostate. J Clin Invest 63:351.

Morgagni GB (1760). "The Seats and Causes of Disease Investigated by Anatomy." Book 3. London, Johnson and Payne, p. 460.

Mostofi FK (1970). Benign hyperplasia of the prostate gland. In Campbell MF, Harrison JH (eds): "Urology" 3rd ed, Philadelphia: W.B. Saunders, p 1065.

Neubauer BL, Mawhinney MG (1981). Actions of androgen and estrogen on guinea pig seminal vesicle epithelium and muscle. Endocrinology 108:680.

Pirke KM, Doerr P (1975) Age related changes in free plasma testosterone, dihydrotestosterone, and oestradiol. Acta Endocrinol 80:171.

Pradhan BK, Chandra K (1975). Morphogenesis of nodular hyperplasia-prostate. J Urol 113:210.

Rotkin ID (1983). Origins, distribution, and risk of benign prostatic hypertrophy. In Himan F. (ed): "Benign Prostatic Hypertrophy", New York: Springer-Verlag, p. 10.

Rubens RM, Dhont M, Vermeulen A (1974). Further studies on Leydig cell function in old age. J Clin Endocrinol Metab 39:40

Scott WW (1953). What makes the prostate grow? J Urol 70:477.

Siiteri PK, Wilson JD (1970). Dihydrotestosterone in prostatic hypertrophy. I. The formation and content of dihydrotestosterone in the hypertrophic prostate of man. J Clin Invest 49:1737.

Swyer GIM (1944). Post-natal growth changes in the human prostate. J Anat 78:130.

Trachtenberg J, Hicks LL, Walsh PC (1980). Androgen-and estrogen-receptor content in spontaneous and experimentally induced canine prostatic hyperplasia. J Clin Invest 65:1051.

Walsh PC, Hutchins GM, Ewing LL (in press). The tissue content of dihydrotestosterone in human prostatic hyperplasia is not supranormal. J Clin Invest.

Walsh PC, Wilson JD (1976). The induction of prostatic hypertrophy in the dog with androstanediol. J Clin Invest 57:1093.

Wendel EF, Brannen GE, Putong PB, Grayhack JT (1972). The effect of orchiectomy and estrogens on benign prostatic hyperplasia. J Urol 108:116.

White JW (1895). The results of double castration in hypertrophy of the prostate. Ann Surg 22:1

Wilson JD (1980). The pathogenesis of benign prostatic hyperplasia. Amer J Med 68:745.

Wilson JD, Gloyna RE (1970). The intranuclear metabolism of testosterone in the accessory organs of reproduction. Recent Prog Horm Res 26:309.

Wilson JD, Gloyna RE, Siiteri PK (1975). Androgen metabolism in the hypertrophic prostate. J Steroid Biochem 6:443.

Zumoff B, Strain GW, Kream J, O'Connor J, Rosenfeld RS, Levin J, Fukushima DK (1982). Age variation of the 24-hour mean plasma concentrations of androgens, estrogens, and gonadotropins in normal adult men. J Clin Endocrinol Metab 54:534.

Discussion

Bhuyan: Is there any work being done comparing the Orientals, who are apparently much less susceptible to BPH, to Western man?

Walsh: We know that the Japanese develop BPH, and that the disease is quite common in the Chinese population in San Francisco. As for the Chinese in their nativeland, it is my understanding that as more of these people live longer, the disease will become more obvious. In direct answer to your question, "Has anyone studied those patients chronologically?" Not to the best of my knowledge.

McNeal: Dr. Bruchovsky and Dr. McLaughlin have published evidence that 5-alpha reductase in the stroma of BPH nodules is increased three-fold while it tends to remain at normal levels in the epithelium of BPH nodules, as compared with normal prostatic tissue. How does that fit into the fascinating series of data that you presented here?

Walsh: I am not certain as to the the source of their normal tissue. In the past they have obtained normal tissue from cadavers; so that in any study in which you are comparing cadaveric tissue with surgically obtained BPH tissue, one has to careful about the significance of the results.

McNeal: I have one more brief question, Dr. Walsh. Why do you refer to the dog hyperplastic lesion as BPH?

Walsh: What would you want me to call it?

McNeal: Dog prostatic hyperplasia. BPH is a colloqulism, unique to the description of the human disease. The similarity hasn't yet been proven between man and the dog. .

Walsh: In the manuscript you will see that we call it canine prostatic hyperplasia.

Ofner: I think you are to be congratulated in throwing this very interesting observation in the works of the DHT involvement is my first comment.

I have a question and two points of comment.

There is a small subset, I believe, of human BPH patients that develop the disease very early - in their 40's. My question is, is there something different about those patients?

I wanted to just talk a little about our work in which we have also used the castrate dog model with short term influences of androgen and estrogen. We found that estrogen, given alone, induces squamous metaplasia with proliferation of basal cells to squamous cells and also produces a squamous phenotype in tonofilament-containing non-proliferating glandular cells. When you give both hormones together, you still have squamous proliferation of the basal cells, but now you have a bidirectional development of morphological phenotypes in the glandular cells, with squamous and secretory characteristics. Under the influence of both hormones, we have seen proliferation in the basal and glandular compartments of the epithelium in the same acinus. It has to be shown whether these effects apply to the human prostate.

The second point I wanted to make refers to Dr. Giorgi's work. He emphasized the medium and low affinity binding sites which may have regulatory importance. That is where estrogen binding may be very important. We found that if you expose canine prostate in organ culture to labelled androgen or estrogen, there is about three or four-fold greater uptake of estrogen than androgen. If circulating estrogen stays the same but those of androgen decrease, there may be a subsequent considerable increase in the uptake of estrogen relative to androgen in the prostate.

Walsh: Let me just comment on those three factors. Peter has made a good point. What about young men with BPH? The converse is also very important. What about the older man who has no BPH? As urologists, when we cystoscope men for various conditions we observe both conditions. It would be very interesting to study the young men that have it and the old men who don't have it, to see what is different about them.

The second question you bring up is about squamous metaplasia. There is no question that in the dog and in other animal species, the development of squamous metaplasia is a marker for estrogenic stimulation. What about in man? In castrated men who have been treated with estrogen, if you examine their prostates, the lining of the urethra and the prostatic ducts has squamous metaplasia, but the acini of BPH do not. This is a further suggestion that at least the acini of BPH do not develop the squamous change typical of an estrogen target tissue, again questioning whether or not the acini of BPH are indeed a target organ for estrogen.

Finally, your comment about low affinity binders, which may augment and heighten androgen stimulation, is an attractive way to think about a mechanism for increasing sensitivity of the prostate to androgen.

Cunha: I wish to comment about a mechanism of hormones on target organs. I think what is called for is not so much a study of the prostate as a whole in the sense of homogenates, but more specifically, I think what we have to do is to look at what are the various components of the prostate in terms of their estrogen receptor activity. It may be that the explanation of this situation just described could be solved by looking at estrogen receptors autoradiographically. It strikes me that very little information is available on estrogen receptors in the various cell types within the prostate. Krieg's work demonstrates that most of the receptor activities are within the stromal compartment, but again, there may be great heterogeneity amongst that, as well. Autoradiographic studies, I think, are needed.

Walsh: We know that it is difficult to separate epithelium and stroma, so many of those studies are left in question. There is

Kreig's study and another study in the rat, that show that although the estrogen receptor content of the intact prostate is very low, when you separate stroma and epithelium, somehow the stromal content of estrogen receptor is quite high. We have not tried to repeat those studies but there is no question that radioautography would be a useful technique to confirm them.

Karr: When you say that the old people don't have BPH, I assume you are referring to clinical BPH. I wonder if in our discussion if we should try to keep aware of the histologic condition? Then add to that whenever we have information on the actual clinical manifestation of the disease as well.

Walsh: I think that is a very important point. John McNeal is going to talk about the location of BPH. This tissue can be visualized during cystoscopy.

Karr: In the autopsy studies of normal patients, did they have any symptoms that suggested any type of BPH?

Walsh: Are you referring to the DHT content measurements?

Karr: Yes.

Walsh: Let me clarify how that study is done. We dissected out the normal peripheral prostate, and the periurethral adenomous tissue. When we talk about normal prostate, we talk about normal peripheral prostate. Some of the patients had normal prostates without any BPH and some of them had BPH. In the clinical study, we had eleven patients who at surgery had both adenomatous tissue and normal peripheral prostate. We measured the content of DHT in those eleven patients simultaneously in peripheral and in BPH tissue. We could find no difference in DHT content in those two compartments within the same patient, taken at the same time.

Lewis: One type of patient that we see in urology that doesn't appear to get BPH as often, are those with urethral stricture disease. Perhaps this would be a patient source that really ought to be studied to see why this particular patient does not get clinical BPH, at least, not as often as those who are the same age and don't have stricture disease.

Bartsch: First of all, what is normal prostatic tissue?

Regarding growth of the prostate we showed by rectal sonometrics that a high percentage of patients do not develop an increase of prostatic weight in the 6th and 7th decades of life. This study is in agreement with the date of Swyer. Do you have any explanation for this phenomena?

Walsh: We only used whole prostates and with the help of the pathologist dissected out normal peripheral prostate. The pathologist examined this tissue histologically to make certain that there was no cancer. This is what we call normal peripheral prostate. The second point is what about the older man with a normal size prostate who has symptoms. Dr. Tissel is going to talk about the normal prostate with aging. He has reported that the prostate in the normal man may not increase in weight with age.

New Approaches to the Study
of Benign Prostatic Hyperplasia, pages 27–53

ANATOMY OF THE PROSTATE AND MORPHOGENESIS OF BPH

John E. McNeal, M.D.

Division of Urology, Stanford Medical Center

Stanford, California 94305

Benign nodular hyperplasia (BPH) develops exclusively within a very small region of the prostate, a region which shows a grouping of anatomic features not found elsewhere in this organ. The details of the anatomic relationships in this region and the morphologic features of the BPH nodules together provide a number of possibly important clues to the biologic nature of this condition. They also provide a standard against which the adequacy of proposed animal models for BPH may be critically evaluated. Despite the potential importance of morphology, the anatomy of the prostate remains controversial (McNeal, 1980), and the implications of BPH nodule histology for understanding the disease have not been fully explored.

The studies reviewed here are based on detailed examination of more than 500 autopsy prostates from all age groups. The earliest lesions of BPH are fully characterized histologically and related to the normal anatomic landmarks found in the prostates of men in the third and fourth decades. From these data, inferences are drawn about the pathogenesis of BPH and its possible relationship to a re-expression of embryonic processes in adult life. Criteria are proposed for an optimal animal model, and these are compared to the morphologic findings in several different species.

ANATOMY OF THE PROSTATE

The functioning glandular prostate is an organ which

is markedly flattened in its antero-posterior dimension. Its main ducts radiate predominantly laterally from the urethra into a coronal plane, with smaller branches deviating posteriorly and to an even lesser degree anteriorly (McNeal 1983a). Much of the tissue anterior to a coronal plane along the long axis of the urethra is not glandular; it consists of an "anterior fibromuscular stroma" which is unrelated to prostatic function but adds considerably to the apparent thickness and bulk of the organ when examined at autopsy.

The anterior fibromuscular stroma is tightly fused to the anterior surface of the glandular prostate, and the different glandular regions are fused to each other. Hence, the anatomic complexity of this organ is not apparent on external inspection, and gross dissections are difficult. Optimum visualization of anatomic relationships requires cut sections which are carefully oriented in coronal planes along the long axis of the prostatic urethra.

The prostatic urethra, therefore, is a key anatomic reference point for study of the glandular tissue. In a sagittal plane of section (Fig. 1), its most important feature is a sharp angulation of the posterior wall at the midpoint of its intraprostatic course (McNeal 1972). The base of the verumontanum rests against the posterior wall at its point of angulation. The verumontanum extends distally from this level and therefore lies entirely in the distal urethral segment. The ejaculatory ducts and the ducts of about 95% of the prostatic glandular tissue also empty entirely into this segment. This tissue can be optimally demonstrated in a single coronal plane of section (C) running along the long axis of the distal urethral segment.

The anatomic relationships of the proximal urethral segment, above the point of urethral angulation, are quite different. In this region, the remaining 5% of the prostatic glandular tissue is intimately related to a cylindrical smooth muscle sphincter, the "preprostatic sphincter" (McNeal 1978). The anatomic relationships of this region are best demonstrated in a single oblique coronal plane of section (OC) running along the long axis of the proximal urethral segement and therefore offset at an angle of about 35° from the plane of the coronal section (C).

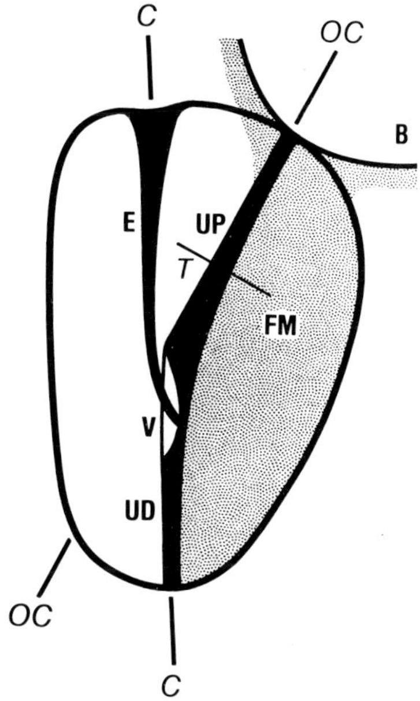

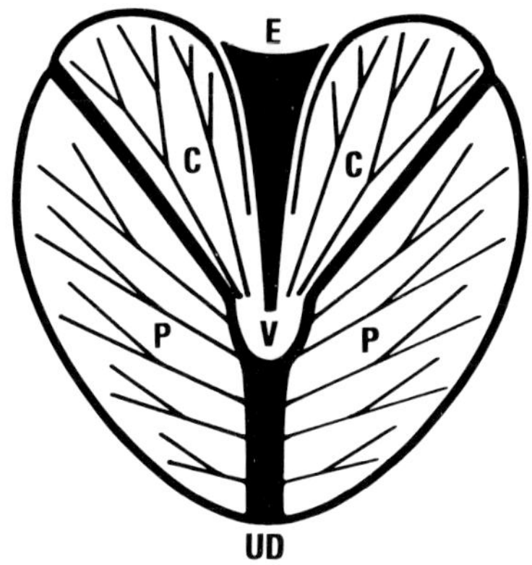

Fig. 1. (left) Sagittal diagram of prostate. Coronal plane of section (C) is related to ejaculatory ducts (E), verumontanum (V) and distal urethral segment (UD). Oblique coronal plane of section (OC) is related to bladder (B) and proximal urethral segment (UP). Anterior fibromuscular stroma (FM). Transverse plane of Fig. 6 (T). (From McNeal JE [1981]. Prostate 2:35 by permission.)

Fig. 2. (right) Diagram of coronal plane of section: Ducts of central zone (C) radiate proximally from verumontanum (V), flanking ejaculatory ducts (E). Ducts of peripheral zone (P) radiate laterally along distal urethral segment (UD). (From McNeal JE [1981]. Prostate 2:35 by permission.)

Anatomic Relationships of the Distal Urethral Segment

Two anatomically separate and histologically different zones of prostatic glandular tissue are identified in the coronal plane (Fig. 2) (McNeal 1968). The "peripheral zone" makes up about 75% of the glandular tissue revealed in this section. Its ducts exit directly laterally from the postero-lateral recess of the urethral wall, and their orifices trace a double lateral line extending from the prostate apex to the base of the verumontanum. Microscopically the architecture of the peripheral zone consists of small, simple, round to oval, acinar structures (Fig. 3) emptying into long narrow ducts and surrounded by a stroma of loosely arranged and randomly interwoven muscle bundles. The ducts and acini are lined by a simple columnar epithelium composed of clear cells with basally placed small, dark nuclei (Fig. 4).

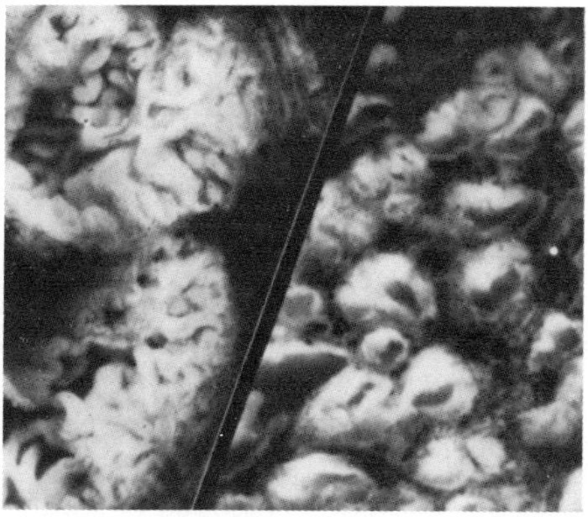

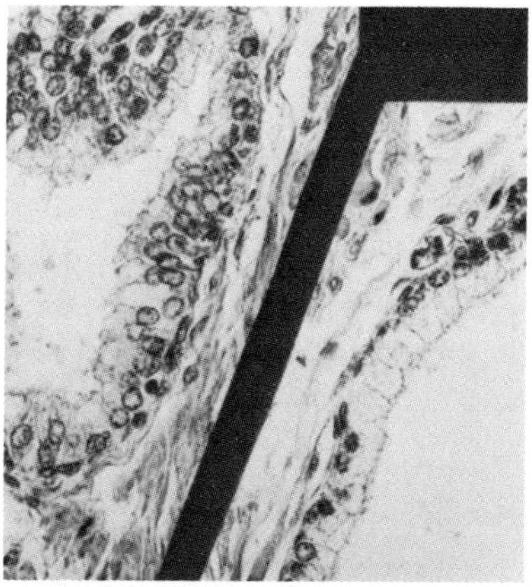

Fig. 3. (left) Cut surface of prostate. Lumens of central zone acini (upper left) are large and irregular, with intraluminal ridges. Lumens of peripheral zone acini (lower right) are small and rounded. (Original magnification x20). (From McNeal JE [1970]. In Griffiths K, Pierrepoint CG [eds]: "Some Aspects of the Aetiology and Biochemistry of Prostatic Cancer". Cardiff: Tenovus, p 23.)

Fig. 4. (right) Epithelium of central zone (upper left), showing large pale crowded nuclei and granular cytoplasm. Peripheral zone epithelium (lower right) has more uniform columnar cells, with pale cytoplasm and basal, small dark nuclei. (Hematoxylin-eosin, original magnification x320). (From McNeal JE [1970]. In Griffiths K, Pierrepoint CG [eds]: "Some Aspects of the Aetiology and Biochemistry of Prostatic Cancer". Cardiff: Tenovus, p 23.)

The proximal sector of the disc of glandular tissue

seen in the coronal plane is the "central zone". Its duct orifices lie on the convexity of the verumontanum immediately surrounding the ejaculatory duct orifices and anatomically separate from the double lateral line of the peripheral zone. The central zone ducts course predominantly proximally, closely following the ejaculatory ducts, which also lie in this coronal plane. The central zone completely surrounds the ejaculatory ducts as a conical mass, which is greatly flattened in its antero-posterior dimension.

The architecture of the central zone is quite different from that of the peripheral zone. Its ducts and acini are much larger and of irregular contour. The acini are polyhedral in cross section, and their walls bear a system of intraluminal ridges (Fig. 3). The lining epithelium appears crowded and pseudostratified, with larger, paler nuclei lying at different levels in columnar cells having granular, opaque cytoplasm (Fig. 4). The muscular stroma is much more compact than that of the peripheral zone.

The histologic differences between these zones are striking. The possibility that these differences may have biologic significance is reinforced by the finding that almost all cases of carcinoma and prostatitis arise in the peripheral zone, while the central zone is nearly immune to disease (McNeal 1968).

The histologic appearance of the central zone has some similarity to that of the seminal vesicle. Furthermore, the central zone is intimately related anatomically to the ejaculatory ducts. On the basis of these facts, it has been proposed that the central zone may be derived from the embryonic Wolffian duct rather than the urogenital sinus (McNeal 1983a).

Anatomic Relationships of the Proximal Urethral Segment

The double lateral line of peripheral zone ducts continues into the proximal urethral segment and there it gives rise to the remaining 5% of the prostatic glandular tissue which is located in the preprostatic region (McNeal 1978). The histology of the duct-acinar system here is identical to that of the peripheral zone. Nevertheless, there are several reasons to consider this a separate region of glandular tissue. First, the preprostatic gland mass is anatomically displaced anteriorly from the coronal plane of greatest extent of the peripheral zone. Secondly, there is an abrupt reduction of an order of magnitude in size and degree of development of the duct system from the peripheral zone to the preprostatic region. Thirdly, the stroma here is different from that of the peripheral zone. Finally, it is within this tissue exclusively that BPH takes origin.

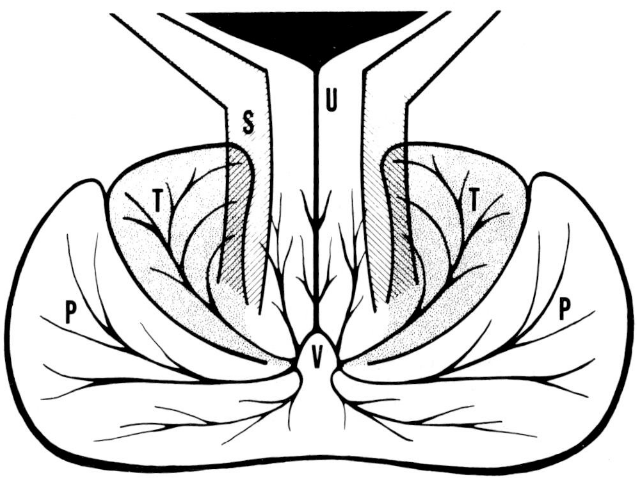

Fig. 5. Diagram of oblique coronal plane of section. Ducts of transition zone (T) exit from urethra just proximal to highest ducts of peripheral zone (P) and lateral to base of verumontanum (V). They follow outer border of preprostatic sphincter (S). Periurethral glands, shown larger than actual size, lie entirely in periurethral stroma (U). (From McNeal JE [1978]. Invest Urol 15:340 by permission.)

The dominant anatomic feature of this region is the preprostatic sphincter extending from the base of the verumontanum to the bladder neck (Fig. 5). This cylindrical sleeve of smooth muscle fibers is most compact and well defined dorsal to the urethra. Extending laterally, its fibers become progressively more widely separated from each other, particularly the most external fibers. Ventral to the urethra the fibers are still more widely separated, and there they interdigitate with the fibers of the anterior fibromuscular stroma (Fig. 6).

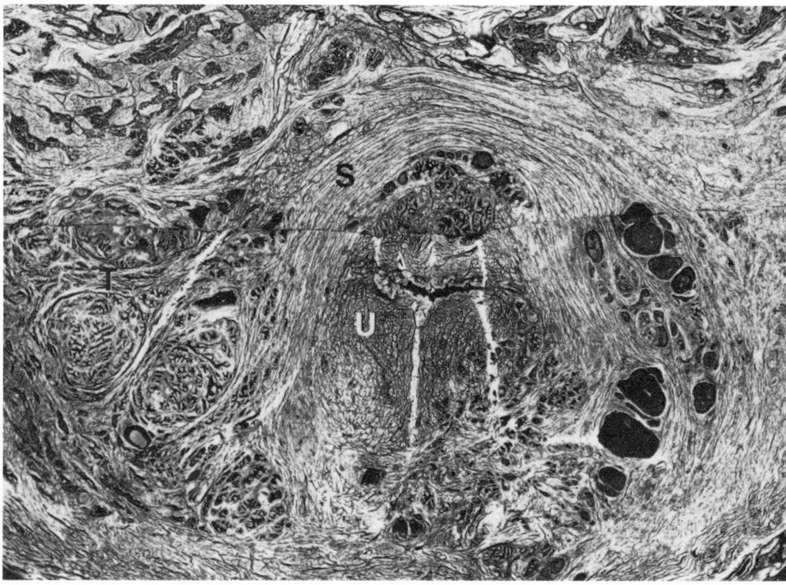

Fig. 6. Tissue section transverse to proximal urethral segment (plane T of Fig. 1). Preprostatic sphincter (S) forms a compact band dorsal to periurethral stroma (U). Sphincter fibers spread apart lateral to urethra and run between acinar clusters of transition zone (T), which have formed small BPH nodules. (Trichrome, original magnification x20.) (From McNeal JE [1978]. Invest Urol 15:340 by permission.)

The glandular tissue of the preprostatic region can be further subdivided into two zones on the basis of differences in relative degree of development of the duct system, location along the urethra, and relationship to the preprostatic sphincter. The "transition zone" is the larger of these two subdivisions (Fig. 5). Its ducts are the most distal, exiting laterally from the urethral wall at a single level, just proximal to the most proximal of the peripheral zone ducts and immediately distal to the lower border of the preprostatic sphincter. The most medial duct branches then curve proximally toward the bladder neck. They run parallel to the long axis of the preprostatic urethral segment and immediately adjacent to the external border of the preprostatic sphincter. The remaining duct branches fan out laterally from the urethra, lying close to the oblique coronal plane or diverging from it ventrally. None of the duct branches extend very far dorsal to the oblique coronal plane.

The most external fibers of the preprostatic sphincter spread laterally away from the main sphincteric mass and penetrate deeply through the transition zone muscular stroma lateral and ventral to the urethra. This interdigitation of sphincteric and transition zone stromas is further accentuated medially. The most medial small ducts and acini of this zone curve toward the midline and penetrate directly into the compact body of the sphincter. Such a blending of stromas associated with different functions is seen nowhere else in the prostate.

A further proximal continuation of the double lateral line of duct orifices into the segment of the urethra surrounded by the sphincter gives rise to the "periurethral gland zone" (Fig. 5). Unable to penetrate the sphincter, these duct branches lie confined inside it, embedded in the longitudinal, periurethral smooth muscle. The duct branches run proximally, directly parallel to the long axis of the preprostatic urethral segment. Their degree of development is abortive; they remain tiny in size with few branches, few acini and apparently no periacinar smooth muscle slings. This region is strung out along most of the preprostatic urethral segment. Its total glandular mass is nearly microscopic in size - - an order of magnitude smaller than the transition zone.

MORPHOLOGY OF BPH

Morphologic Features of BPH origin

In prostates with few BPH nodules, the anatomic coordinates of very early nodules can be clearly identified. The area of greatest predilection to nodule formation is the medial transition zone, either within or immediately adjacent to the preprostatic sphincter and directly lateral or somewhat ventral to the urethral lumen (Fig. 7) (McNeal 1978). Within this narrow zone, nodule formation is more common distally near the base of the verumontanum than

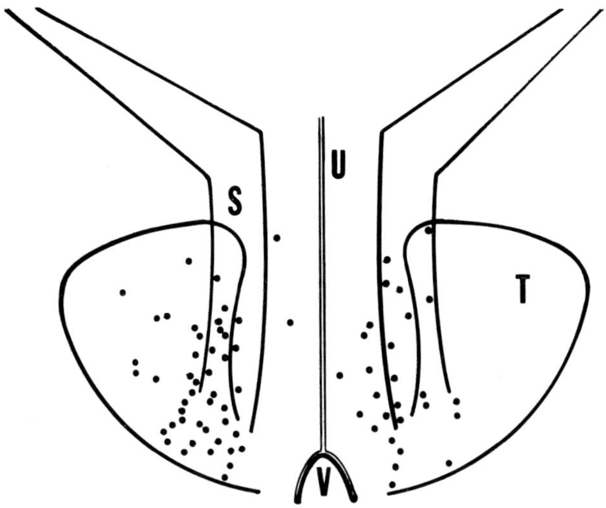

Fig. 7. Sites of origin of BPH nodules less than 3 mm in diameter projected onto modified diagram of OC plane (Fig. 5). Urethral lumen (U), verumontanum (V), preprostatic sphincter (S), transition zone (T). All glandular nodules are shown to left of urethra; all stromal nodules are shown to right of urethra. (From McNeal JE [1978]. Invest Urol 15:340 by permission.)

proximally toward the bladder neck. A second area of strong predilection for nodule formation is the periurethral stroma inside the confines of the preprostatic sphincter. In this location the distribution of small nodules is relatively uniform along the proximal urethral segment between the bladder neck and the base of the verumontanum. Here nodules occur with nearly equal frequency dorsally, laterally and ventrally to the urethral lumen. There is, therefore, an extraordinarily sharp focusing of the sites of nodule origin within the prostate into a region comprising perhaps less than 2% of its total mass.

Within this tiny volume, however, the locations of individual nodules appear to be randomly determined.

In prostates with somewhat larger and more numerous BPH nodules, which represent an older age group, the anatomic focusing is the same but is not as restricted. Small early nodules are now found occasionally in almost any portion of the transition zone. If the areas of the transition zone nodules in these prostates are subtracted from the total transition zone area, there is evidence that the uninvolved transition zone is modestly larger in prostates with more nodules. This suggests that a diffuse increase in the size of the transition zone accompanies advancing age or the development of more nodules, even though its morphology is not significantly altered.

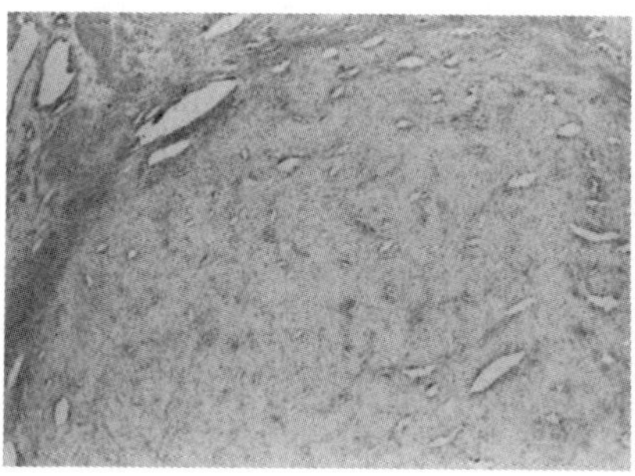

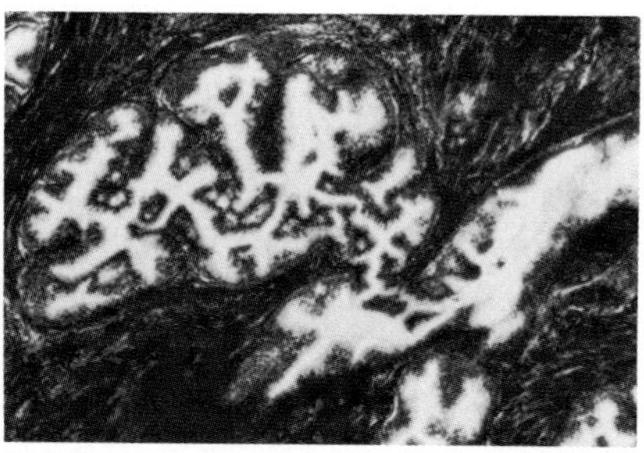

Fig. 8. (left) Morphology of small stromal nodule. Loose pale stroma of nodule lacks glands. It forms sharp expansile border with mature periurethral stroma at upper left. (Hematoxylin-eosin, original magnification x20.) (From McNeal JE [1983]. Monographs in Urology 4:3.)

Fig. 9. (right) Morphology of small glandular nodule. Branch from a medium-sized duct at lower right arborizes into a nodular cluster of small ducts and acini. (Trichrome, original magnification x20.) (From McNeal JE [1983]. Monographs in Urology 4:3.

The great majority of periurethral nodules are purely stromal in character or show only a few small glands penetrating from the periphery. The stroma of these nodules is unique. It is distinctively reminisent of embryonic mesenchyme, with an abundance of pale ground substance and only a few fine collagen fibers (Fig. 8). Partial maturation of some of the fibroblast-like cells into smooth muscle is occasionally seen.

Most transition zone nodules are histologically quite different. The earliest lesion is a proliferation of glandular tissue with a relative reduction in the amount of stroma. The stroma usually consists of mature smooth muscle like that of the uninvolved transition zone. The glandular tissue of these nodules is derived from newly formed small duct branches which bud off of pre-existing ducts and grow into the adjacent stroma, repeatedly re-branching to create a new architectural system within the nodule (Fig. 9). A given nodule often contains new branches from more than one small duct in the vicinity. Branches from opposite sides of a nodule may send twigs directly toward each other; their acini meet near the center of the nodule, with only a narrow band of stroma between them.

While they remain small, glandular nodules lack a well defined expansile border and are more difficult to recognize than stromal nodules, which stand out because of their uniquely different mesenchymal composition. The distinctive features of glandular nodules are the abrupt increase in closeness of acinar packing in a focus where small ducts branch directly toward each other. Also the lining epithelium is often taller within the nodule than in the immediate vicinity. This hypertrophy of individual epithelial cells is characteristic of glandular nodules and can frequently be demonstrated in a striking manner in ducts which pass close to the border of a nodule. The wall of the duct closest to the nodule shows a marked increase in the height of the columnar epithelial cells, while the more distant duct wall shows a normal to atrophic epithelium (Fig. 10). Also the nearer wall of the duct often sends several branches directly into the nodule, but no branches are found on the opposite wall. (Fig. 11). Eccentric branching from the inner walls of tangent ducts can be seen at the borders of the largest glandular nodules, suggesting that their growth at all stages of development is accomplished by accretion from beyond the nodule periphery as well as expansion from within.

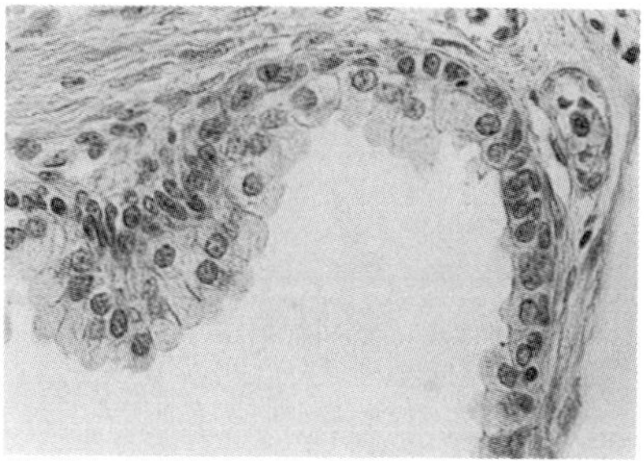

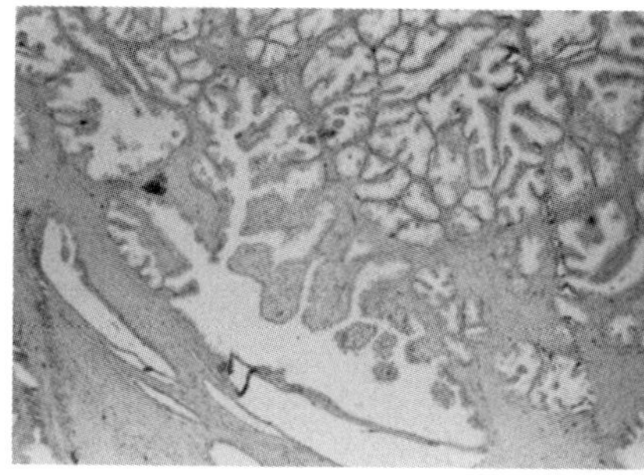

Fig. 10. (left) Border duct of glandular nodule cut tangentially. Duct wall facing nodule shows cell enlargement and crowding, whereas duct wall away from nodule at right shows mild epithelial atrophy. (Hema-toxylin-eosin, original magnification x320.) (From McNeal JE [1983]. Monographs in Urology 4:3.)

Fig. 11. (right) Border of large glandular nodule. Duct adjacent to nodule sends out branches exclusively on the nodule side, and these grow into the glandular mass. (Hematoxylin-eosin, original magnification x20.) (From McNeal JE [1983]. Monographs in Urology 4:3.

Morphologic Features of BPH Evolution

Occasional small glandular and stromal nodules can be found in the transition zone and periurethral zone even in men in the fourth decade. Their numbers increase in a linear progression with age, but large nodules are uncommon in most prostates until well into the seventh decade. Thus for about 30 years, the progression of BPH is represented predominantly by increase in nodule numbers, while the subsequent growth of each newly formed nodule is generally slow. Then between the late years of the seventh decade and the first half of the eighth decade there is a second phase of evolution, characterized by a rather abrupt and marked increase in the number of prostates having nodules of large mass.

Throughout the first phase of BPH evolution there is a tendency for glandular nodules to be somewhat larger than stromal nodules. In the second phase of nodule expansion, this difference is further accentuated. Marked increase in size is overwhelmingly a complication affecting glandular nodules, and consequently is a process which in most men is limited to the transition zone. The typical "lateral lobes" of the usual case of clinical BPH lie in precisely the anatomic location of the normal transition zone.

In a distinct minority of cases, prominent periurethral nodule expansion is found. In these prostates almost invariably the enlarged nodules are found to be glandular. This suggests that exuberant gland invasion of periurethral stromal nodules is a prerequisite for marked enlargement. The commonest location for periurethral nodules of clinically significant size is dorsal to the urethral at the bladder neck. Such "middle lobe" BPH is always periurethral since there is no transition zone tissue dorsal to the urethra at any level.

In the second phase of BPH evolution, it is uncommon to find that marked nodule enlargement has affected only a few out of a large number of nodules in a gland. Most often there appears to be coordinated growth of the majority of the nodules in any given prostate. Also, early in the eighth decade those prostates with the largest BPH mass often show an increase in glandular activity within their nodules to well above the mean level which is characteristic of nodules in earlier decades. The picture of exuberant epithelial hyperplasia, with numerous, closely packed small glands and little stroma is usually shared by most of the enlarged nodules within any prostate.

BIOLOGY OF BPH - INFERENCES FROM MORPHOLOGY

In the observations presented above there are a number of clues to the dynamic processes underlying the origin and evolution of BPH. These observations are assembled here into an integrated hypothesis of the nature of this disease, one which emphasizes the probability of a critical role for the operation of embryonic processes reawakened in a distorted form in adult life.

The developmental course of the transition zone, the main substrate for BPH development, suggests that it may be a region which is unusually susceptible to disturbances of growth control. In the prepubertal prostate, complete morphogenesis of the transition zone appears to lag behind that of the rest of the organ. Then in the adult the normal post-pubertal repression of further growth potential may be less completely imposed here, as evidenced by the gradual increase in transition zone mass with age. Also the mingling of transition zone tissue with a foreign sphincteric stroma might be expected to increase the chances for disturbances of the epithelial-stromal interactions which contribute to the maintenance of the normal adult state. Indeed, the portion of the transition zone which is most susceptible to BPH is that which is closest to the sphincter.

The genesis of the BPH nodule probably results from a disturbance arising entirely at the local tissue level within this susceptible region. Nodule genesis by definition is sharply focal, and its distribution is random within the area of susceptibility. A primary endocrine imbalance would probably be expressed diffusely, at least throughout a given region. Furthermore, no endocrine imbalance has been described as early as the fourth decade, when nodules begin to appear.

There are several lines of evidence supporting the postulate that the initial abnormality in nodule genesis is a spontaneous reversion of a clone of stromal cells to the embryonic state. One important piece of evidence supporting this proposition is the mesenchymal appearance of the periurethral zone nodule.

The absence of such a morphologic stromal abnormality in the more actively proliferative transition zone glandular nodule might appear to negate this hypothesis. In fact, it strongly supports the concept if the principles of normal embryonic development are kept in mind. The stromas of embryonic glandular organs normally have a limited capacity for self-stimulation of growth. Full actualization of growth potential is achieved only through coordinated interactions -- inductions -- between epithelium and stroma. So most nodules, like most embryonic organs, grow well only if the stroma can stimulate adjacent epithelium. This is more likely to occur in the gland-rich transition zone than in the gland-poor periurethral zone. Furthermore, in normal embryonic development, epithelium provides the inductive stimulus for the stroma to mature into adult smooth muscle. Consequently, if embryonic principles are followed in BPH nodules, sufficient epithelial participation would insure that stroma would not accumulate in excessive amounts and would not remain embryonic in character. On the other hand, the stromal nodule, lacking epithelium, would be arrested in both growth and maturation.

The ratio of stroma to glands is extremely variable among glandular nodules, and stereological analysis of a series of suprapubic prostatectomies has shown that on the average the proportion of stroma is greater than in normal prostatic tissue (Rohr 1980). It should be noted that the validity of the hypothesis of stromal induction as presented here does not depend on the ratio of stroma to glands in the nodule. In fact, early nodules of microscopic size most often show exuberant gland proliferation with a relative reduction in the proportion of stroma. There is evidence that at least some larger nodules with a high ratio of stroma to glands may be the result of secondary involution of the epithelial component. Of greater significance in supporting the hypothesis of a primary stromal abnormality in BPH, is the recent finding of a threefold increase in the concentration of 5 alpha reductase in the nodule stroma, while the epithelial concentration of the enzyme is not significantly elevated (McLoughlin 1983).

Some of the inductive interactions of embryonic development are mediated by diffusible inducers. That these may operate to stimulate epithelial activity in BPH is suggested by the morphologic peculiarities seen in ducts which are tangent to nodule borders. They often show epithelial cell hyperplasia and budding of new duct branches exclusively on the duct wall which faces the nodule center. Such an eccentric effect on a single duct strongly implies that one side of the duct is exposed to an influence which is not felt by the opposite wall. Of course, this interpretation is valid only if normal adult epithelium retains the capacity to respond to embryonic inducers. In support of this critical point, it has recently been shown that adult bladder epithelium, a tissue of urogenital sinus derivation, will proliferate to form mature prostatic ducts and acini when exposed to embryonic prostatic mesenchyme (Cunha 1980).

The process of formation of new architecture by budding from pre-existing ducts must be considered to be the basic, definitive morphologic feature of the glandular nodule. It is the initial abnormality seen in the incipient lesion, and it is found in tangent ducts adjacent to larger nodules throughout the natural history of the disease. Since the formation of new architecture is a central feature of embryonic development and is consistently repressed in adult life, this is perhaps the strongest evidence of all that the development of BPH nodules is driven by an embryonic program.

The concept that the genesis of BPH nodules results from alterations at the local tissue level does not negate the possibility that hormones play a role in pathogenesis. Androgens are necessary for the activation of the embryonic developmental program of the prostate and are presumably necessary for the expression of reawakened embryonic capacities in the adult. However, androgenic stimulation can elicit the formation of new gland architecture only in tissues which already have that capacity. Therefore, the initial pathogenetic event must be a deviation of the androgen responsiveness of the target tissue away from that of the normal adult state. In this perspective, it is probable that the quantitative level of androgenic stimulation may have little additional promoting effect on the process so long as it exceeds a threshold value.

In addition to a probable permissive role for androgens in nodule genesis, there are indications that another type of endocrine influence may be involved in the marked enlargement of nodules which is seen in the second stage of BPH evolution. Acceleration of nodule growth appears to affect multiple nodules at nearly the same time and is often accompanied by evidence of enhanced epithelial proliferation. Also its time of onset in most men falls in a rather narrow age range between the seventh and eighth decades. This pattern suggests the possibility that some rather marked alteration in endocrine status occurs in most men in the seventh decade. No dramatic change in the levels of any steroid hormones has been identified in this age range. It is possible, therefore, that non-steroidal hormones may be involved. It is also possible that the triggering event may be the removal of a growth repressing effect rather than a direct stimulus. To date there has been no investigation of the effect of pineal hormones on the prostate in adult life, even though the pineal gland is known to have a dramatic repressing effect on sexual development before puberty. The pineal continues to secrete during adult life, and its functional atrophy in the seventh decade might remove important restraints to growth. The release effect should be felt diffusely, but it might only become manifest in areas such as the BPH nodule where growth control is already partially lost. In an age range where some degree of atrophy in many organs is not unexpected, this hypothesis has logical appeal.

ANIMAL MODELS FOR NODULAR HYPERPLASIA OF THE PROSTATE

An ideal animal model for BPH would be one in which the morphologic details of the BPH nodule occur spontaneously or are induced in a region of the animal prostate which corresponds in its anatomic relationships to the area in which the human disease develops. Nothing close to this ideal has yet been found. Less than optimal models must be used, and much valuable information can be gained from them. It is important, however, for us to be aware of the exact nature and degree of the differences so that the findings from animal studies will be extrapolated to the human disease with appropriate reservations.

The dog is a popular animal model for BPH because prostatic hyperplasia often occurs spontaneously in older animals of this species. But unlike the human gland, the dog prostate is grossly and microscopically homogenous (McNeal 1983b). The entire organ corresponds most closely in its anatomic relationships to the human peripheral zone. The seminal vesicles and any tissue resembling the human central zone are absent. This may represent an arrest in the development of Wollfian duct derived tissues. All ducts extend from the urethra to the capsule; there is no "periurethral organ". No ducts arise from the urethra proximal to the verumontanum, and there is no area of admixture of glandular and sphincteric tissue.

Canine hyperplasia arises diffusely throughout all areas of the prostate, and tissue closer to the urethra may often be less involved than the subcapsular tissue. There are no nodules in canine hyperplasia, and there is no alteration of stroma to resemble embryonic mesenchyme. Perhaps, most importantly, there does not appear to be any formation of new gland architecture. There is, therefore, no morphologic evidence that embryonic processes are involved in the pathogenesis of canine prostatic hyperplasia.

Prostatic hyperplasia in the dog appears to consist purely of a proliferation of epithelial cells. The prostate accomodates to the increased epithelial cell population by enlargement of pre-existing ducts and acini and by displacement of the crowded epithelium into tufts and papillations which partly fill gland lumens. Stereologic analysis confirms the visual impression of a primary epithelial hyperplasia without stromal involvement (Rohr 1983). A similar histologic picture is produced in the human prostate by prolonged administration of high doses of testosterone.

It remains to be proven how important these morphologic differeneces may be to the interpretation of results from canine investigations. Until such proof is available, it seems inappropriate to use the term "canine BPH", which appears to imply that a significant homology to the human disease is already established.

The non-human primate may be a good candidate for an animal model because of close genetic relationship to the human species. The cranial and caudal lobes of the rhesus and baboon prostate are probably directly homologous to the human central and peripheral zones (Blacklock 1977). These two lobes are clearly identifiable on external examination because the anterior fibromuscular stroma is absent, and the two zones are not welded together as they are in the human (Fig. 12). The preprostatic sphincter is also not contained within the prostate, and it can be seen on external examination. No glandular tissue appears to arise from the urethra proximal to the base of the verumontanum, and the transition zone and periurethral zone are probably absent. It remains to be seen whether anything closely resembling BPH can be induced in the prostates of other primates.

The anatomic differences between the human, canine and non-human primate prostates are representative of a general pattern of great interspecies anatomic diversity. The full range of this diversity is not known because the prostates of relatively few species have been studied in detail. Accordingly, while further research on the canine and primate models may yield important findings, a search should

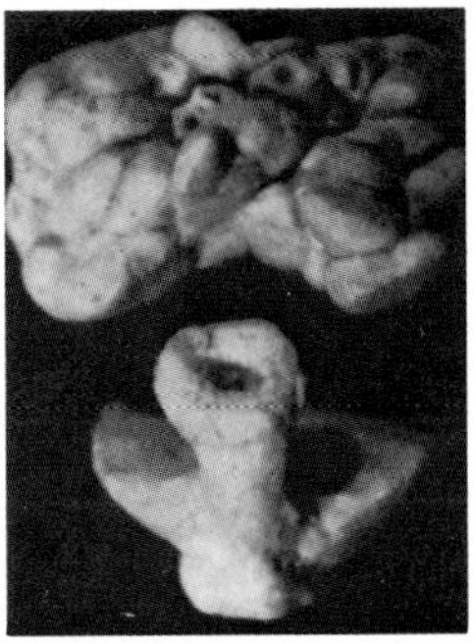

Fig. 12. Baboon prostate, frontal view. Cranial lobe detached and displaced superiorly. Caudal lobe is adherent to distal urethral segment and extends mainly posteriorly. Proximal urethral segment to bladder neck is not embedded in prostate. (From McNeal JE [1981]. Prostate 2:35 by permission.)

probably continue for some species in which prostatic anatomy more closely resembles that of the human gland.

REFERENCES

Blacklock NJ, Bouskill, K (1977). The zonal anatomy of the prostate in man and in the rhesus monkey. Urol Res 5:163.

Cunha GR, et al (1980). Glandular epithelial induction by embryonic mesenchyme in adult bladder epithelium of BALB/C mice. Invest Urol 17:302.

McLoughlin MG, Bruchovsky, N (1983). Stromal-epithelial interaction. In Hinman F (Ed) "Benign Prostatic Hypertrophy". New York:Springer-Verlag, p. 130.

McNeal, JE (1968). Regional morphology and pathology of the prostate. Amer J Clin Pathol 49:347.

McNeal, JE (1972). The prostate and prostatic urethra: a morphologic synthesis. J Urol 107:1008.

McNeal, JE (1978). Origin and evolution of benign prostatic enlargement. Invest Urol 15:340.

McNeal, JE (1980). Anatomy of the prostate: an historical survey of divergent views. Prostate 1:3.

McNeal, JE (1983a). The prostate gland: morphology and pathobiology. Monographs in Urology 4:3.
McNeal, JE (1983b). Relationship of the origin of benign prostatic hypertrophy to prostatic structure of man and other animals. In Hinman F (Ed). "Benign Prostatic Hypertrophy", New York: Springer-Verlag, p. 152.
Rohr HP, Bartsch G (1980). Human benign prostatic hyperplasia: A stromal disease; new perspectives by quantitative morphology. Urology 16:625.
Rohr HP, Bartsch G (1983). Stereological analysis: An approach to the pathogenesis of benign prostatic hyperplasia. In Hinman F (Ed). "Benign Prostatic Hypertrophy", New York: Springer-Verlag, p 112.

Discussion

Katzenellenbogen: You propose a very interesting hypothesis. What factors do you feel are important in this reactivation of the embryonic program in the stromal component?

McNeal: Well, that gets us to a very speculative level. I can't resist having my fantasies about this, so that's what this is, a fantasy. Everytime cells divide, they entertain a risk of error. We know that the division process is not error free. It is my proposal that, as the stromal cells divide very slowly during adult life, occasionally an error occurs. That error is simply a shift, one gene backward on the chromosome from the adult stromal program to the embryonic stromal program. I think this occurs purely at the local level. Embryonic inductions similar to those of the BPH nodule are seen in other diseases in other organs. They are seen in adenomyosis of the uterus, Warthin's tumor of the salivary gland and the fibroadenoma of the breast. There are other conditions in which the same rules seem to apply that apply here. I think this reversion to an embryonic program on the part of the stroma with induction of epithelium is something that occurs much more commonly in adult life than we realize.

Katzenellenbogen: You think, that this would be a normal correlate of aging of the gland?

McNeal: I think of it as time dependent. Maybe in a time frame, or perspective, of the numbers of cell divisions, rather than aging in terms of deterioration of body tissues. That is speculative, too.

Katzenellenbogen: Why do you think that this transitional stroma is particularly susceptible.

McNeal: The transition zone is late to complete organogenesis. Organogenesis seems never to be complete and the transition zone continues to enlarge in later adult life. Also, there is an admixture of inappropriately combined stromas. These are just hints, and I can't go from there to specific mechanisms. No one knows enough.

Katzenellebogen: Is there any evidence for the expression of any fetal antigens in this stroma?

McNeal: That would be interesting to find out. I don't think anyone has tried.

Mawhinney: You're saying that benign prostatic hypertrophy involves neither the peripheral prostate nor the central zone. A critical question is whether or not the peripheral prostate glands or glands of the central zone, which may have a different embryonic origin, ever come in contact with the periurethral sphincteric material. Might you assume that if there was such a mixture of these other compounds, similar to that of the transitional zone and sphincteric stroma, that they would likely respond with adenomatous growth?

McNeal: Definitely the peripheral zone and the central zone never show any intimate relationship of sphincteric to glandular tissue. The glandular tissue of the central zone is close to the external portion of the sphincter in small areas but not as close as the transitional zone. However there doesn't seem to be any effect. I think your observation is very interesting and pertinent. Beyond that I can't add further.

Mawhinney: When you mention species here, have you looked among any other species where we might search for a relationship that looks like that of the human transitional zone and sphincteric muscle? We need a species that we could work with in a laboratory, where we could control age and hormone environment.

McNeal: I have looked at some other species, including sheep, pigs, cats, and a variety of small primates. The glands look strikingly different from one species to another. It is very difficult to pick out homologies, but I think we ought to try. I think looking at more primates is definitely in order. The monkeys that I have looked at are so tiny that one has to do the gross examination under a microscope. Under those circumstances I haven't had enough material to be sure about homologies one way or the other.

Mawhinney: I have seen comments about the fact that the basal part of a lot accessory sex organs respond differently to hormones than the part that is more distant to the urethra. For example, maximal estrogenic response is in the basal part of a seminal vesicle. In the prostate the region around the urethra may show more proliferative response than the more distal areas. I wonder if this is something your are addressing here. I really think what we need to know what would be an appropriate system in animals to duplicate what you are talking about.

McNeal: I wish I could answer the questions you have raised.

Li: I enjoyed your talk very much. One thing I liked about it was that you don't think that hormonal responses are the total problem in BPH. I think we ought to look at all the possibilities. Your hypothesis is reasonable, namely that dedifferentation of the stroma may be one of the causes of BPH. Why is BPH limited to old age? Can it randomly occur at any age in the male population?

McNeal: I'm glad you brought that up. The earliest BPH nodules are found not rarely in men in their 30's. I know that they are not always reported to be found so early. If one does careful serial sections in the oblique coronal plane one can pick up small nodules occurring in men in their 30's. I think nodules begin to appear not long after the full postpubertal development of the prostate is complete. The nodules seem to progress in linear fashion throughout the remainder of life. I don't know whether that progression accelerates with old age, which would lead me to think of an aging process, or whether the progression is simply time dependent. This is a question which ought to be answered. Your initial statement is important: we should stop limiting ourselves to looking at BPH as a disease with one cause, since it is more likely a complex multifactorial thing. Maybe the causal factors I presented here aren't all there are, and maybe a lot of them aren't the right ones, but the possibility that there are several should be explored.

Li: Has the immunological status of a virus related phenomena been explored in the area?

McNeal: Not to my knowledge. Good point.

Cunha: I really enjoyed your talk, John. Just a couple of comments and then a question. In order for the neoformation of glandular tissue to occur in adult, we really have to satisfy two requirements. One, there must be a mesenchymal inductor, and secondly, there also must be an epithelium present that is capable of responding. Both of those requirements have to be fulfilled, or else we do not get a morphogenetic process. The comment I would like to make is that we have been exploring the possible existence of those types of properties within the adult prostatic components. In the case of the epithelium, the evidence is very clearcut. The adult prostatic epithelium is, indeed, responsive to an embryonic prostatic inductor. These data have been developed in our laboratory by one technique, and more recently in Leland Chung's laboratory through a different technique. This conclusion is on very solid ground at this point in time. In addition, we have preliminary data that suggest that adult prostatic stromal cells may be able to function with an embryonic epithelium in a morphogenetic sense. This is preliminary finding which needs clarification, but we do have data that adult stromal cells have the ability to induce or participate in morphogenetic processes. Conversely, the epithelium is clearly responsive.

I have another comment. You mentioned the differentiation of mesenchymal cells in some of the pure stromal nodules into smooth muscle and how that, in turn, they might be affected by the invading epithelium. There are some studies buried back in the literature on epithelium-mesenchymal interactions on the developing lung. The lung mesenchyme must give rise to a variety of derivatives: cartilage, smooth muscle, and just connective tissue. In that particular system, the differentiation of the mesenchymal cells from the undifferentiated state to those end products requires contact with epithelium. This fits very nicely with what you are considering as well.

The questions I have relate to what type of nodule appears first. Does the stromal nodule appear first and then later are there epithelial nodules? In any given prostate, how many nodules are going to be stromal and how many are going to be epithelial? In BPH, are we dealing with clinical symptoms that are generated primarily by purely stromal nodules, or symptoms that are generated by nodules of mixed epithelial and stromal content?

McNeal: You brought up a number of things that I didn't make clear. First I meant to mention your work, which I think is an extraordinarily important confirmation of what I have suggested. Secondly, as far as nodules are concerned, stromal and glandular nodules begin appearing at about the same age -- in the 30's. They both increase in numbers in linear fashion. The glandular nodules tend to be more numerous and a bit larger in any age group all the way along the line. Later, when nodules begin to accelerate their growth, that acceleration and massive enlargement is almost always limited to the glandular nodules. So the early nodules which are small, and which remain small for decades, don't cause clinical symptomotology. When the nodules begin to become massively enlarged and are then associated with clinical disease, these are almost exclusively the glandular nodules, although some overgrown stromal nodules may be mixed in with them.

Cunha: One other comment, I think it may be very important for all of us to consider. I think I am restating something you said, John. BPH is a nodular disease and there is a big difference between the tissue from a TUR operation, and BPH. Any given chip is not necessarily BPH unless it can be shown to be part of a nodule, is this correct?

McNeal: Yes, that is an excellent, practical point. In the first place TURs almost invariably reach out and remove a portion of the peripheral zone. When you are dealing with a TUR chip, you may be dealing with BPH nodule, with peripheral zone tissue at the margins of the resection, or or you may be dealing with non-nodular urethral and bladder neck tissue from the beginning of the resection. In addition, there are men in other age groups with urethral obstruction who do not have significant BPH. Their symptoms are naturally relieved when the sphincter and bladder neck tissue are removed, even though that tissue under the microscope does not show the histologic features of BPH. So, you are quite right, Gerry. When you've got this tissue from a transurethral resection, you need to confirm under the microscope exactly which tissue component you are looking at before you take that tissue and subject it to more sophisticated analysis.

Bhuyan: Your talk brings to mind the similarity between BPH and the growth of neoplastic cells. First, you are saying that there is a focal development, in the same way that neoplastic cells apparently develop from a mutation. Second, as the nodule grows, it is diffusing something into its environment, so that the gland is sending out branches towards it. In the same way, when the tumor grows it is diffusing something that allows blood vessels to grow towards it. Finally, there is an increase with the number of cancer patients with age, in the same way that the number of nodules or the number of BPH increase with age. If all of these similarities are true, then would you suggest this could be an original mutation process in which the hormones might be acting as promotional agents?

McNeal: I think the analogy which you have drawn has a very limited validity. I don't think that BPH is intrinsically the same process that we are dealing with in neoplasia, certainly not malignant neoplasia. There isn't time to go into all the thoughts that I have about this, or the evidence. I just want to mention a few things very briefly. First, and perhaps most importantly, in the BPH nodule differentiation of the epithelial and stromal components is complete and perfect in terms of normal adult tissue. I don't believe it can be said of any neoplasm, that it completely capitulates the appearance of normal tissue. Secondly, although I can't give you evidence of this, but I feel that the difference between neoplasia and this process is that BPH is under a very tightly controlled growth program. It simply is a growth program that is playing by different rules than the growth program of the rest of the body. In BPH, the track the train is going down is a different track. In neoplasia the train has gone off the track, and there is loss of the growth control program. At least in BPH there is a substitution of one growth control program for another.

Walsh: Are there any changes in the peripheral zone of the prostate with aging? We know there is a difference in the hormonal milieu with aging, is this reflected in anyway in morphological changes in the peripheral lobe?

McNeal: There are tremendous morphologic changes in the peripheral zone. One of the things that has kept me so fascinated with prostate glands for so long is that after you get past the age of 40 years, no two prostate glands look alike. The peripheral zone is subjected to a variety of atrophic and hyperplastic changes, which at this point haven't yet been fully and adequately classified. Many of the hyperplastic changes represent the progressive initial stages of growth autonomy, many of which lead years later to malignancy.

Walsh: But when you see hyperplastic changes, are they like the hyperplastic changes in the dog prostate?

McNeal: Some of them are.

Walsh: Do they correlate with the growth of the nodules in the transition zone?

McNeal: Only in that both correlate with time and age. They are both so common that it's impossible to separate their correlations; the correlation of both with the passage of time and of aging. One could separate the correlations if either or preferably both processes were less frequent. But they are both occurring in the majority of men and so statistically it isn't possible to separate them.

Ofner: Could you consider the periurethral zone a Mullerian remnant and is there cross talk between it and the transitional zone? How do you feel that the two affect each other?

McNeal: I don't think that the Mullerian duct embryonic tissue plays any particular part in any anatomical area of the prostate, except perhaps the utricle. I even have some suspicions that in the cavity of the utricle the Mullerian system there has been replaced or overgrown by tissue which is non-Mullerian in origin. Thus, there remains no remnant of Mullerian tissue.

Lewis: I appreciate what you have seen in the coronal cuts and the oblique coronal cuts. If you cut across transversely at the preprostatic area, you should be able to distinguish three areas: the central, transitional and peripheral. Yet, I have never seen this type of cut in any of your publications. I am sure you must have done this, and I think that this would really help to visualize what you are saying conceptually.

McNeal The cut and the location you describe will show all the things you are talking about. However, it will show a central zone only where all the acini are gone and the smaller duct branches are collecting into the larger ducts immediately before they empty onto the verumontanum. You won't see anything that is histologically distinctive, just a small collection of big ducts coming down to join the urethra. With other cuts that you make, you invariably find that you cannot follow the ducts system in profile of all three of these zones at the same time. This is because they are going out in three different directions. To gain something, you're going to lose something. You can show them all right, and the best section to show all three is a parasagittal section. If you look at a parasagittal section, it is very difficult to know what you are looking at because none of the three duct systems show their branches in profile.

J. Isaacs: You were just suggesting that in BPH the nodules recapitulate normal morphology and morphogenesis. Many years ago, and he has stated it many times since, L.M. Franks made the point that the stromal tissue in BPH is relatively unique compared with normal stroma nodules in that the elastin fibers are apparently lacking in BPH nodules. Do you ever see this?

McNeal: That is a very interesting observation. It is hard for me to attach significance to it. I haven't studied it myself, and I apparently overlooked that Dr. Franks made that observation.

J. Isaacs: The reason why I bring it up is that several people at this meeting have talked about collagens. As we are now aware, the collagens are not of one, but multiple types. While morphologically stromal tissue in BPH nodules may look like normal stroma from an inductive or biochemical standpoint, the two may be very different.

McNeal: Yes, you are getting into an area that goes beyond morphology, and I think it is appropriate at this point for us to go beyond morphology. I have shown you what morphology can do. All that it can do is provide clues, and you are starting to follow up on the clues with your suggestions that require other techniques - Dr. Cunha's work and Dr. Chung's work are examples along those lines. I think that is where we will find the answers. I think one can carry morphology too far and beat it into the ground. I think looking at the elastic tissue and speculating on its meaning may be a dead end. I think it is a time for nonmorphologic studies and more sophisticated morphologic studies.

Marks: You rejected the idea of a similarity between BPH and tumors, but I wanted to offer one other possibility. If you look on a cancerous growth as a derepression rather than a mutational event and a return to embryonic growth in an unnatural adult situation, would you also consider the possibility that maybe BPH is a return to embryonic growth due to a derepression?

McNeal: I agree with you that malignancies involve, at least in some facet of their development, derepressions of embryonic programs. I think we just have to be cautious, since we know so little about BPH, so little about neoplasia, and so little about malignancy. If we find a derepression of embryonic-like programs in one condition and another derepression in another condition we shouldn't generalize and say they are all the same thing or that they are closely related. We just don't have enough information to make those generalizations.

New Approaches to the Study
of Benign Prostatic Hyperplasia, pages 55–65

ANATOMY OF THE HUMAN PROSTATE AND ITS THREE PAIRED LOBES

Lars E Tisell[1] and Håkan Salander

[1]Associate Professor of Surgery

Sahlgren's hospital, Göteborg, Sweden

In 1912 Lowsley published his description of the anatomy of the human prostate. His concept of the prostatic anatomy was founded on careful studies on embryonic and fetal glands. He described a dorsal or posterior lobe, a median and two lateral lobes and also a ventral lobe which, however, atrophied after birth.

The fact that these lobes could not be defined by dissection in the adult man explains why we have so many different views on the anatomy of the human prostate (Franks 1954, Hutch, Rambo 1970, McNeal 1968).

In the rat we know that the prostatic lobes can be anatomically separated. The prostatic lobes in rat also differ as to histology and physiology (Price, Williams-Ashman 1961). The lobe from which the sample was taken is always mentioned in research reports concerning the rat prostate. This seems self-evident, and should be so also in works concerning the human prostate.

That the adult human prostate is not a homogenous organ was substantiated by the findings of Saigraeff in 1928. He observed that the cranial part of the human prostate located below the seminal vesicles was delimited from the rest of the prostate by connective tissue. He named this part of the prostate "Nebenlappen" and noted that it had larger acini than the rest of the prostate. He also stressed the analogy between the anatomical location of this part of the human prostate and the cranial lobe of the monkey prostate as well as the coagulating glands of the rat. The observations of Saigraeff were forgotten but have later been confirmed and extended by the work of McNeal (1968, 1972).

After performing a lot of studies concerning the hormonal dependency of the prostatic lobes in rat (Tisell 1972) we draw the conclusion that it must be important to identify the lobes of the human prostate. It was indeed a very good thing that Saigraeff (1928) and McNeal (1968) had demonstrated that the prostate was histologically inhomogenous. However, the finding of only two subdivisions is not in keeping with the results of the careful embryological studies of Lowsley (1912). We therefore decided to try to identify and delimit the prostatic lobes of the human prostate. For this purpose we used fresh prostatic glands obtained from autopsy cases which were between 20 and 40 years of age (Tisell, Salander 1975). For the histological studies we also used prostates obtained from patients operated on with total cystoprostatectomies ranging in age from 43 to 73 years (Salander, Johansson, Tisell 1981).

Our anatomical findings concerning the human prostate is illustrated by the following sequence of figures.

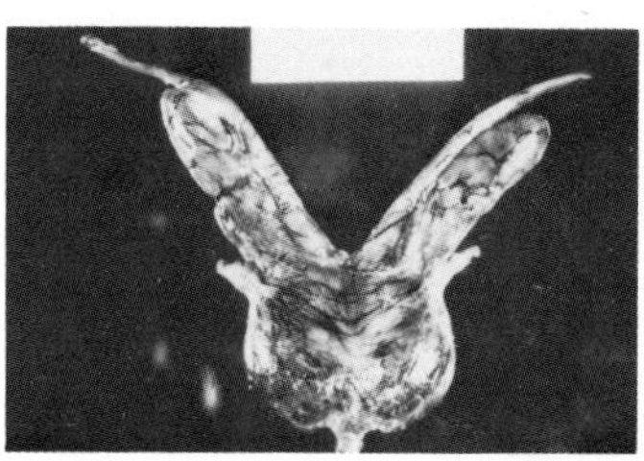

Fig. 1. This is an intact prostate seen from behind with seminal vesicles and deferential ducts. Note the prostatic vessels reaching the prostatic gland at its upper lateral corners.

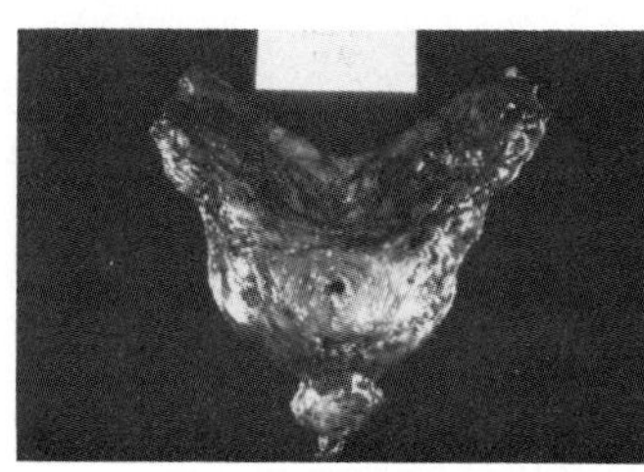

Fig. 2. Anterior view of intact prostate with seminal vesicles. In the center is the urethral lumen with an abundance of periurethral tissue. Some of the external sphincter muscle remains caudally around the urethra.

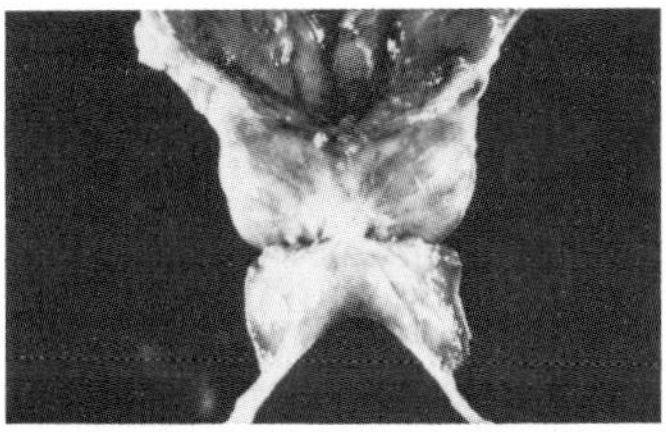

Fig. 3. View from behind. The dorsal lobes have been mobilized and turned downwards exposing the dorsal surfaces of the lateral lobes. Ducts from the dorsal lobes can be seen penetrating between the two lateral lobes to reach the urethra near the midline.

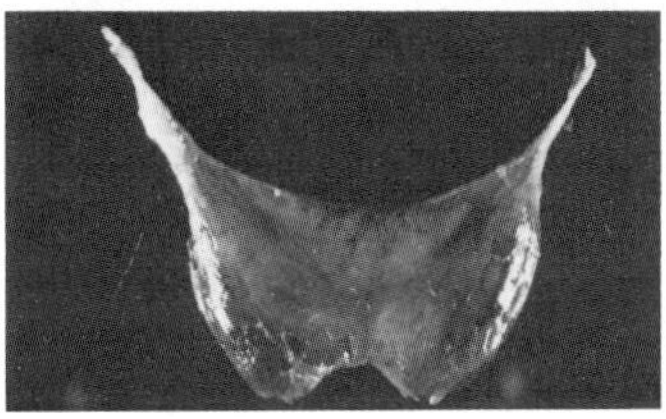

Fig. 4. The isolated dorsal lobes viewed from behind. The lobes are covered by a thin capsule and are united in the midline.

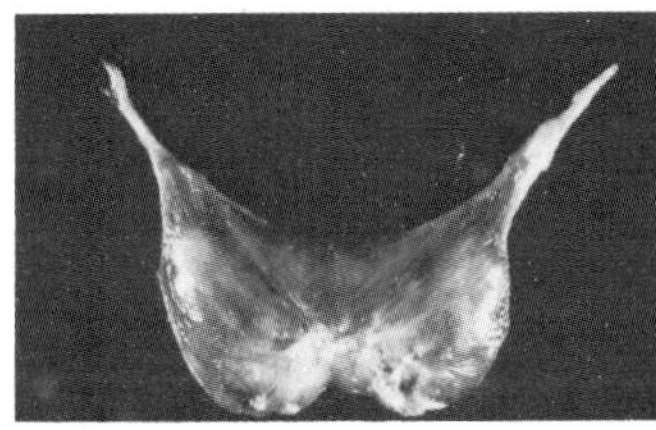

Fig. 5. Anterior view of the same isolated dorsal lobes as in fig 4. In the centre some cut ducts can be seen. Note the thin capsule.

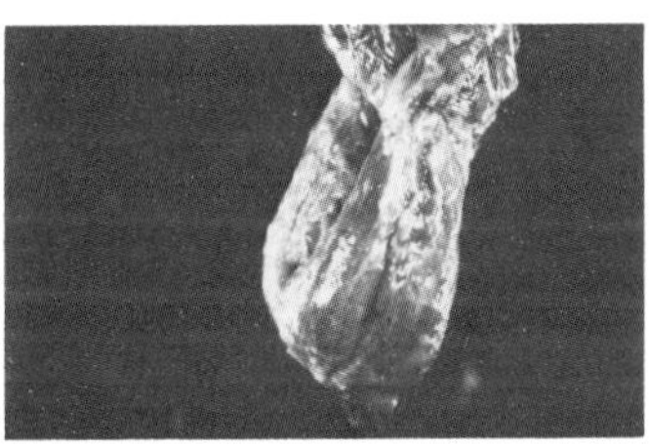

Fig. 6. Left lateral view of the prostate. The borderline between the dorsal and lateral lobes has been accentuated through dissection. Note that the dorsal lobes forms a considerable part of the lateral surface of the prostate and also forms the apex of the gland

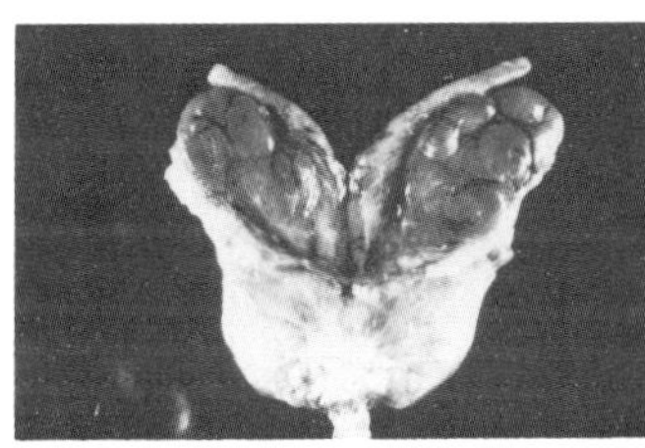

Fig. 7. The prostate after the dorsal lobes have been removed so that the lateral lobes are exposed from behind. Distally in the midline the defect can be seen where the ducts from the dorsal lobes went through to reach the urethra.

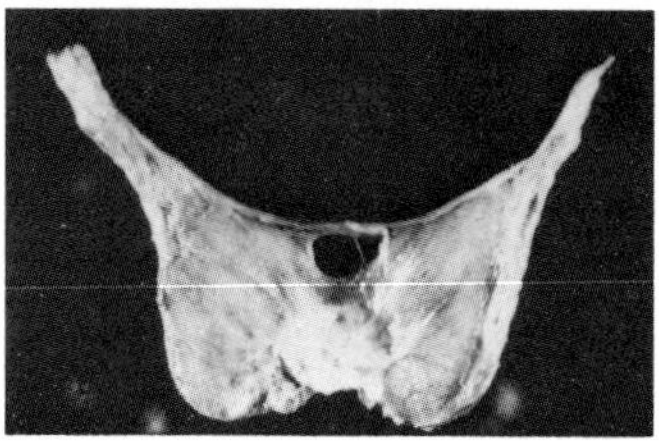

Fig. 8. The isolated lateral lobes seen from behind. The parenchyma is located laterally but the lobes are joined together in the midline behind the ejaculatory ducts.

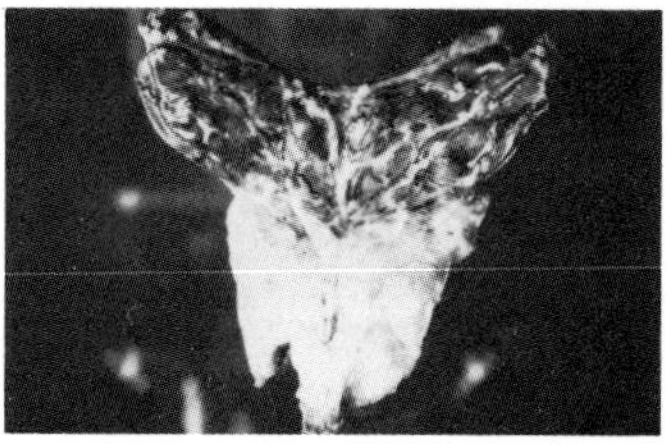

Fig. 9. Here the medial lobes are seen from behind after both the dorsal and lateral lobes have been removed. On the right side periurethral tissue can be seen below the arched lower border of the medial lobe. On the left side the periurethral tissue has been removed. There is no medial lobe parenchyma dorsally in the midline but the two medial lobes are joined togehter by connective tissue.

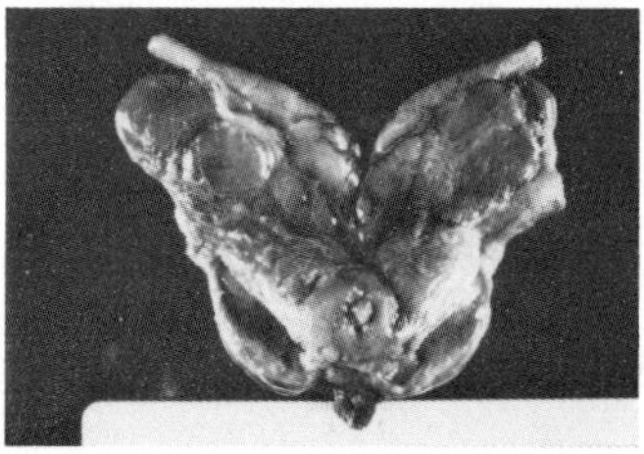

Fig. 10. Anterior view of the prostate and seminal vesicles. Centrally is the urethra with periurethral tissue. The medial lobes surround the urethra dorsolaterally. Lateral and posterior to the medial lobes are the freed lateral lobes.

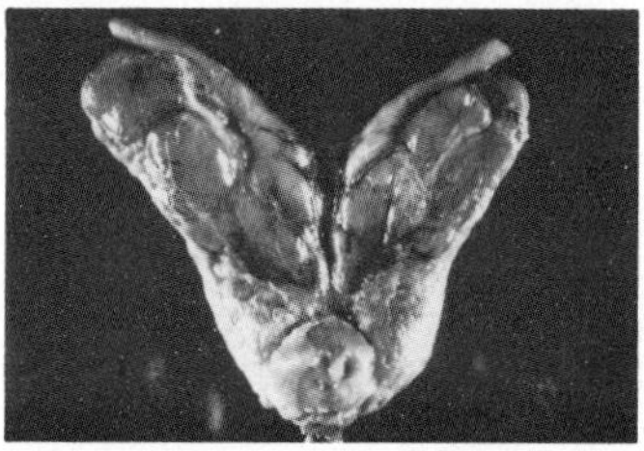

Fig. 11. Anterior view of the same prostate as in fig. 10 after the dorsal and lateral lobes haves been removed. Note that the medial lobes are closely attached to the seminal vesicles.

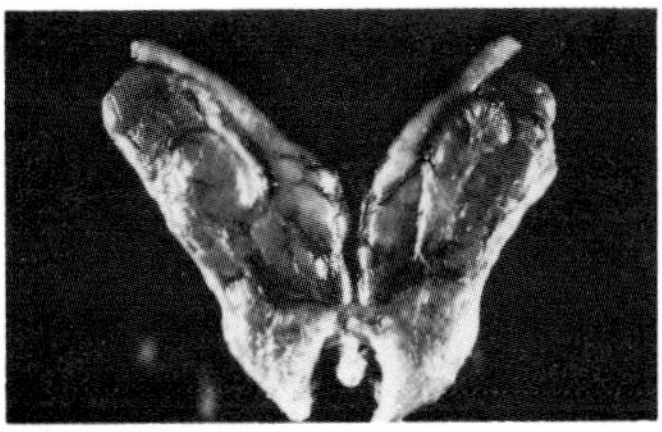

Fig. 12. Compared to fig. 11 urethra with periurethral tissue has been removed. The seminal colliculus, however, has been left in place.

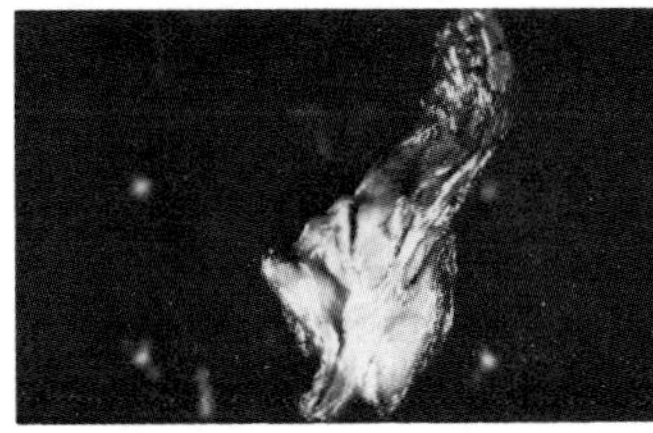

Fig. 13. Left lateral view of a sagittal section through the prostate. Note the ejaculatory duct opening on the seminal colliculus. In this section almost all of the prostatic parenchyma dorsal to the ejaculatory duct belongs to the dorsal lobe and only a narrow strip can be seen of the lateral lobe. Anterior to the ejaculatory duct is the cut-surface of the medial lobe. There is no prostatic parenchyma anterior to the urethra.

Histologically the three prostatic lobes differ from each other (Figs. 14 and 15). The medial lobes have the most unique histology with large acini arranged in a lobular pattern. The acini are divided into several parts by connective tissue. There are prominent papillary formations with ramifications. The stroma of the medial lobes is relatively dense. Transverse sections just above the seminal colliculus showed two areas with typical medial lobe acini, separated from each other by connective tisue. This finding is explained by the fact that the lower border of the medial lobes is arched (Fig. 9). A transverse section above the seminal colliculus therefore first passes through the medial lobes, then through periurethral tissue and then again through the medial lobe. These observations illustrate that the concept of the gross anatomy of the prostate cannot be based only on light microscopic studies. The acini of the dorsal lobes were smaller and more evenly distributed than in the medial lobes. The epithelium formed some simple papillary formations projecting towards the center of the acini. The acini of the lateral lobe were often dilated and cystlike.

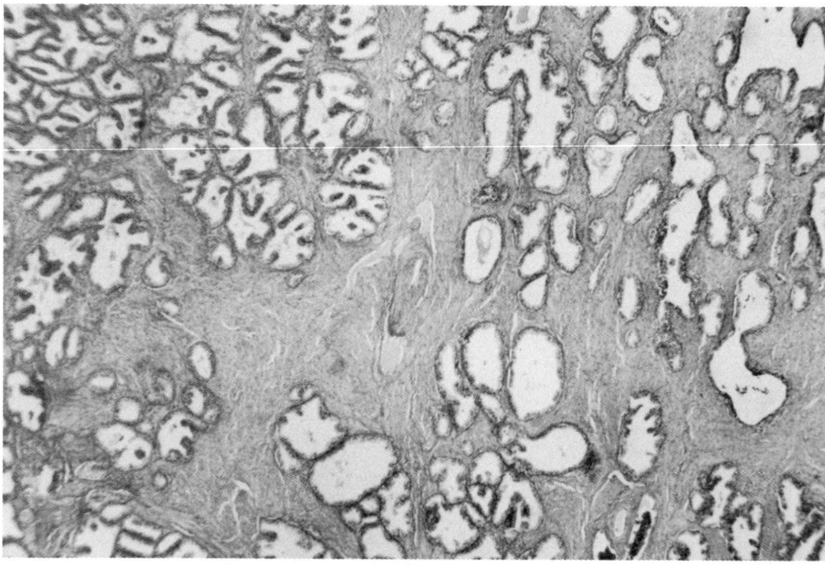

Fig. 14. This section illustrates the boundary zone between the medial lobe to the left and the lateral lobe to the right. The lobes are separated by sheets of fibrous tissue. Note the large artery.

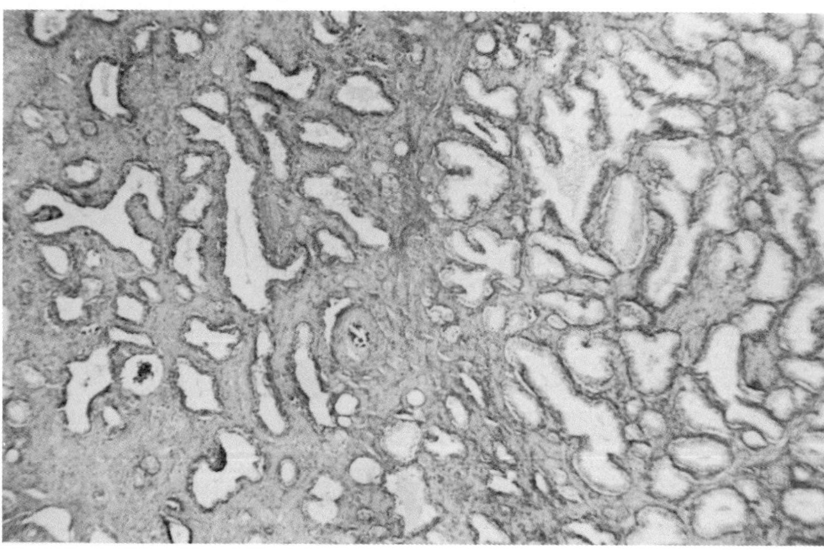

Fig. 15. This section illustrates the boundary zone between the lateral lobe to the left and the dorsal lobe to the right.

For further illustrations concerning the histology of the prostatic lobes see Salander, Johansson, Tisell (1981).

Our anatomical and histological studies have demonstrated that the human prostate is composed of three paired lobes. The medial lobes have a very distinct histological appearance but in a few cases it can be difficult to distinguish between the dorsal and lateral lobes in cases with very proliferent epithelium. On the other hand, in the macroscopic dissection of the prostate the most obvious demarcation was found between the dorsal and lateral lobes. Thus the histological and macro-anatomical methods are complementary to each other when to distinguish the separate prostatic lobes of the human prostate.

Our findings concerning the prostatic anatomy are not totally consistent with those of Lowsley (1912). An important difference is that we found that the two lateral lobes were joined together dorsally to the ejaculatory ducts. Some of the differences as to the lobe distribution within the prostate may be the result of the growth that occurs from embryonic life. It is to be remembered that the prostate increases in weight more than twenty times from birth to adultness (Leissner, Tisell 1979).

McNeal (1968) has proposed a new terminology for the division of the prostate, the central and peripheral zones. We have used the same terminology as Lowsley (1912) because his and our findings did not differ greatly from each other. We consider a zone a region without a sharp anatomical demarcation and therefore convenient to describe for instance the different layers of the adrenal cortex. A lobe on the other hand is a part of an organ demarcated by fissures or fibrous capsules. Therefore the different regions of the human prostate should be called lobes as they can be anatomically separated. This term is also used for the various regions of the monkey and rodent prostate. Using the same terminology in all species with discrete prostatic regions facilitates comparisons between homologous structures. The terms medial, lateral and dorsal don't entirely correspond to the position of the prostatic lobes in the adult man. However, we don't think it is appropriate to have different terminology for prostatic regions in embryos and adults.

Franks LM (1954). Benign nodular hyperplasia of the prostate: A review. Ann R Coll Surg 14:92.
Hutch JA, Rambo ON (1970). A study of the anatomy of the prostate, prostatic urethra and the urinary sphincter system. J Urol 105:443.
Leissner KH, Tisell LE (1979). The weight of the human prostate. Scand J Urol Nephrol 13:137.
Lowsley O (1912). The development of the human prostate gland with reference to the development of other structures of the neck of the urinary bladder. Am J Anat 13:299.
McNeal JE (1968). Regional morphology and pathology of the prostate. Am J Clin Pathol 49:347.
McNeal JE (1972). The prostate and prostatic urethra: A morphologic synthesis. J Urol 107:1008.
Price D, Williams-Ashman HG (1961). The accessory reproductive glands of mammals. In Sex and Internal Secretions (ed. W.C. Young) 3rd ed. Williams & Wilkins, Baltimore. vol. 1 pp. 366-448.
Saigraeff M (1928). Zur Frage der Histotopographie der Vorsteherdrüse und der Samenblasen. Z Urol Chir 24-25:389.
Salander H, Johansson S, Tisell LE (1981). The histology of the dorsal, lateral and medial prostatic lobes in man. Invest Urol 18:479.
Tisell LE (1972). Morphological studies of hormonal effects on the ventral and dorsolateral prostate, the coagulating glands and the seminal vesicles in rats. Thesis. University of Göteborg, Sweden.
Tisell LE, Salander H (1975). The lobes of the human prostate. Scand J Urol Nephrol 9:185.

The authors wish to acknowledge the editor of Scand J Urol Nephrol for permission to publish figures 1 to 13.

Discussion

McNeal: Dr. Tisell, I think we agreed previously that the very distinctive histologic appearance you show for your medial lobe is the same as the histologic appearance I have described for the central zone. Is that correct?

Tisell: Yes, this is correct.

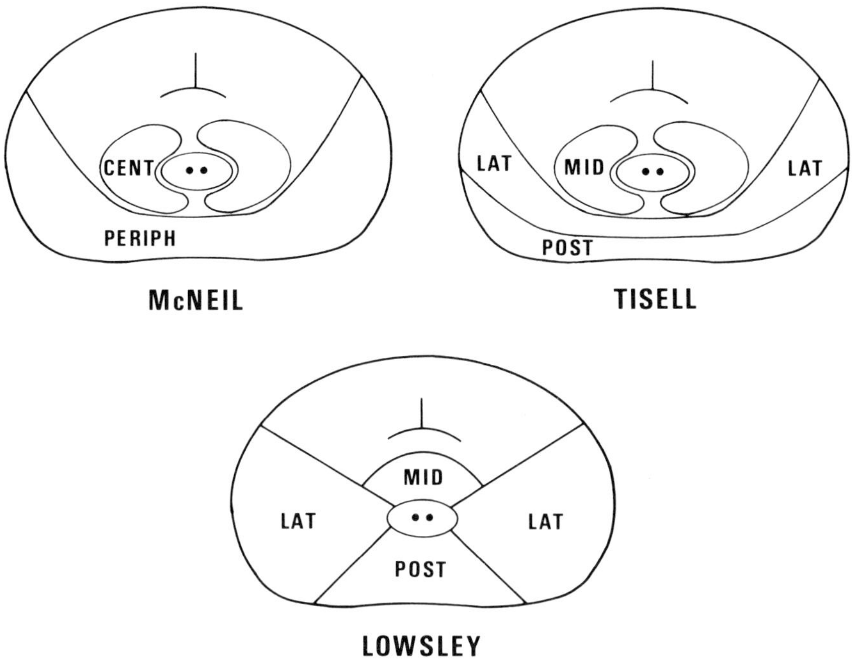

McNeal: I wanted to ask you a couple of semantic questions. I have asked the projectionist to project a slide for me. Does the figure labelled Tisell look like your representation of the anatomy? I admire your gross dissections. For pathologists, accustomed as I am to the microscopic section, it should be possible to lay these out on one plane of section. I made the mistake, Dr. Tisell, in calling this the posterior lobe rather than the dorsal lobe. This figure is a transverse section somewhat proximal to the verumontanum with the ejaculatory ducts in the center, the urethra up at the top, and the rectal surface of the prostate down at the bottom. Is that approximately your representation of the medial, lateral and dorsal lobes?

Tisell: In what plane?

McNeal: This is in a transverse plane. The colliculus is below this plane of section toward the base of the prostate. This is towards the bladder neck.

Tisell: I don't think this is exactly correct. I think that the dorsal lobes have a wider distribution than this and you have a thinner connection here for the lateral lobe parenchyma. The lateral lobe is situated more laterally. As I showed previously in that anatomical slide, I think we have another portion of the medial lobe parenchyma here lateral to the urethra.

McNeal: Lowsley's description of the lobes is approximately as shown in the figure labelled Lowsley's, is that correct?

Tisell: Yes.

McNeal: The ejaculatory ducts for Lowsley are the reference point. The medial lobe is anterior to the ejaculatory ducts, the dorsal or posterior lobe is of course posterior to the ejaculatory ducts, the two lateral lobes are lateral to the ejaculatory ducts and do not meet in the center.

Tisell: The prostate grows greatly, at least 20 times from birth to adulthood. I think it is possible for the posterior lobe to grow out in this direction. When you look in Lowsley's paper you see a few epithelial buddings here below the seminal vesicles and they are situated anterior to the ejaculatory ducts. I think they grow up along the seminal vesicles. It must be possible for them to do that. We didn't find any medial lobe parenchyma in the midline dorsally.

McNeal: I see what you're saying about the difference between the embryo and the adult, Dr. Tisell, but this is what Dr. Lowsley described in the embryo, is it not?

This figure shows my view on the left, your view on the right, and Lowsley's view at the bottom. My central zone corresponds just about in its size and location to your medial lobe. The rest of the tissue, your lateral and posterior lobes correspond to the area taken up by my peripheral zone. The differences histologically between the lateral and posterior lobe are less as you described them than the difference between the medial lobe and the lateral lobe of the prostate. I question as to whether the difference between lateral and posterior lobes is significant. I think this is something that remains to be proved by more sophisticated techniques. If you used my terminology, it would seem that the peripheral zone is simply divided into a dorsal and lateral portion and none of the other lines cross each other. In comparing your view of the prostate with Lowsley's view of the embryonic prostate, which, has been challenged as to its validity repeatedly, all the lines seem to cross each other. May I ask you why, since we're dealing with adults, you chose Lowsley's terminology which requires a complete dislocation of our reference points for the lobes between the embryo and the adult, and not my terminology on the right which, in fact, seems to coincide with what you've found with the exception of one subdivision. Why have you chosen the terminology of Lowsley?

Tisell: My first purpose with this work was to identify the lobes of the human prostate. I thought this was important because I have worked with the rat and found that there was different hormonal dependency for the different lobes. Then, the primary purpose must have been to identify all the lobes. I have used Lowsley's terminology because the number of lobes he described are the same number I can find in the adult human prostate. If there are some differences between his and my concept of the anatomy, I think it is of minor importance. His description concerns embryonic and fetal glands and my description the adult prostate. Even if there are some differences you must have the same terminology for the fetal and adult prostate.

Chung: I have a question about whether there is a homology between the lobes of human prostate and the prostatic lobes that you find in rats and mice. If there is a homology, then what is the basis?

Tisell: I think there is a homology, at least between the coagulating glands and the medial lobes. I think that Dr. McNeal has proposed that they both originate from the Wolffian ducts and there are a lot of similarities between these two structures. The other lobes, I don't know.

Lewis: From your studies, can you say from what area in the lobe structure that you describe that BPH arises?

Tisell: In none. We have never seen the transitional zone.

New Approaches to the Study
of Benign Prostatic Hyperplasia, pages 67–79

BENIGN PROSTATIC HYPERTROPHY AND UTERINE LEIOMYOMAS: ANALOGOUS OR DISSIMILAR DISEASES?

Stanley J. Robboy, M.D.[1]
W. Dwayne Lawrence, M.D.

James Homer Wright Pathology Laboratory
Massachusetts General Hospital
Boston, MA 02114 and

Department of Pathology
Harvard Medical School

Gerald R. Cunha, Ph.D.

Department of Anatomy
University of California Medical School
San Francisco, CA 94143

INTRODUCTION

The subject Dr. Allen Buhl asked us to address, namely, whether uterine leiomyomas and benign prostatic hypertrophy (BPH) might be analgous conditions, was accepted as a challenge for discussion, but not necessarily for solution. Certain similarities seem quite obvious. Both disorders occur in organs of the genital tract, begin in middle reproductive life, and in some yet undefined manner require specific hormonal milieus. The question of analogy is not new. In a workshop on BPH held in 1975 and sponsored by the National Institutes of Health, Dr. Oscar Hechter (1975) queried in his closing statement whether the two disease processes had similarities. One striking similarity was our lack of understanding of the etiologies involved. This essay will reflect on similarities and dissimilarities.

[1]Supported in part by grants 1-670 and 1-837 from the National Foundation and HD-17491 from the National Institutes of Health.

EMBRYOLOGY

The uterus and prostate are both genital tract organs, but their embryologic origins differ. The uterus is an organ of mullerian derivation, while the prostate derives from the urogenital sinus and possibly also from the wolffian duct. During normal development of the female fetus, the mullerian ducts appear circa day 37 as funnel shaped openings of the coelomic epithelium and grow as paired undifferentiated tubes that fuse at about day 54 to become the utero-ovaginal canal (primordia of the uterine corpus and cervix and vagina) (Koff 1933; Robboy et al in press). During early development, the uterus is a simple, thinbore, straight tube lined by a single layer of columnar epithelium. Throughout fetal life the uterine corpus constitutes only a small (1/6th) portion of the entire uterovaginal canal. The wall of the uterus is composed of two distinct zones of mesenchyme. The inner layer, which becomes the definitive endometrial stroma, is characterized by a loose arrangement of cells with extensive extracellular matrix (Robboy et al 1982). The outer layer of mesenchyme, which is composed of more compact cells, takes on microscopic properties at about the 16th week that are distinctive of smooth muscle (myometrium) (Taguchi et al 1983).

The origin of the prostate is more complex (Bengmark 1958, Cunha, Lung 1979; Jirasek 1980; Kellokumpu-Lehtinen 1980; McNeal 1975; McNeal 1978; Zondek, Zondek 1980). The most widely accepted concept holds that the 5 lobes of the prostate, the anterior, middle, posterior, and 2 lateral, are of urogenital sinus origin (Lowsley 1912). More recent studies suggest that the wolffian duct may also contribute. According to McNeal (1975), the central structure is the pelvic urethra, which itself is heterogeneous in composition. Most of the urethra is derived from endodermal urogenital sinus. The posterior wall of the upper half of the urethra may also contain epithelium of mesodermal origin derived from resorption and incorporation of the proximal portions of the wolffian ducts. No sharp demarcations or histologic differences among the different epithelia are apparent (Bengmark 1958).

In contrast to the developmental sequence traced by Lowsley (1912), McNeal (1975) has proposed that the central, compact zone of prostate is of wolffian duct origin. A cluster of prostatic buds on the verumontanum are oriented to form a small circle, which completely encompass the junction of the wolffian ducts and urethral mucosa and which radiate upward from the verumontanum to course along the wolffian duct superiorly and appear as a rosette about the ejaculatory ducts. The remainder of the prostate proper, the outer zone, develops from the prostatic ducts that have arisen in the lower half of the pelvic urethra from tissue of urogenital sinus origin.

Postnatally, changes occur along the urethra cranial to the verumontanum. A zone of periurethral glands appear, which McNeal (1975) believes is the region from which BPH arises in later life. It is not certain at present whether the glands which give rise to BPH are present at birth or are those which arise postnatally.

Consideration has been given to whether the mullerian tissues present in the vestigial prostatic utricle (male uterus) in the verumontanum may contribute to the development of prostate. We believe this unlikely. The first buds of prostate begin to develop circa the 12th week of human fetal formation. By this time the embryonic mullerian ducts in the male should already have been irreversibly destroyed. We have shown recently that by the 51st day of fetal life, the mullerian ducts already exhibit substantial inhibition (Taguchi et al in press). The key target of the mullerian inhibiting substance (MIS) seems to be mesenchyme. By the 63rd day the inhibition is complete.

MORPHOLOGY

Prostate

Although benign prostatic hyperplasia is often considered to be a disorder of proliferating glandular nodules, growing evidence points to stroma as the chief target tissue for nodular growth. Franks (1975) has described 5 types of nodular growth, based on the relative compositions within nodules of stromal (collagen and elastic tissue), smooth muscle, and epithelial proliferation. These include: 1) the stromal (fibrous) nodule; 2) the fibromuscular nodule; 3) the muscular nodule ("leiomyoma"); 4) the fibroadenomatous nodule; and 5) the fibromyoadenomatous (fibromyoepithelial) nodule. Based on stereological studies, which provide precise quantitation of tissue elements, Rohr and Bartsch (Bartsch et al 1979a; Bartsch et al 1979b; Rohr, Bartsch 1980) have suggested that human BPH may be predominantly a stromal disease. Based on a study of prostates from patients who underwent suprapubic prostatectomies, the stromal to glandular epithelial ratio increased more than twofold from 2:1 in the normal prostate to 5:1 in the hyperplastic gland.

Uterine Leiomyoma

Uterine leiomyomas may range in size from millimeters to as much as 25 cm in greatest diameter. Most are solid, rubbery and white. The muscle fibers are usually arranged in a whorled pattern which is often appreciated on gross examination of the cut surface. On microscopical examination, they are composed of bundles of smooth muscle enveloped within a thin, delicate connective tissue layer.

Hyperplasia Versus Neoplasm

Smooth muscle and stromal proliferation and the glandular growth in prostatic nodules represent both hypertrophy and hyperplasia in BPH. By contrast, studies using glucose-6-phosphate dehydrogenase (G6PD) isoenzymes as cell markers have demonstrated that leiomyomas of the uterus are benign neoplasms as they appear to have a clonal origin (Townsend et al 1970). The gene responsible for G6PD production which is located on the X chromosome, produces two isoenzymes. In a uterus with multiple leiomyomas, each smooth muscle nodule possesses one or the other isoenzyme, but not both, which argues for a unicellular (clonal) origin of each nodule.

NATURAL HISTORY AND AGING

Both BPH and uterine leiomyomas appear to be diseases related to aging. It is estimated that at least 20% of all women and as many as 40% of women over the age of 40 harbor uterine leiomyomas (Hendrickson, Kempson 1980)

BPH is seldom seen before age 40 (Brendler 1975). The incidence of BPH increases with advancing age so that hyperplastic nodules are present in more than 3/4ths of prostate glands of men who reach the age of 80 years. It is thought that the evolution of a nodule from initiation to a size capable of producing symptoms requires roughly 15-20 years.

PERTINENT RELATED CONDITIONS

Peritoneal leiomyomatosis (leiomyomatous peritonealis disseminata) is a rare condition which occurs in women of reproductive age (Nogales et al 1978; Tavassoli, Norris 1982). It is characterized by the presence of tens to hundreds of tiny leiomyomas scattered throughout the peritoneal cavity. The pertinence of this condition to our general thesis is that peritoneal leiomyomatosis almost always occurs on a background of hormonal stimulation (see below). Of the 20 women reported with this condition through 1982, 10 were pregnant or immediately postpartum, and 7 had been taking oral contraceptive steroids. On microscopical examination, the peritoneal nodules contained smooth muscle cells. Some were composed exclusively of smooth muscle; most contained some admixture of myofibroblasts, altered smooth muscle cells or fibroblasts. Most of the women with this condition have been treated conservatively. In no one has it proved wise to act in a clinically aggressive fashion. A small number of these women underwent a subsequent laparotomy at sometime after the pregnancy had ended or the oral contraceptive medication stopped. In 4 of 5 cases the peritoneal tumors had disappeared or had partially regressed. These findings suggest that removal of the hormonal stimulation can result in tumor atrophy.

ETIOLOGY AND HORMONES

Several lines of evidence suggest that sex hormones play a critical role in the pathogenesis of both lesions under discussion. In the uterus one line of circumstantial evidence is that leiomyomas develop after menarche, grow and enlarge during pregnancy (Emge 1934; Mixson, Hammond 1961) and regress after menopause.

A second line concerns hormone and hormone binding protein analyses. Leiomyomas, in comparison to normal myometrium, contain substantially higher concentrations of both estrogen receptors (Wilson et al 1980) and 17 β-estradiol (Otubu et al 1982), lower than normal rates of conversion of estradiol to estrone (Pollow et al 1978), and low levels of activity of 17β-hydroxysteroid dehydrogenase (Pollow et al 1978), an enzyme that is responsible for the conversion of estradiol to estrone. Otubu et al (1982) postulate that these findings represent a selective retention of estradiol by the tumor or a relative deficiency of the tumor's ability to metabolize estrogen. Sutherland et al (1980) performed receptor studies in a case of peritoneal leiomyomatosis in a women who had taken oral contraceptives for 12 years and found in comparison to the patient's normal myometrium that the estrogen and progesterone binding was markedly elevated. Because estrogen increases both estrogen and progesterone cytoplasmic binding (Janne 1975), it was reasoned that a high-estrogen milieu by either endogenous or exogenous means may cause some target cells to acquire more cytoplasmic receptors. Because progesterone receptor concentration is presumed to be regulated by estrogen in the human uterus (Janne 1975), the inability to detect progesterone binding in the tumor tissue of the patient 6 months after oophorectomy, which coincided with tumor regression, was interpreted to suggest that a hormonal stimulus was instrumental in the etiology of peritoneal leiomyomatosis (Sutherland et al 1980). Recently 5-alpha reductase was also shown to be present in leiomyomas in greater concentrations than in normal myometrium, raising the possibility that androgens may also play a role in the pathophysiology of uterine smooth muscle lesions (Buttram, Reiter 1981; Jasonni et al 1982; Reddy, Rose 1979). The role of estrogen and androgen receptors in normal and hyperplastic prostate are the subjects of several other presentations in this symposium, and will not be covered herein.

A third and more direct line of evidence concerns the experimental production of smooth muscle lesions by the administration of estrogens, progesterone, or combinations thereof. Ross and Klebanoff (1967) have demonstrated that injections with 17β-estradiol will activate smooth muscle cells in the prepubertal rat uterus. Three days of estrogen injections in young female virgin mice increase the number of cell organelles (Rohr, Jurukova 1968). Autoradiographic electron microscopic studies have demonstrated that the uterine smooth muscle cells incorporate radiosulphate and tritiated proline, indicating that smooth muscle cells participate in the synthesis of connective ground substances under defined experimental conditions. Similarly in prostrate, administration of estrogens (diethylstilbestrol) in Strong A/J mice produced predominantly stromal enlargement and growth of smooth muscle cells (Fingerhut, Veenema 1966). In beagle dogs (Rohr in press) and humans (Bolton et al 1981; Kozak et al 1982) estrogens have also been found to preferentially reside in prostate smooth muscle nuclei, also suggesting that estrogens possibly play a role in the induction of smooth muscle growth in prostate.

Prolonged estrogen or combined estrogen and progestin stimulation has also resulted in the production of lesions histologically similar to uterine leiomyomas and peritoneal leiomyomatosis in the guinea pig. As far back as 1941 Lipshutz and Vargas (1941) demonstrated that peritoneal leiomyomas could be induced to develop experimentally if large doses of estrogens were administered; the nodules regressed once the steroid stimulant was discontinued (Lipschutz, Schwarz 1944). However, the presence of greater numbers of fibroblasts than smooth muscle cells had led others to negate the findings.

More recently Fujii et al (1981) showed that treatment with estradiol benzoate for a minimum of 3 months leads to the development of disseminated peritoneal nodules. The cells resembled fibroblasts by ultrastructural analysis. After the addition of progesterone and administration of the combination for at least another month, the nodules resembled smooth muscle and decidual cells. The investigators postulated that estrogen elicited differentiation and proliferation of fibroblast-like cells from the subcoelomic mesenchyme. These cells subsequently are thought to differentiate into smooth muscle-like cells and decidual-like cells under the influence of both estrogen and progesterone. An interesting concept linking the mullerian duct with the coelom is the acknowledged fact that the mullerian duct arises as an outpouching of the coelom itself (Koff 1933; Sutherland et al 1980). These conclusions from experiments in guinea pigs are in keeping with the clinical and pathological features of peritoneal leiomyomatosis found in the human.

In addition to the data presented above about the role of hormonal stimulation of leiomyomas in the uterus or peritoneum, there is evidence that sex hormones are also instrumental in the pathogenesis of BPH (Mawhinney, Neubauer 1979; Wilson 1980). According to Wilson's working hypothesis (Wilson 1980), dihydrotestosterone (DHT) accumulates within the prostate gland and serves as the hormonal mediator for the hyperplasia. The accumulation occurs because of both decreased catabolism of DHT with increasing age and also because with increasing age there is enhanced intracellular binding of the molecule. Estrogen accelerates the process which in turn enhances the level of androgen receptors in the prostate. Thus, there is an increase in the androgen receptor levels which allows for androgen mediated growth even in the face of declining androgen production in advanced age. The work by Bartsch et al (1982) refines the preferential site of androgen metabolism to the stroma.

Considering that there is an underlying hormonal basis for BPH, then we might muse about Hechter's (1975) consideration if men underwent menopause at age 45 to 50 years, like women, secretion of their sex hormones would be arrested. From this it would follow that BPH might be much less a problem than it now represents.

STROMAL INDUCTION OF GLADULAR EPITHELIUM

The property of stroma to induce the formation of specific types of epithelium has been demonstrated by Cunha and co-workers (Cunha et al 1980; Cunha et al 1983). Elsewhere in this symposium, Cunha addresses the subject of stromal-epithelial interactions in the prostate. Recent studies indicate that in the female genital tract the stroma may also play a key role in the induction of specific epithelial forms. For example, vaginal stroma grown with uterine epithelium induces a keratinized squamous epithelium reminiscent of vaginal epithelium (Cunha, Fujii 1981; Cunha et al 1982). In reciprocal recombinants, uterine stroma grown together with neonatal vaginal epithelium induces the growth of a columnar epithelium resembling that of the uterine corpus. Of particular interest, we have seen cases where uterine leiomyomas contain small growths of endometrial glands. While it is possible that the glands are entrapped by the growing neoplasms, it is also likely that the growth may have been induced by the smooth muscle cells themselves. Of interest, glands with mullerian-type epithelium (ciliated and mucinous) have been found in peritoneal leiomyomas in human (Kaplan et al 1980; Kuo et al 1980) and in guinea pigs exposed to estrogens and progestogens (Fujii et al 1983).

CONCLUSIONS

Similarities exist, as expected between uterine leiomyomas and BPH. Substantial differences also exist. Both disorders arise in organs of the genital tract, but the embryology of the organs substantially differ. The prostate arises from the endodermal urogenital sinus and also possibly in part from the wolffian duct. The uterus is mullerian. Peritoneal leiomyomas, which are mesodermal, arise from the subcelomic mesenchyme, which is also the tissue from which the mullerian duct derives. Leiomyomas of the uterus are benign neoplasms composed of smooth muscle. BPH is a disease of hyperplastic nodules that may possess a diversity of cell types, but predominantly stroma, in various ratios. Substantial evidence points to a hormonal milieu as a key factor in the pathogenesis of these lesions. Both conditions can be produced experimentally with hormone administration and both conditions are characterized by the presence of estrogen receptors and the enzymes requisite for estrogen and androgen metabolism. As both conditions are thought to require 15 to 25 years to develop before they become clinically symptomatic in the middle to late reproductive years at earliest, then it might be postulated that the initiating stimulus for the development of uterine leiomyomas and BPH is operative shortly after the onset of puberty or in early childhood.

REFERENCES

Bartsch, G, Frick J, Ruegg I, Bucher M, Holliger O, Oberholzer M, Rohr HP (1979a). Electronmicroscopic stereological analysis of the normal human prostate and benign prostatic hyperplasia. J Urol 122:481.

Bartsch G, Muller HR, Oberholzer M, Rohr HP (1979b). Light microscopic stereological analysis of the normal human prostate and of benign prostatic hyperplasia. J Urol 122:487.

Bartsch W, Krieg M, Becker H, Mohrmann J, Voigt KD (1982). Endogenous androgen levels in epithelium and stroma of human benign prostatic hyperplasia and normal prostate. Acta Endocrinol 100:634.

Bengmark S (1958). "The prostatic urethra and prostatic glands. Their derivation and embryonic development studied in the rat with morphologic and experimental methods." Lund, Sweden: Berlingska Boktryckeriet, p l.

Bolton NJ, Lahtonen R, Hammond GL, Vihko R (1981). Distribution and concentrations of androgens in epithelial and stromal compartments of the human benign hypertrophic prostate. J Endocrinol 90:125.

Brendler H (1975). Benign prostatic hyperplasia: natural history. In Grayhack JT, Wilson JD, Scherbenske MJ (eds): "Benign Prostatic Hyperplasia," Washington, DC: DHEW Publication No. (NIH) 76-1113, p 101.

Buttram VS Jr, Reiter RC (1981). Uterine leiomyomata: etiology, symptomatology, and management. Fertil Steril 36:433.

Cunha GR, Chung LWK, Shannon JM, Reese BA (1980) Stromal-epithelial interactions in sex differentiation. Biol Reprod 22:19.

Cunha GR, Chung LWK, Shannon JM, Taguchi O, Fujii H (1983). Hormone-induced morphogenesis and growth: Role of mesenchymal-epithelial interactions. Recent Prog Horm Res 39:599.

Cunha GR, Fujii H (1981). Stromal-parenchyml interactions in normal and abnormal development of the genital tract. In Herbst AL and Bern HA (eds): "Developmental Effects of Diethylstilbestrol (DES) in Pregnancy," New York: Theime Stratton, p 179.

Cunha GR, Lung B (1979). Development of male accessory glands. In Spring-Mills E, Hafez ESE (eds): "Accessory Glands in the Male Reproductive Tract," Michigan: Ann Arbor Sci 6:1.

Cunha GR, Shannon JM, Taguchi O, Fujii H, Chung LWK (1982). Mesenchymal-epithelial interactions in hormone-induced development. J Animal Sci 55:14.

Emge LA (1934). The influence of pregnancy on tumor growth. Am J Obstet Gynecol 28:682.

Fingerhut B, Veenema RJ (1966). Histology and radioautography of induced benign enlargement of mouse prostate. Invest Urol 4:112.

Franks LA (1975). Gross and microscopic anatomy. In Grayhack JT, Wilson JD, Scherbenske MJ (eds): "Benign Prostatic Hyperplasia," Washington DC: DHEW Publication No. (NIH) 76-1113, p 63.

Fujii S, Konishi I, Ban C, Okamura H (1983). Adenomatoid tumor-like structures in the subperitoneal nodules produced by sex steroids. Am J Obstet Gynecol 145:850.

Fujii S, Nakashima N, Okamura H, Takenaka A, Kanzaki H, Okuda Y, Morimoto K, Nishimura T (1981). Progesterone-induced smooth muscle-like cells in the subperitoneal nodules produced by estrogen. Experimental approach to leiomyomatosis peritonealis disseminata. Am J Obstet Gynecol 139:164.

Hechter O. Reflections on the NIH workshop on BPH (1975). In Grayhack JT, Wilson JD, Scherbenske MJ (eds): "Benign Prostatic Hyperplasia." Washington, DC: DHEW Publicaiton No. (NIH) 76-1113, p. 269.

Hendrickson MR, Kempson RL (1980). "Surgical Pathology of The Uterine Corpus." Philadelphia: Saunders.

Janne O, Kontula K, Luukkainen T, Vihko R (1975). Oestrogen-induced progesterone receptor in human uterus. J Steroid Biochem 6:501.

Jasonni VM, Bonavi AM, Lodi S, Preti S, Bulletti C, Falmigni C (1982). Androstenedione metabolism in human uterine tissues: endometrium, myometrium and leiomyoma. J Steroid Biochem 17:547.

Jirasek JE (1980). Normal development of the male accessory glands. In Springs-Mills E, Hafez ESE (eds): "Male Accessory Sex Glands," New York: Elsevier/North-Holland Biomedical Press, p. 3.

Kaplan C, Benierschke K, Johnson KC (1980). Leiomyomatosis peritonealis disseminata within endometrium. Obstet Gynecol 55:119.

Kellokumpu-Lehtinen P (1980). Embryonic development of human prostate. Thesis. University of Turku, Finland.

Koff AK (1933). Development of the vagina in the human fetus. Contrib. Embryol 24: (#140)59.

Kozak I, Bartsch W, Krieg M, Voigt KD (1982). Nuclei of stroma: site of highest estrogen concentration in human benign prostatic hyperplasia. Prostate 3:433.

Kuo T, London SN, Dinh TV (1980). Endometriosis occurring in leiomyomatosis peritonealis disseminata. Ultrastructural study and histogenetic consideration. Amer J Surg Pathol 4:197.

Lipschutz A, Schwarz J (1944). Microscopic structure of estrogen induced uterine and other abdominal fibroids treated with progesterone. Cancer Res 4:24.

Lipschutz A, Vargas L Jr (1941). Structure and origin of uterine and extragenital fibroids induced experimentally in the guinea pig by prolonged administration of estrogens. Cancer Res 1:236.

Lowsley OS (1912). The development of the human prostate gland with reference to the development of other structures at the neck of the urinary bladder. Amer J Anat 13:299.

Mawhinney MG, Neubauer BL (1979). Actions of estrogen in the male. Invest Urol 16:409.

McNeal JE (1975). Developmental and comparative anatomy of the prostate. In Grayhack JT, Wilson JD, Scherbenske MJ (eds): "Benign Prostatic Hyperplasia," Washington DC: DHEW Publication No. (NIH) 76-1113, p 1.

McNeal JE (1978). Origin and evolution of benign prostatic enlargement. Invest Urol 15:340.

Mixson WT, Hammond DO (1961). Response of fibromyomas to a progestin. Am J Obstet Gynecol 82:754.

Nogales FF, Matilla A, Carrascal E (1978). Leiomyomatosis peritonealis disseminata. An ultrastructural study. Amer J Clin Pathol 69:452.

Otubu JA, Buttram VC, Besch NF, Besch PK (1982). Unconjugated steroids in leiomyomas and tumor-bearing myometrium. Am J Obstet Gynecol 143:130.

Pollow K, Sinnecke G, Boquoi E, Pollow B (1978). In vitro conversion of estradiol-17β into estrone in normal human myometrium and leiomyoma. J Clin Chem Clin Biochem 16:493.

Reddy VV, Rose LI (1979). Delta 4-3-ketosteroid 5 alpha-oxidoreductase in human uterine leiomyoma. Am J Obstet Gynecol 135:415.

Robboy SJ, Taguchi O, Cunha GR (1982). Normal development of the human female reproductive tract and alterations resulting from experimental exposure to diethylstilbestrol. Human Pathol 13:190.

Robboy SJ, Welch WR, Cunha GR. Pathological basis of intersex. In Fox H (ed): "Haines & Taylor's Gynaecological and Obstetrical Pathology," London: Churchill Livingstone, in press.

Rohr HP, Bartsch G (1980). Human benign prostatic hyperplasia. A stromal disease? Urol 16:625.

Rohr HP, Jurukova Z (1968). Beitrag zur Bildung bendegewebiger Matrix in glatten Muskelzellen. Elecktron mikroskopisch-autoradiographische Untersuchungen mit 3H-Prolin und 35 S-Sulfat am Oestrogen-stimulierten Mauseuterus. Pathol Europ 3:571.

Rohr HP. The effect of estrogen on stromal growth of the dog prostate (quantitative ultrastructural study). Urol Euro In Press.

Ross R, Klebanoff SJ (1967). Fine structural changes in uterine smooth muscle and fibroblasts in response to estrogen. J Cell Biol 32:155.

Sutherland JA, Wilson EA, Edger DE, Powell D (1980). Ultrastructure and steroid-binding studies in leiomyomatosis peritonealis disseminata. Am J Obstet Gynecol 136:992.

Taguchi O, Cunha GR, Lawrence WD, Robboy SJ. Mullerian inhibiting substance (MIS) irreversibly inhibits the development of the human female reproductive tract. Submitted.

Taguchi O, Cunha GR, Robboy SJ (1983). Experimental study of the effect of diethylstilbestrol (DES) on the development of the human female reproductive tract. Biol Res Pr 4:56.

Tavassoli FA, Norris HJ (1982). Peritoneal leiomyomatosis (leiomyomatosis peritonealis disseminata): A clinicopathologic study of 20 cases with ultrastructural observations. Int J Gynecol Path 1:59.

Townsend DE, Sparkes RS, Baluda MC, McClelland G (1970). Unicellular histogenesis of uterine leiomyomas as determined by electrophoresis of glucose-6-phosphate dehydrogenase. Amer J Obstet Gynecol 107:1168.

Wilson EA, Yang F, Rees ED (1980). Estradiol and progesterone binding in uterine leiomyomata and in normal uterine tissues. Obstet Gynecol 55:20.

Wilson JD (1980). The pathogenesis of benign prostatic hyperplasia. Am J Med 68:745.

Zondek LH, Zondek T. Congenital malformations of the male accessory sex glands in the fetus and neonate. In Spring-Mills E, Hafez ESE (eds): "Male Accessory Sex Glands," New York: Elsevier/North Holland Biomedical Press, p 17.

Discussion

McNeal: As you were describing leiomyomas which can contain glands, you showed a photograph which showed the Mullerian epithelium, beneath which was a very loose stroma which looked like endometrial stroma, and beneath that was smooth muscle. This is the sort of lesion which the usual term is adenomyosis, is that correct, as opposed to leiomyoma?

Robboy: Yes, or sometimes adenomyoma. A difficulty with the terminology is that adenomyosis is believed to represent downgrowths of the endometrial epithelium and stroma into the myometrium. In the present situation, the endometrial type glands appear to be integrated to the leiomyoma rather than a downgrowth. In that case the term adenomyosis is inappropriate.

McNeal: Now an idle question. Leiomyomas are pure white. The myometrium is a tan coloration. Adenomyosis generally has a tan coloration and the nodules of BPH generally have a tan coloration. Is there any meaning to this? Why are leiomyomas white when they derive from a tan colored tissue?

Robboy: You have me on that one.

Bartsch: If you look at a prostatic nodule it is a multicellular system. There are fibroblasts, smooth muscle cells, glandular cells, and a lot of extracellular matrix. If you look to a leiomyoma you have a unicellular system. There are smooth muscle cells and a very low amount of extracellular matrix. So, do you think this is a model for human benign prostatic hyperplasia?

Robboy: Uterine leiomyomas and BPH may be entirely different diseases. The purpose of this talk was to examine whether there might be any features in common. According to Lipschtz's work in 1981 and Fujii's recent work, the nodules in the peritoneal leiomyomatosis are composed of smooth muscle fibroblasts and have a component of extracellular matrix. The amount of each depends on the hormonal background.

Bartsch: Do you have use of markers to determine whether these are fibroblasts or smooth muscle cells, or have you done EM studies to determine this?

Robboy: Electron microscopic studies would be helpful here.

New Approaches to the Study
of Benign Prostatic Hyperplasia, pages 81–102

Androgenic effects upon prostatic epithelium are mediated via trophic influences from stroma

Gerald R. Cunha

Department of Anatomy
University of California
San Francisco, California 94143

Development of the prostate from the embryonic urogenital sinus as well as regulation of its adult structure and function are dependent upon androgens. Dihydrotestosterone (DHT), produced within the embryonic urogenital sinus thru metabolic reduction of testosterone (Wilson, Lasnitzki 1971), elicits the coordinated and harmonious expression of (1) epithelial morphogenesis (development of ductal-acinar architecture), (2) epithelial proliferation, and (3) epithelial cytodifferentiation, which culminates in the formation of secretory prostatic epithelial cells. In adulthood these epithelial cells continue to require androgens to maintain normal cytological features and for expression of functional activity (Farnsworth 1980; Brandes 1974; Liao 1976; Price, Williams-Ashman 1961; Mainwaring 1977). Androgen-deprivation results in reduction of prostatic weight, cessation of secretory activity, considerable epithelial cell death, and atrophy of the remaining epithelial cells (Lee 1980; Brandes 1974; Farnsworth 1980; Coffey 1978). Administration of androgens to castrates elicits prostatic epithelial and stromal cell proliferation and restores epithelial cytodifferentiation and function to the pre-castrate condition (Price, Williams-Ashman 1961; DeKlerk, Coffey 1978). All of these androgen-induced effects on prostatic epithelial morphology and function are thought to be mediated via androgen receptors, which have been characterized in extracts of prostates from a wide variety of species (Liao 1976; Walsh, Hicks 1979; Mainwaring 1978; Karr et al 1978). Autoradiographic and biochemical studies have demonstrated that androgen receptors are present in both the epithelial and stromal cells of the adult prostate (Stumpf and Sar 1976; Shannon and Cunha 1983a; Lahtonen et al 1983).

Investigation of the testicular feminization syndrome (Tfm) provides particularly strong support for the essential role of androgen receptors in prostatic development. Despite an adequate production of testosterone in Tfm individuals, prostatic tissue never develops. Instead the urogenital sinus forms a shortened vagina (Lyon et al 1981; Cunha 1975; Onno 1979). The molecular explanation of this androgen-resistant syndrome is based upon a mutation affecting androgen receptor activity which may be undetectable, reduced to low levels, or abnormal (Attardi, Ohno 1974; Weiland, Fox 1979; Wilson et al 1981).

Despite the undeniable importance of androgens and androgen receptors in prostatic development and function, it is unclear whether intra-epithelial androgen receptors play any role what so ever in growth of adult prostatic epithelial cells. To illustrate this problem, we note that administration of androgens to castrated males elicits growth of prostatic epithelium. This proliferative effect is thought to be mediated via androgen receptors, which are present in both the epithelial and stromal cells of the prostate. The presence of androgen receptors in both cell types raises the possibilities that prostatic epithelial growth (1) may be elicited directly within the epithelium via intra-epithelial androgen receptors, (2) may be elicited indirectly within prostatic epithelial cells via growth factors produced by androgen-receptor-positive stromal cells, or (3) may require simultaneous action of androgens upon both epithelial and stromal cells via their respective androgen receptors. The fortuitous association of androgen-induced epithelial growth with intra-epithelial androgen receptors does not in and of itself prove that androgen-induced prostatic epithelial growth is mediated via androgen receptors within the responding epithelial cells themselves. As yet it has not been possible to distinguish between these possible mechanisms by biochemical studies which destroy the architectural complexity of the prostate. However, the fundamental questions raised above are amenable to cell biological analysis of tissue recombinants composed of epithelium and mesenchyme derived from Tfm and wild-type mice. Progress in this area of research will be summarized below.

The pioneering work of Klaus Kratochwil and this colleagues established the idea that embryonic mammary mesenchyme is the actual target and mediator of androgenic effects upon the developing mouse mammary gland whose epithelial component degenerates in response to testosterone (Kratochwil, Schwartz 1976; Kratochwil et al 1979). The relevance of this basic idea to the prostate was confirmed thru similar experiments (Cunha, Lung

1978; Lasnitzki, Mizuno 1980) in which epithelium and mesenchyme from urogenital sinuses of Tfm and wild-type mouse embryos were recombined as indicated below (Fig. 1).

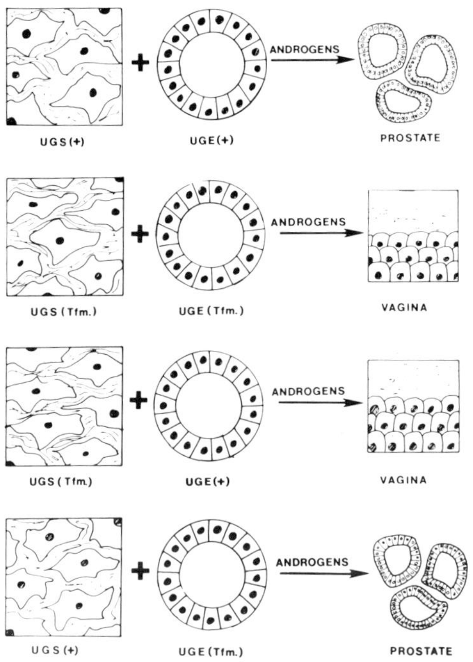

Fig. 1. Recombination experiments between urogenital sinus epithelium and mesenchyme from Tfm and wild-type mouse embryos. Prostatic morphogenesis occurs only when wild-type mesenchyme is utilized irrespective of the source of the epithelium (wild-type or Tfm). Conversely, vaginal differentiation occurs when either wild-type or Tfm epithelium is grown in association with Tfm mesenchyme. (From Cunha et al 1980b).

From these studies it is evident that prostatic development occurs only in those tissue recombinants prepared with wild-type mesenchyme (androgen-receptor-positive) irrespective of the source of the epithelium (wild-type or Tfm). Conversely, prostatic development does not occur under any circumstance when Tfm mesenchyme is utilized. These studies in both the developing prostate and mammary gland establish the idea that mesenchyme is the actual target and mediator of androgen-induced glandular development. This concept is supported by the finding that in wild-type mice androgen receptors (nuclear ^{3}H-DHT binding sites) are

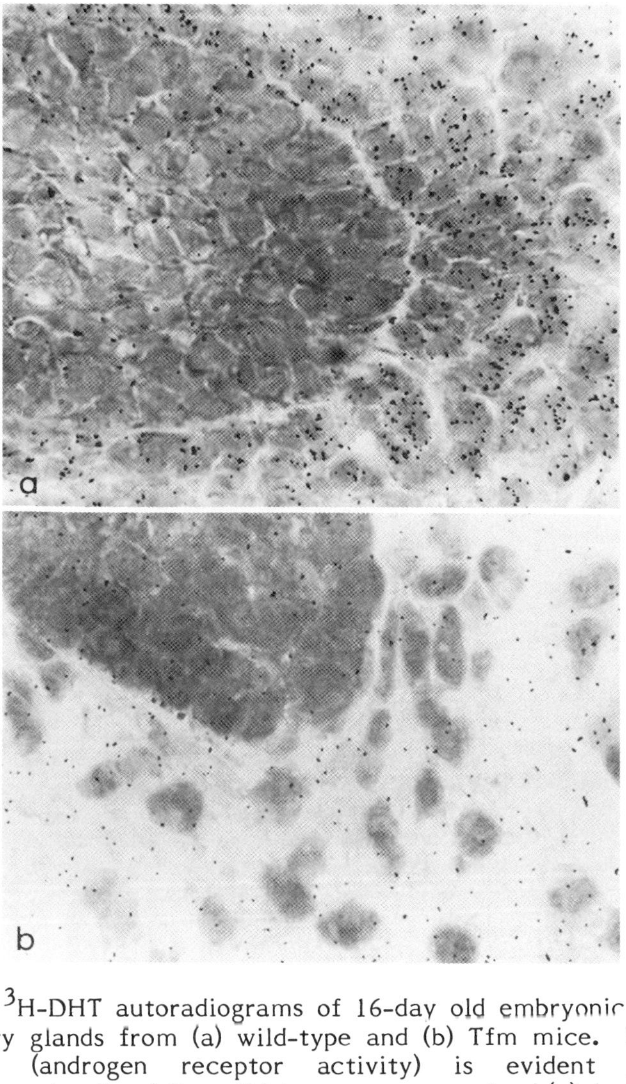

Fig. 2. ^{3}H-DHT autoradiograms of 16-day old embryonic female mammary glands from (a) wild-type and (b) Tfm mice. Nuclear labelling (androgen receptor activity) is evident in the mesenchymal cells of the wild-type mammary gland (a), but absent in mesenchymal cells of Tfm embryos (b). Note that epithelial labelling is essentially at background in the epithelium of both Tfm and wild-type glands. 800x. (a) is from Cunha et al (1981).

found in mesenchymal cells of both the developing prostate and mammary glands (Cunha et al 1981; 1982; Shannon et al 1981; Shannon, Cunha 1983a; Heuberger et al 1982). Surprisingly, the epithelial cells of these developing wild-type glands appear devoid of androgen-receptors. Moreover, the only obvious difference in nuclear DHT binding sites in Tfm versus wild-type mammary glands and urogenital sinuses (embryonic prostate) was observed in the mesenchyme. Nuclear androgen receptors were present in mesenchymal cells of wild-type fetuses but not in Tfm fetuses, while the epithelial cells of these organ rudiments were completely devoid of nuclear androgen receptors in both Tfm and wild-type embryos (Fig. 2). Specificity of nuclear androgen binding in these studies was demonstrated by processing non-target tissues (urinary bladder and intestine, which fail to exhibit nuclear ^{3}H-DHT binding), and by performing competition studies with other classes of steroids. Only radioinert DHT, and not estradiol, progesterone, or dexamethasone reduced nuclear binding (Shannon, Cunha 1983a). We have concluded that nuclear ^{3}H-DHT binding in mesenchymal cells of the developing prostate and mammary gland is a true manifestation of androgen receptor activity. Thus, data from Tfm/wild-type recombinations and steroid autoradiographic studies indicate that androgenic effects on developing prostatic and mammary epithelium is the consequence of trophic influences from mesenchyme which is the actual target and mediator of androgenic effects upon these epithelia. As yet there is no evidence that suggests a direct action of androgens upon epithelial morphogenesis and proliferation.

Another approach for exploring the importance of mesenchymal tissue in prostatic growth is based upon the analysis of tissue recombinants of urogenital sinus mesenchyme and epithelium (UGM + UGE) in which the ratio of tissue mass was experimentally altered (Chung, Cunha 1983). For this experiment 16 day embryonic mouse urogenital sinuses were used. Total mesenchyme and epithelium from 16 day urogenital sinuses were designated as 1X. UGM + UGE recombinants were constructed of 1X UGM and variable amounts of UGE (1X to 0.01X) or alternatively 1X UGE and variable amounts of UGM (0.1X to 2X) (Fig. 3). Tissue recombinants were then grown for 1 month in intact male hosts after which prostatic growth was assessed histologically and through analysis of wet weights and DNA contents of the harvested grafts. Prostatic growth was found to be dependent upon the mass of UGM used. When the amount of UGM was 1X, variation in UGE from 1X to 0.01X did not affect total prostatic growth attained in 1 month. By contrast, in recombinants prepared with 1X UGE and variable amounts of UGM (2X to 0.1X), total growth after 1 month reflected the amount of UGM utilized (Fig. 3).

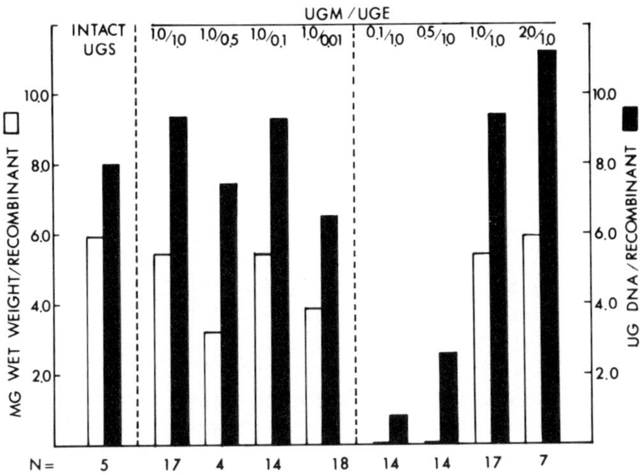

Fig. 3. Effect of varying the ratio of mesenchyme to epithelium in homotypic recombinants prepared with 16 day embryonic mouse urogenital sinuses. Urogenital sinus recombinants were prepared in which the amounts of epithelium and mesenchyme were varied from 2X to 0.01X. Prostatic growth (DNA content and wet weight) was measured at the end of a 1 month growth period in intact male hosts. Data represent the average wet weights and DNA contents from 4 to 18 recombinants/group (N=number of recombinants). (From Chung, Cunha 1983)

Thus, conclusions drawn from steroid autoradiographic and Tfm/wild-type experiments demonstrating that mesenchyme is the actual target and mediator of androgenic effects upon the epithelium, are complemented by the finding that total prostatic growth is regulated by the mass of urogenital sinus mesenchyme present (Chung, Cunha 1983). These observations suggest that future studies on prostatic epithelial growth should focus upon the stromal cell and its putative growth stimulating activity.

An important observation that has facilitated our analysis of prostatic epithelial growth and differentiation has been the finding that prostatic development can be induced by urogenital sinus mesenchyme in epithelium of the adult urinary bladder of either wild-type or Tfm mice (Cunha et al 1980a, b; Cunha, Chung 1981). In tissue recombinants prepared solely with wild-type tissues, the induced bladder epithelium was shown to exhibit a multitude of morphological and biochemical features indicative of prostatic differentiation (Cunha et al 1980b; Cunha et al 1983a; Neubauer et al 1983). The availability of relatively large quantities of adult Tfm bladder epithelial cells has been a key factor in our continued analyses of Tfm/wild-type prostatic inductions (see below).

The development of mature prostatic acini, which occurs in recombinants of wild-type urogenital sinus mesenchyme and Tfm bladder epithelium (UGM + Tfm BLE), is androgen-dependent (occurs only in intact male hosts) and is the culmination of the coordinated expression of androgen-induced epithelial morphogenesis, epithelial growth, and secretory cytodifferentiation. Simple histological examination of the starting Tfm bladder epithelium versus the induced prostatic acini (which develop in UGM + Tfm BLE recombinants) illustrates the profound morphogenetic and cytodifferentiative changes elicited in Tfm BLE by UGM. To demonstrate directly that Tfm epithelial cells undergo androgen-dependent DNA synthesis during prostatic morphogenesis, twenty UGM + Tfm BLE recombinants were prepared and grown for seven days as grafts in intact (10) or castrated adult male mice (10). Two hours before sacrifice the male hosts (mice) were injected with ^{3}H-thymidine (1 uCi/g body weight). Paraffin sections were prepared and processed autoradiographically to assess DNA synthesis (nuclear labelling). In UGM + Tfm BLE tissue recombinants grown in castrated male hosts, the bladder epithelium remained unchanged demonstrating that the inductive process is androgen-dependent. Labelling of the un-induced Tfm BLE was virtually nil (Fig 4a). By contrast, UGM + Tfm BLE recombinants grown in intact male hosts exhibited ductal-acinar morphogenesis and considerable epithelial labelling (Fig 4b). Thus, in the presence of androgens (intact hosts), Tfm epithelial cells express glandular morphogenesis, a high rate of DNA synthesis, and ultimately secretory cytodifferentiation which culminates in the formation of glands that are distinctly prostatic (Cunha et al 1983b; Shannon, Cunha 1983b). These androgen-induced processes are expressed in Tfm epithelial cells that continue to lack androgen receptors (Fig. 5) as demonstrated autoradiographically (Cunha et al 1983b; Shannon, Cunha 1983b).

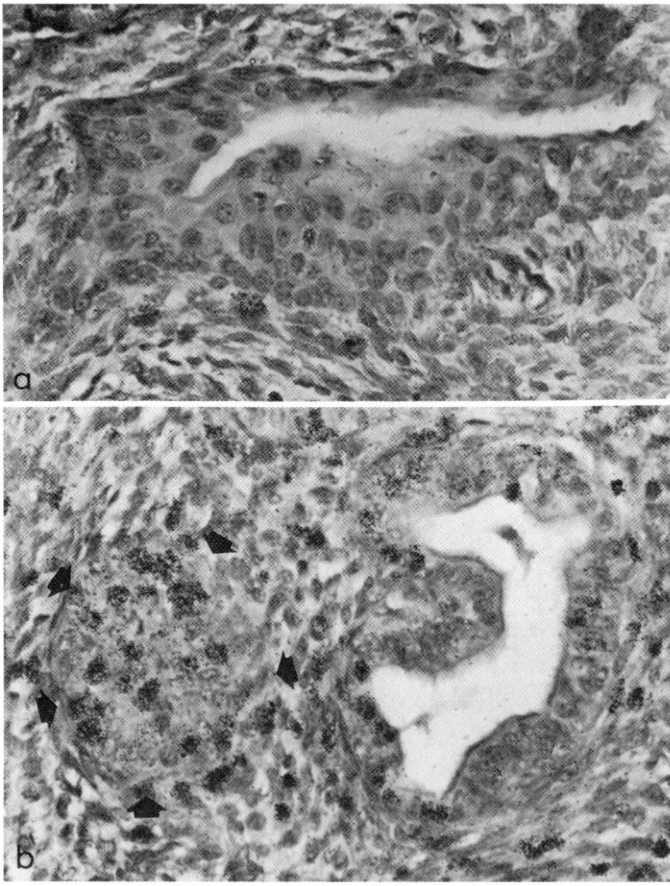

Fig. 4. Autoradiographs of ^{3}H thymidine incorporation in recombinants composed of wild-type UGM + Tfm BLE. (a) Recombinants grown in castrated male hosts do not undergo prostatic morphogenesis. Instead the epithelium remains unchanged and labelling is essentially nil. (b) UGM + Tfm BLE recombinant grown in an intact male host. Note the solid (arrows) and canalized prostatic ducts, which demonstrate that prostatic morphogenesis and cytodifferentiation is occurring in the Tfm epithelium. Labelling of the Tfm epithelium with ^{3}H-Thymidine is substantial. 400X. (From Cunha et al 1983b).

Androgen receptors are expressed in the wild-type mesenchymal cells of these tissue recombinants.

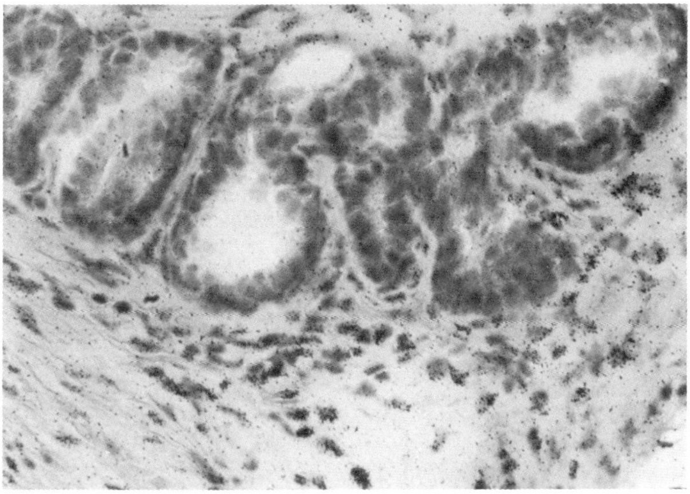

Fig 5. ^{3}H dihydrotestosterone localization indicative of androgen receptor activity in tissue recombinants composed of wild-type UGM and Tfm bladder epithelium. Androgen receptors are undetectable in prostatic acini induced in Tfm epithelium, whereas androgen receptor activity is prominently displayed in the surrounding wild-type mesenchymal cells. X400. (From Cunha et al 1983b).

Therefore, the androgenic sensitivity of these UGM + Tfm BLE recombinants is presumably due to the presence of mesenchymal androgen receptors. We conclude that androgen-induced prostatic epithelial morphogenesis, growth, and secretory cytodifferentiation are elicited via trophic factors emanating from androgen-receptor-positive mesenchymal cells. Direct interaction of testosterone or DHT with intra-epithelial androgen receptors does not seem to be required for eliciting androgenic effects within prostatic epithelium.

To explore androgenic action in UGM + Tfm BLE recombinants that have been grown to adult-like maturity (1 month in intact male hosts), protein and DNA synthesis have been investigated. Androgen-induced protein synthesis in UGM + Tfm BLE recombinants analyzed in 2 dimensional gels exhibits a remarkable similarity to that of wild-type prostate (Cunha, Chung 1981). Nonetheless, subtle differences were observed between wild-type prostate and UGM + Tfm BLE recombinants. Biochemical analysis of DNA synthesis in UGM + Tfm BLE recombinants demonstrates that incorporation of ^{3}H-thymidine into DNA is inducible by androgens, an effect that can be blocked by co-administration of the anti-androgen, cyproterone acetate (Cunha, Chung 1981). To verify that androgen-induced DNA synthesis measured biochemically is actually an accurate manifestation of DNA synthesis in the induced Tfm BLE, parallel autoradiographic studies of ^{3}H-thymidine labelling have been recently performed (Cunha unpublished). Comparable epithelial labelling was observed in epithelial cells of UGM + Tfm BLE recombinants and in epithelial cells of wild-type prostate (Fig. 6). Finally, cytological features of acinar cells of UGM + Tfm BLE recombinants display predictable changes in response to androgen-deprivation and androgen stimulation. Under the influence of androgens (intact male hosts), the induced Tfm prostatic epithelial cells are tall and exhibit prominent apical cytoplasm characteristic of secretory cells. These Tfm prostatic epithelial cells atrophy to low columnar cells upon castration, but are restored to a tall secretory state when testosterone is administered to the castrated male hosts. This later change can be blocked by co-administration of cyproterone acetate (Cunha, Chung 1981). To date the only difference (relative to wild-type prostate) observed in the androgenic response of UGM + Tfm BLE recombinants are the subtle differences in protein synthesis mentioned above. It is apparent, therefore, that many androgenic effects (morphogenesis, growth and cytodifferentiation) expressed within prostatic epithelial cells are mediated via trophic factors from stromal cells and not by direct (androgen-receptor-mediated) action of androgens upon the epithelium. Several observations support this idea. Franks and Barton (1960) demonstrated that maintenance in vitro of normal prostatic ultrastructure by exogenous testosterone was dependent upon continued association of epithelium with stroma. Incorporation of tritiated thymidine and amino acids into prostatic epithelium was greatly reduced following separation of the epithelium from stroma (Franks et al 1970). Recently, McGrath (1983) has demonstrated augmentation of growth response of mammary epithelial cells to estradiol by mammary stroma. The fact that epithelial cells from male and female genital tracts and the mammary gland are stimulated in vivo to proliferate by estrogens or androgens, but in cell culture fail to respond to these same hormones also argues against a direct receptor-mediated mitogenic effect of estrogens and androgens upon epithelial cells (Sirbasku, 1980; Sonnenschein and Soto, 1980). Failure to stimulate epithelial proliferation in epithelial monolayers may be due to an absence of stromal cells and stroma-produced growth factors, or to changes in epithelial cell shape, which is known to influence epithelial response to growth factors (Gospodarowicz et al 1981).

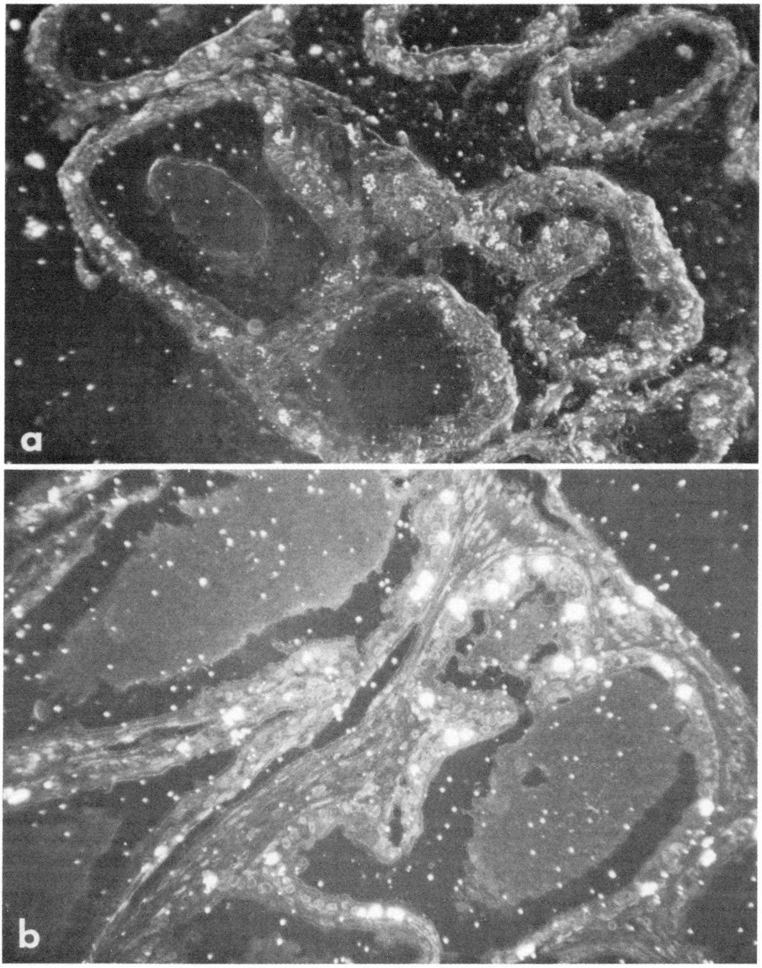

Fig. 6. Autoradiograms of ^{3}H-thymidine in (a) wild-type prostate and (b) wild-type UGM + Tfm BLE recombinants. Recombinants were grown for 1 month in intact male hosts, which were then castrated. Two weeks post-castration, the hosts were injected daily with testosterone propionate (TP). Seventy hours after initiation of TP treatment the host mice were injected with ^{3}H-thymidine (1uCi/g body weight) and sacrificed 2 hours later. Paraffin sections were prepared and processed autoradiographically. (a) is the wild-type prostate of the host bearing the grafted UGM + Tfm BLE recombinant (b). Note that nuclear labelling is similar in both specimens (400X). (From Cunha et al 1983b)

Future examination of stromal cell products may elucidate the mechanism of hormone-induced epithelial growth.

Acknowledgements: The author is indebted to Leland W.K. Chung, John M. Shannon, and Blake L. Neubauer, colleagues who have contributed greatly to this project. This work was funded by NIH Grants AM25266, CA27418, and AMCA 16570.

References:

Attardi B, and Ohno S (1974). Cytosol androgen receptor from kidney of normal and testicular femininized (Tfm) mice. Cell 2: 205.

Brandes D (1974). Hormonal regulation of fine structure. In Brandes D (ed): "Male Accesory Sex Organs: Structure and Function in Mammals", New York: Academic Press, p 184.

Chung LWK, Cunha GR (1983). Stromal-epithelial interactions II. Regulation of prostatic growth by embryonic urogenital sinus mesenchyme. Prostate (In Press).

Coffey DS (1978). The biochemistry and physiology of the prostate and seminal vesicles. In Harrison JH, Gittes RF, Perlmutter AD, Stamey TA, Walsh PC, (eds): "Campbell's Urology", 4th ed., Philadelphia: Saunders, p 161.

Cunha GR (1975). The dual origin of vaginal epithelium. Am. J. Anat 143:387.

Cunha GR, Chung LWK (1981). Stromal-epithelial interactions: Induction of prostatic phenotype in urothelium of testicular feminized (Tfm/Y) mice. J Steroid Biochem 14:1317.

Cunha GR, Lung B (1978). The possible influence of temporal factors in androgenic responsiveness of urogenital tissue recombinants from wild-type and androgen-insensitive (Tfm) mice. J Exptl Zool 205:181.

Cunha GR, Lung B, Reese B (1980a). Glandular epithelial induction by embryonic mesenchyme in adult bladder epithelium of Balb/c mice. Invest Urol 17:302.

Cunha GR, Chung LWK, Shannon JM, Reese BA (1980b). Stromal-epithelial interactions in sex differentiation. Biol of Reprod 22:19.

Cunha GR, Shannon JM, Neubauer BL, Sawyer LM, Fujii H, Taguchi O, Chung LWK (1981). Mesenchymal-epithelial interactions in sex differentiation. Human Genetics 56:68.

Cunha GR, Shannon JM, Taguchi O, Fujii H, Chung LWK, (1982). Mesenchymal-epithelial interactions in hormone-induced development. J Animal Science 55 (Suppl.):14.

Cunha GR, Fujii H, Neubauer BL, Shannon JM, Sawyer L, Reese BA (1983a). Epithelial-mesenchymal interactions in prostatic development. I. Morphological observations of prostatic induction by urogenial sinus mesenchyme in epithelium of the adult rodent urinary bladder. J Cell Biol 96:1662.

Cunha GR, Chung LWK, Shannon JM, Taguchi O, Fujii H (1983b). Hormone-induced morphogenesis and growth: Role of mesenchymal-epithelial interactions. Recent Prog Hormone Res 39:559.

DeKlerk DP, Coffey DS (1978). Quantitative determination of prostatic epithelial and stromal hyperplasia by a new technique: Bio-morphometrics. Invest Urol 16:240.

Farnsworth WE (1980). Functional biochemistry of the prostate. In Spring-Mills E, Hafez ESE, (eds): "Male Accessory Sex Glands", New York: Elsevier/No Holland, p 155.

Franks LM, Barton AA (1960). The effects of testosterone on the ultrastructure of the mouse prostate *in vivo* and in organ culture. Exp Cell Res **19**: 35.

Franks LM, Riddle PN, Carbonell AW, Gey GO (1970). A comparative study of the ultrastructure and lack of growth capacity of adult human prostate epithelium mechanically separated from its stroma. J Pathol 100:113.

Gospodarowicz D, Fujii DK, Giguere L, Savion L, Tauber JP, Vlodavsky I (1981). In Murphy GP, Sandberg AA, Karr JP (eds): "The Prostatic Cell: Structure and Function", Part A, New York, AR Liss, p 95.

Heuberger B, Fitzka I, Wasner G, Kratochwil K (1982). Induction of androgen receptor formation by epithelium-mesenchyme interaction in embryonic mouse mammary gland. Proc Natl Acad Sci 79:2957.

Karr JP, Kirdani RY, Murphy GP, Sandberg AA, (1979). The baboon prostate as a model for steroid hormone receptors in the human gland. In Murphy GP, Sandberg AA (eds): "Prostatic Cancer and Hormone Receptors", New York: AR Liss, p 165.

Kratochwil K, Schwartz P (1976). Tissue interaction in androgen response of embryonic mammary rudiment of mouse: Identification of target tissue of testosterone. Proc Natl Acad Sci USA 73:4041.

Kratochwil KH, Durnberger H, Heuberger B, Wasner G (1979). Hormone-induced cell and tissue interaction in the embryonic mammary gland. Cold Spring Harbor Conference on Cell Proliferation 6:717.

Lahtonen R, Bolton NJ, Kontturi M, Vihko R (1983). Nuclear androgen receptors in the epithelium and stroma of human benign prostatic hypertrophic glands. Prostate 4:129.

Lasnitzki I, Mizuno T (1980). Prostatic induction: Interaction of epithelium and mesenchyme from normal wild-type and androgen-insensitive mice with testicular feminization. J Endoc 85:423.

Lee C (1981). Physiology of castration-induced regresion in rat prostate. In Murphy GP, Sandberg AA, Karr JP, (eds): "The Prostatic Cell: Structure and Function", Part A, New York: AR Liss Inc, p 145.

Liao S, (1976). Receptors and the mechanism of action of androgens. In JR Pasqualini (ed): "Receptors and Mechanisms of Actions of Steroid Hormones", New York: Marcel Dekker, p 159.

Lyon MF, Cattanach BM, Charlton HM (1981). Genes affecting sex differentiation in mammals. In Austin CR, Edwards RG, (eds): "Mechanisms of Sex Differentiation in Animals and Man", New York: Academic Press, p 339.

Mainwaring WIP (1977). The mechanism of action of androgens Springer-Verlag, New York.

Mainwaring WIP (1978). Androgen receptors and biologic responses: A survey. In O'Malley BW, Birnbaumer L (eds): "Receptors and Hormone Action", Vol II, New York: Academic Press, p. 105.

McGrath CM (1983). Augmentation of the response of normal mammary epithelial cells to estradiol by mammary stroma. Cancer Res 43:1355.

Neubauer BL, Chung LWK, McCormick K, Shannon JM, Cunha GR (1983). Epithelial-mesenchymal interactions in prostatic development. II Biochemical observations of prostatic induction by urogenital sinus mesenchyme in epithelium of the adult rodent urinary bladder. J Cell Biol 96:1671.

Ohno, S (1979). Major Sex Determining Genes. Springer-Verlag, New York.

Price D, Williams-Ashman HG (1961). The accessory reproductive glands of mammals. In Young WC (ed): "Sex and Internal Secretions", 3rd ed., Baltimore: Williams and Wilkins, p 366.

Shannon JM, Cunha GR, Vanderslice KD (1981). Autoradiographic localization of androgen receptors in the developing urogenital tract and mammary glands. Anat Rec 199:232A.

Shannon JM, Cunha GR (1983a). Autoradiographic localization of androgen binding in the developing mouse prostate. Prostate 4:367.

Shannon JM, Cunha GR (1983b). Stromal-epithelial interactions: II Characterization of androgen binding and DNA synthesis in prostate-like structures induced in testicular feminized (Tfm/Y) mice. Biol Reprod (Submitted).

Sirbasku, DA (1980). Estromedins: Uterine-derived growth factors for estrogen-responsive tumor cells. In Jimenez de Asua, (ed): "Control mechanisms in animal cells", New York: Raven Press, p 293.

Sonnenschein C, Soto SM (1980). But are estrogens per se growth promoting hormones? J Nat'l Cancer Inst 64:211.

Stumpf WE, Sar M (1976). Autoradiographic localization of estrogen, androgen, progestin, and glucocorticosteroid in "target tissues" and "non-target tissues". In Pasqualini JR (ed): "Receptors and mechanism of action of steroid hormones", New York: Marcel Dekker Inc, p 41.

Walsh PC, Hicks LL (1979). Characterization and measurement of androgen receptors in human prostatic tissue. In Murphy GP,

Sandberg AA, (eds): "Prostatic Cancer and Hormone Receptors," New York: AR Liss, p 51.

Wieland SJ, Fox TO (1979). Putative androgen receptors distinguished in wild-type and testicular feminized (Tfm) mice. Cell 17:781.

Wilson JD, Lasnitzki I (1981). Dihydrotestosterone formation in the fetal tissue of the rabbit and rat. Endocrinol 89:659.

Wilson JD, JE Griffin, Leshin M, George FW (1981). Role of gonadal hormones in development of the sexual phenotypes. Human Genetics 58:78.

Discussion

J. Issacs: I have two questions. You have clearly shown the inductive effect of urogenital sinus mesenchyme on urogenital epithelium in fetal prostate. Are you implying that these same inductive interactions occur in postpubertal adult animals?

Cunha: I think that adult stromal cells are involved in maintaining both epithelial morphology and function and they are also involved in the morphological changes during adulthood. In particular for the prostate, inductive activities come into play during androgen induced regrowth of the prostate after castration.

J. Isaacs: But you're postulating very specific types of mesenchymal-epithelial interactions during prostatic development. In prostatic cancer it's very common to get bony metastases. At these metastatic sites, prostate cancer cells are presumably surrounded by stromal cells derived from bone not prostate. These metastatic lesions are often, however, still androgen sensitive. Therefore, you have to postulate that prostatic cancer represents fundamentally different mechanism of hormonal responsiveness since these cancer cells don't require unique prostatic stromal cells to be hormonally sensitive.

Cunha: I think that the fundamental difference, between normal prostatic epithelial cells and a prostatic adenocarcinoma is that the normal prostatic cells are dependent upon a specific mesenchyme for their development and probably also for their continued function. Whereas, tumor cells have evolved to a state of independence from a specific mesenchyme and therefore exist, proliferate and form new acini in sites far away from prostatic stroma. In fact, the specific kind of stroma that is required for prostate morphogenesis is a urogenital stroma probably in proximity to the urogenital sinus. Most importantly, I think prostatic stroma must have androgen receptors, since the Tfm urogenital sinus mesenchym is incapable of promoting prostatic morphogenesis.

J. Isaacs: Do you think that epithelial cells in the normal prostate have the ability after they have gone through morphogenesis to respond directly to hormones themselves?

Cunha: We know that epithelial cells of the adult wild type prostate have androgen receptors. We have to infer that it may be possible for them to respond directly to androgens since they have androgen receptors. We don't know what those epithelial receptors are involved in. Are they involved in growth? I rather doubt it. Because if we isolate adult prostatic epithelial cells from their mesenchyme and put them in culture, they grow equally fast whether androgens are present or absent. These cells will synthesize protein in response to androgens. They are androgen responsive, and therein may be the function of the epithelial receptor. My point is that any study in which a prostate has been homogenized is irrelevant to the issue we are discussing right now. The only way we're going to understand the function of the androgen receptor within a prostatic epithelial cells is from a cell biochemical approach.

Katzellenbogen: I have a question that relates to tissue specificity of the mesenchyme. Is the only important criterion that it have an androgen receptor? For example, could one do recombinations of the Tfm epithelium with a mammary stromal population that had androgen receptors? Would one then get appropriate differentiation into the prostate? Obviously these would not be easy to do and I'm not even sure if the androgen receptor would be quantitatively sufficient.

Cunha: I'm not sure, those experiments haven't been done; not all of them, anyway. In order to get prostatic development the use of a glandular inducer is required. You're not ever going to get prostate by using urinary bladder or skin mesenchyme, because those mesenchymes just do not induce glands. In addition, the only types of glandular inducers that have worked have been glandular inducers that have androgen receptors within their mesenchymal cells.

Katzenellenbogen: I wonder whether a mammary stromal population would be a reasonable one with which to test this, because there is good evidence for similar sorts of interactions in mammary gland?

Cunha: That would be a beautiful experiment because the embryonic mammary mesenchyme is one of the few non-urogenital mesenchymes that also has androgen receptors. The sub-mammary mesenchyme might also seem to be a possibility, but I suspect that it doesn't have androgen receptors. No one has looked at that.

Mawhinney: I'm reminded of some work you did in the early 1970's on epithelial-stromal interactions. You were isolating epithelium and mesenchyme and exposing them to *in vitro* androgen and making then various recombinations. If I recall correctly, you felt at that time that it was important that the epithelium be exposed to androgen but it really wasn't important that the mesenchyme be exposed. I wonder if in this particular set of experiments that design might be very telling. You could expose the Tfm epithelium to androgen *in vitro* and then recombine them with wild type mesenchyme not exposed to androgen. This way you could determine if the Tfm epithelium was capable of responding directly to the hormone.

Cunha: I think those experiments certainly could be done today. I don't talk very much about particular experiment you alluded to because I think that the experiments weren't done correctly. In that particular experiment the levels of androgen were very, very high and we didn't take precaution to wash out all the androgen before we recombined. So, I really don't think that particular experiment would be really valid and applicable to the issues today. A few years later a rather similar experiment by was done by Lasnitzki who concluded that the effect of the androgen on the mesenchyme was the key event. That result is more in line with the Tfm wild-type recombinations that have been performed by us and others both in the developing prostate and the mammary gland.

Mawhinney: I could also interpret your data to mean that the mesenchyme confers upon the epithelium the ability to respond to androgen. If you did those experiments like you did previously but with "more reasonable amounts of androgen," you might be be able to discriminate whether the epithelium responds directly or indirectly to androgen.

Cunha: We have looked at the developing prostate as well as the developing female genital tract of the mouse using autoradiography. As I showed in the case of the mammary gland, we found early stages in which the androgen receptors in the case of the male targets, or the estrogen receptors in the case of the female targets, are present only in the mesenchymal component of those organs. We've been trying to confirm this biochemically. I would like to know the answer to the question "what mesenchymal conditions are required for the ultimate expression of either epithelial androgen or estrogen receptors in these systems?" My guess is that you need the appropriate kind of mesenchyme for expression of epithelial hormone receptor which then confer upon the epithelium the ability to respond to the appropriate hormone later in life. These are experiments that can be easily done.

Wicha: Do you have any information regarding the nature of the signal that's transferred between the mesenchyme and the epithelium? Can you approach these problems using in vitro transfilter experiments?

Cunha: I think we can and we're definitely interested in pursuing that sort of thing. We need to mount an effort on mechanistic studies to identify an early marker of fetal prostate. We've been able to show that you can take a bladder epithelium and induce it to form something that is morphologically and biochemically prostate. However, all the endpoints that we've used to define that change are essentially adult endpoints. What we need is an endpoint indicative of fetal prostate and we don't have that yet. We also have systems where we can look at induction, as Stan Robboy indicated, of uterus and vagina. There again, we need those early markers. That's what we're pursuing right now. Once we develop those markers, the transfilter studies will come and those studies hopefully will define whether we're talking about diffusable molecules, extracellular matrix interactions, or direct cell contacts. I don't believe direct cell contacts are involved because we and others have looked very carefully with the electron microscope at the interface between those two tissues. We've never seen gaps in the basal membrane or direct cell contacts.

W. Isaacs: If you take Tfm transitional bladder epithelium and put it on the urogenital mesenchyme, let that form prostatic type epithelium and then castrate, do you then get cells that look like atrophic prostate or do you get transitional epithelium?

Cunha: It atrophies back to something that looks like atrophic prostate. If we then give androgen, we can bring back nice, tall cells. We can then remove androgen and go back and forth at will, but it's all within the context of prostatic morphology.

W. Isaacs: I have another question. Henry Sun at NYU has recently shown that if you take bladder epithelium, treat with NMU, put the cells in culture then subsequently put them back in the nude mouse, they will form glandular epithelium. Do you think that's due to the transformed cells not needing a mesenchyme to induce them?

Cunha: Where does he put them?

W. Isaacs: I'm not sure, I think its subcutaneously.

Cunha: It's been known for quite some time that the bladder is capable of three types of differentiation. One is the transitional phenotype. It will also undergo squamous metaplasia and under rare instances also can form glands. So, the glandular phenotype is definitely within the developmental repertoire of the epithelium. I suppose that's occurring as a result of NMU and the selective pressures of in vitro culture as well as selection based upon transplantation into a variety of sites, I think it's possible to get that particular phenotype, independent of mesenchyme, if the cell has evolved all the way to that state.

Li: I'd like to ask you a very basic question on the two controls. If you inject only the mesenchyme cells into the animal or only the epithelial cells, what happens to the prostate formation, androgen receptors and DNA synthesis?

Cunha: When we transplant just the wild type urogenital sinus mesenchyme, and we've done alot of that, which is a necessary control, for every hundred specimens of urogenital sinus mesenchyme that are grafted, greater than 99% of those give us a mass of fibromuscular tissue. We find no epithelium whatsoever. At the time of transplantation, mesenchymal cells have the androgen receptors and after they've been grown for one month, they still have androgen receptors. If we take that mesenchyme that's been grown for one month, combine it with urogenital sinus mesenchyme, we find that it still preserves the ability to induce epithelium. If we graft just the epithelium by itself, prostatic morphogenesis does not occur and epithelial survival is very, very low. We haven't looked at the ability of those specimens to incorporate tritiated thymidine.

One other comment about controls: in the past, the validity of this kind of study was really based on an inference. That is, if we graft a hundred pieces of mesenchyme and 99 pieces have no epithelium in them, we infer that 99% of the experimental mesenchyme is clean, as well. Now there's a new way that proving that an induction has taken place and one recombination is all that's required. We developed a method that allows us to differentially stain the nucleus of a mouse cell and distinguish that cell from rat cells or cells from other species. This is based upon the use of the Hoechst dye, 33258, that's been used for C-banning studies for years. From those studies it has been shown that mouse chromosomes show very intense staining near the centromeric region. This allowed cytogeneticists, who were doing somatic cell hybridization, to identify mouse chromosomes from chromosomes from other species in their hybrid cells. Mouse interface nucleus seen in section contains a very large number of brightly fluorescent spots whereas rat nuclei do not. So we've prepared these recombinations in which, as an example, we use a Tfm mouse bladder epithelium and rat urogenital sinus mesenchyme. When we stain that preparation with the Hoechst dye, we find that all the acini within such a preparation are derived from mouse cells. This indicates that indeed the Tfm mouse bladder epithelium is the source of those prostatic acini.

Bartsch: I have a question about your autoradiographic findings. Is this focal labelling of the glandular cell, or is this a diffused labelling of all stromal cells?

Cunha: The labelling within the stroma is quite variable. The particular specimen that you saw here was one in which the labelled cells seemed to be farther away. I could show you another autoradiogram in which the cells immediately subadjacent to the epithelium are heavily labelled. We don't know why there is this heterogeneity in labelling. Some cells, as you also saw in the autoradiograms, have many more silver grains than other cells. We don't know whether this is due to some technical situation or whether indeed there may be heterogeneity with respect to levels of androgen receptors within stromal cells. I can't answer these questions yet.

Bartsch: In the breast and the studies of Kratochuil, the labelling is always just a very focal labelling of the stromal cells just around the glandular cells. That means that the glandular cells that first signal the stromal cells are the ones that are labelled.

Cunha: In the case of the developing prostate, the labelled mesenchymal cells extend essentially the full thickness of the mesenchyme. Initially the interaction is only with a small percentage of those cells; those cells immediately subadjacent to the epithelium. But as the prostate develops, the epithelial buds penetrate the full thickness of the mesenchyme. Prior to that the full thickness of the mesenchyme has androgen receptors. In the adult prostate there is heterogeneity of labelling; some cells with high labelling activity, some with low activity. I'm not sure how to interpret that.

New Approaches to the Study
of Benign Prostatic Hyperplasia, pages 103–128

EXTRACELLULAR MATRICES AND THE CONTROL OF CELL PROLIFERATION AND DIFFERENTIATION IN VITRO

Denis J. Gospodarowicz

Cancer Research Institute
Univ. of Calif. Medical Center
San Francisco, CA 94143

Recent investigations suggest that, in vitro, cell-substratum interactions may play other roles in addition to cell anchorage (Hay 1981; Kleinman et al 1981). The extracellular matrix (ECM) that cells can produce and upon which they rest can be held responsible for the final shape the cells will adopt (Hay 1981; Kleinman et al 1981; Folkman, Greenspan 1975). This shape in turn may play a role in the cell's response to serum factors (Folkman, Moscona 1978) and its differential response to various growth factors (Gospodarowicz et al 1978; Gospodarowicz et al 1979; Gospodarowicz, Tauber 1980). Components of the ECM produced by cells have also been shown to be involved in cell differentiation and the control of gene expression, as well as in cell attachment (Hay 1981; Kleinman et al 1981). Even soluble matrix components can affect cell shape and metabolism through a redistribution of cytoskeletal elements associated with the abluminal cell surface as well as by stimulating the new formation of ECM (Sugrue, Hay 1981).

One of the major limitations of tissue culture techniques currently in use is that cells rest on plastic. Unless cultured cells can produce their own ECM, the possibility exists that contact with plastic could inhibit them from proliferating or could cause them to lose rapidly their ability to express their correct phenotype. In the present review, we will outline recent studies of the behavior of cells maintained on dishes coated with ECM of known composition. The use of such a substrate for the long-term culture of normal diploid and tumor cells will be described.

I. The production of extracellular matrices by cultured corneal endothelial and PF-HR-9 teratocarcinoma cells

The ECM is an organized complex of collagens, proteoglycans, and glycoproteins, all interacting to produce a highly stable structure of whose area only a very small portion is in contact with the cell surface. Elucidation of the components of the ECM involved in controlling cell proliferation either *in vivo* or *in vitro* has been made difficult mostly by its intricate nature. Because the correct *in vitro* reconstruction of the ECM from its isolated native components into the highly ordered structure that it represents would be a formidable task, advantage was taken of the fact that cultured bovine corneal endothelial (BCE) and PF-HR-9 teratocarcinoma cells have the ability to produce, underneath their basal surface, a thick ECM that adheres strongly to plastic (Figs. 1 & 2). The matrix produced by BCE cells is composed of elastin, basement-membrane collagen types IV and V and insterstitial collagen type III (Gospodarowicz 1983), heparin sulfate and dermatan sulfate proteoglycans, and fibronectin and laminin (Gospodarowicz 1983). The ECM produced by PF-HR-9 cells is composed only of basement membrane collagen type IV, heparin sulfate proteoglycans, laminin and entactin (reviewed in Gospodarowicz 1983). Both of these matrices can easily be denuded using either detergent (0.5% Triton-X in water) or base (20 mM NH_4OH) treatment (Gospodarowicz 1983) (Figs. 1 & 2).

II. Identification of growth-promoting agents for normal diploid mesenchymal cells maintained on BCE-ECM instead of plastic

Since plastic can adversely affect the proliferation and phenotypic expression of various cultured cell types, we first sought to determine if maintaining normal diploid cells on BCE-ECM-coated dishes could improve their growth rate and differentiation. Previous studies (Gospodarowicz et al 1980; Gospodarowicz et al 1981) have shown that corneal or vascular endothelial cells passaged repeatedly at low density in serum-supplemented medium have a declining growth rate. This correlates with morphological and structural alterations caused primarily by changes in the composition and distribution of the ECM (Gospodarowicz, Tauber 1980; Gospodarowicz et al 1980; Gospodarowicz et al 1981). The possibility therefore arose that the matrix produced by these cells could have an effect on their ability to proliferate and to express their normal phenotype at confluence (Gospodarowicz, Tauber 1980).

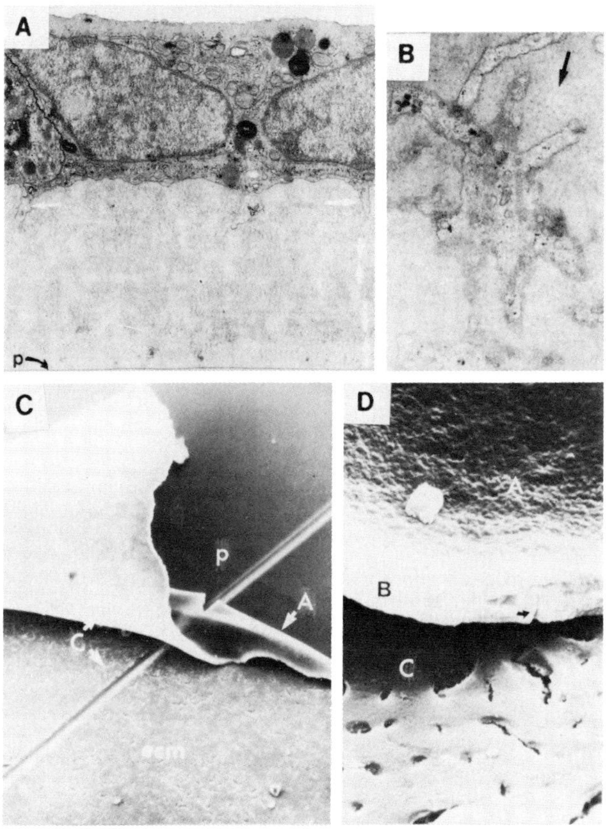

Fig. 1. Transmission and scanning electron micrograph of corneal endothelial cells after 3 weeks in culture.

(A) Cross-section showing the cells resting on a membrane 5 μ thick deposited on the plastic surface (p) of the tissue culture dish. In the basal part of the cells, small cytoplasmic processes are entering into the basement membrane (arrows) and are responsible for the pitted surface observed in (D). (B) Front view of the basement membrane at the level where small processes sent by the cells enter into it (apical surface of the basement membrane).

Numerous nodes (arrow) interconnected with 15 to 17 mm wide filaments can be seen. Similar node distribution can be seen in the upper part of the basement membrane deposited by BCE cells when seen in cross-section.

(C) Low power (X 200) scanning electron micrograph of the ECM. The plastic (p) has been exposed, and the trace of the needle running through the ECM (ecm) and the denuded plastic can be seen. (A) was the ECM side originally attached to the plastic, while (C) was the side on which cells were originally attached. This side is pitted, the pits corresponding to cell processes entering into the ECM. These pits were probably the sites where the cells were originally anchored to the ECM. (D) The ECM can be observed at a higher magnification (X 3000). The fracture edge of the ECM (B) can be seen, as can the transverse section (arrow) of a pit in which a cellular process was present before denudation. The ECM side to which the cells were attached is covered with numerous small empty pits.

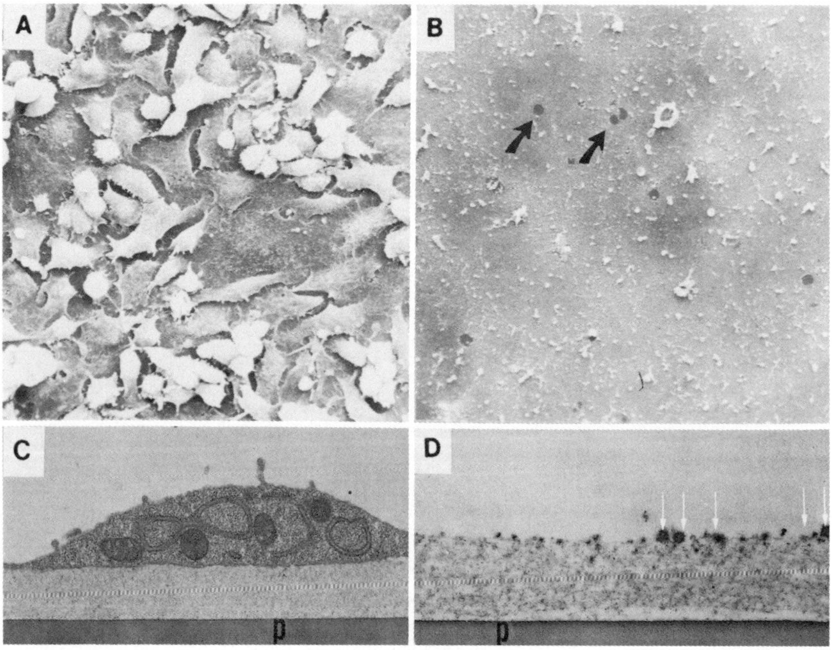

Fig. 2. Scanning and transmission micrographs of HR-9 cell cultures and their extracellular matrix.

(A) Confluent culture of HR-9 cells before treatment with 20 mM NH_4OH (B). After treatment, the cell monolayer has disappeared and the ECM produced by the cells is denuded. In contrast to the corneal epithelial cell extracellular matrix, a bit of cellular debris adhering firmly to the ECM can be seen. The arrows point to a hole in the matrix where the plastic can be seen. (C) Micrograph showing a cross-section of confluent HR-9 cells resting on the extracellular matrix they have produced (plastic, p). (D) Extracellular matrix after denudation of the cell layer by treatment with 20 mM NH_4OH in water. A bit of cell debris can be seen on top of the matrix (arrow) (plastic, p).

This was analyzed by comparing the growth of vascular and corneal endothelial cells seeded at low density on plastic versus BCE-ECM-coated dishes (Gospodarowicz, Ill 1980a; Gospodarowicz, Ill 1980b). Regardless of the initial seeding density, cells maintained on ECM and exposed to plasma-supplemented media divided extremely rapidly (average doubling time 18 hours) and expressed their proper phenotype once confluent. In contrast, similar cultures maintained on plastic and exposed to plasma proliferated poorly (average doubling time 48 to 72 hours) and did not become confluent. A similar observation was made for various other mesenchyme-derived cells which required fibroblast growth factor (FGF) in order to show an optimal growth rate when maintained on plastic and exposed to either serum or plasma-supplemented medium (Gospodarowicz 1983; Gospodarowicz et al 1982a).

Although one might have thought that the BCE-ECM has a direct mitogenic effect on the cells similar to that of FGF, this was shown not to be the case, since the rate of proliferation of these various cell types maintained on ECM-coated dishes was a direct function of the plasma concentration to which cells were exposed (Gospodarowicz, Tauber 1980; Gospodarowicz, Ill 1980a; Gospodarowicz, Ill 1980b). It is therefore likely that the final effect of the ECM on cell proliferation is a permissive one that results in an increased cell sensitivity to plasma factor(s).

Among the plasma factors which could be held directly or indirectly responsible for the active proliferation of these various cell types are plasma lipoproteins (Gospodarowicz, Tauber 1980), insulin or somatomedin C, and epidermal or fibroblast growth factor (Gospodarowicz, Ill 1980b). Preliminary studies demonstrated that transferrin, the main iron-carrying protein in the bloodstream, had to be present, as with most cell types studied to date, if cells were to respond to plasma factors. This absolute requirement for transferrin could either reflect its role in delivering iron to the cells or its ability to detoxify the medium by removing toxic traces of metals.

In addition to transferrin, the plasma factor requirements of the various normal diploid cell types grown on BCE-ECM fell into three broad categories. The first category, represented by vascular endothelial cells, and kidney epithelial cells required only the presence of high density lipoproteins (HDL) in order to proliferate actively (review in Gospodarowicz 1983; Gospodarowicz, Ill 1980b). The second category, to which corneal endothelial cells, lens epithelial cells, vascular smooth muscle cells and fibroblasts belong, required, in addition to HDL, the presence of insulin or somatomedin C, as well as that of EGF or FGF (Gospodarowicz 1983; Gospodarowicz, Ill 1980b). For both of these categories HDL is the main factor, since in its absence cells could not be triggered to divide when exposed to transferrin, insulin, somatomedin C, and FGF or EGF added alone or in combination. While it is presently unknown by what mechanisms of action insulin, somatomedin C, or FGF or EGF trigger cell proliferation, the ways in which HDL could support cell proliferation have been shown to correlate with its ability to activate cellular HMG CoA reductase (Cohen et al 1982a; Cohen et al 1982b). This enzyme is responsible for the synthesis of mevalonic acid, which is later utilized for the synthesis of dolichol, ubiquinone, isopentenyl adenyl adenine, and cholesterol (reviewed in Brown, Goldstein 1980). Of these compounds, the non-sterol products are probably required for cell proliferation as well as for cell survival (Quesney-Huneeus et al 1980).

The third cell category was represented by steroid-producing cells such as adrenal cortex or ovarian granulosa cells. Both of these cell types showed only a minor response to HDL, which at concentrations above 50 µg protein/ml became cytotoxic (Gospodarowicz 1983; Gospodarowicz, Ill 1980b). A major proliferative response of these two cell types to HDL would not have been expected, since these cells produce steroid and have an active HMG CoA reductase pathway. Instead, insulin was the main mitogenic factor for both granulosa and adrenal cortex cells and, although addition of HDL and EGF or FGF improved the final cell density of the cultures exposed to a defined medium, the improvements were slight (Gospodarowicz 1983; Gospodarowicz, Ill 1980b).

The substrate upon which cultures were maintained was found to be of crucial importance if a significant response to HDL or insulin (depending on the cell type) was to be observed, since it was not observed with cells maintained on plastic dishes. This suggests that, in vivo, the integrity of the ECM upon which cells rest and migrate is an important factor in determining the cells' response to lipoproteins and insulin-like activity present in plasma (Gospodarowicz, Tauber 1980; Gospodarowicz 1983; Gospodarowicz, Ill 1980b).

III. Effect of BCE-ECM on tumor cell attachment, migration and proliferation

A central issue in tumor biology is the understanding of the interactions between tumor cells and their environment. It is of interest in this regard to study the tumor cells' interaction with the ECM, since this could throw light on the need for stromal and fibroblastic support for tumor cell growth, on the ability of tumor cells to reorganize their local environment in order to grow and invade, and on the mechanisms through which various artificial substrates that are introduced in vivo into an animal result in the production of malignant mesothelioma and fibrosarcoma.

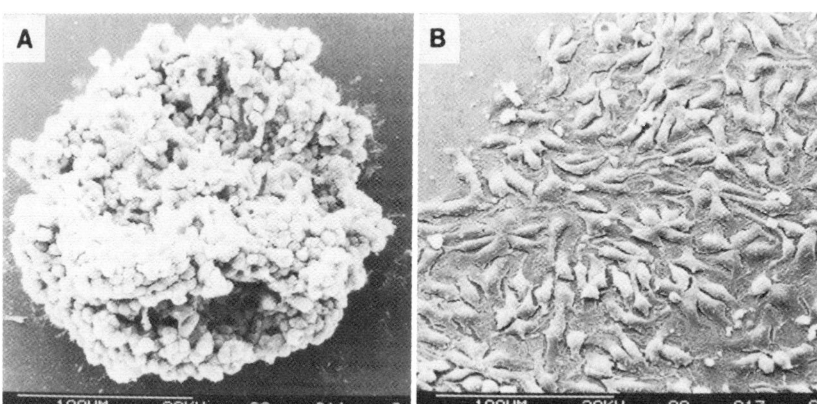

Fig. 3. Scanning electron microscopy of colon carcinoma cells maintained in tissue culture on either a plastic substratum (A) or ECM-coated dishes (B). While on plastic, cells grew as an aggregate that did not adhere to the substratum (A); when maintained on basement lamina, the cells flattened and grew as a monolayer (B).

When the attachment of colon carcinoma cells and Ewing tumor cells to ECM-coated dishes was compared to that observed on plastic, these cells were observed to attach firmly and rapidly to the ECM, but not to plastic dishes (Vlodavsky et al 1980) (Fig. 3). The rapid attachment of colon carcinoma cells and Ewing sarcoma cells was shown in subsequent studies (Vlodavsky, Gospodarowicz 1980) to be mediated by different adhesion factors present in the ECM. While colon carcinoma cells attached through their interaction with laminin, the Ewing cells interacted with fibronectin. The presence of specific adhesion factors in the ECM, as well as the ability or inability of tumor cells to produce and/or interact with such factors, may therefore determine the localization of given tumor cell types to specific ECM's (Vlodavsky et al 1980; Vlodavsky, Gospodarowicz 1980).

After their initial attachment to the ECM surface, cells were observed to migrate rapidly out from cellular aggregates (Vlodavsky et al 1980). This rapid cell migration could be relevant to tumor growth and invasiveness. Contact of the tumor cells with an ECM may favor migration of tumor cells along defined routes, and it is also likely that cell movement and its velocity are controlled by alterations in the extracellular environment and not solely by regulation of the locomotive machinery itself. Migration of cells from aggregates may simply reflect the much stronger adhesive forces between the cells and the ECM versus those existing between cells and plastic or among cells associated in an aggregate. This migratory effect might also be responsible in part for the stimulation of cell growth observed in dishes coated with an ECM versus plastic alone.

Since cell shape has been shown to be a major factor in regulating cell growth, the growth-rate of tumor cells plated on plastic (spherical configuration) was compared to that of cells plated on ECM which adopt a flattened morphology. Although differences in growth rate were observed, both the Ewing and colon carcinoma cells proliferated in either configuration (Vlodavsky et al 1980). This demonstrated that adhesion of the cells to the ECM and their subsequent flattening did not impose a restriction on their ability to proliferate. On the contrary, when cells flattened out, a stimulation of cell growth which depended on the cell type and culture conditions was observed (Fig. 4A). This was best seen with Ewing's sarcoma cells, since active proliferation of attached cells was observed only in dishes coated with an ECM (Fig. 4B). This resulted in an infinite increase in the final density of cells attached to such a substrate versus those attached on plastic (Vlodavsky et al 1980). Cultured Ewing tumor cells can therefore proliferate either when they are highly flattened and firmly attached to the ECM or when they are in suspension. Cell adhesion to the ECM, however, results in a stimulation of cell growth, which is best observed with cells growing in the anchorage-dependent configuration, but not in the floating configuration, thereby indicating a need for an actual contact between the cells and the ECM.

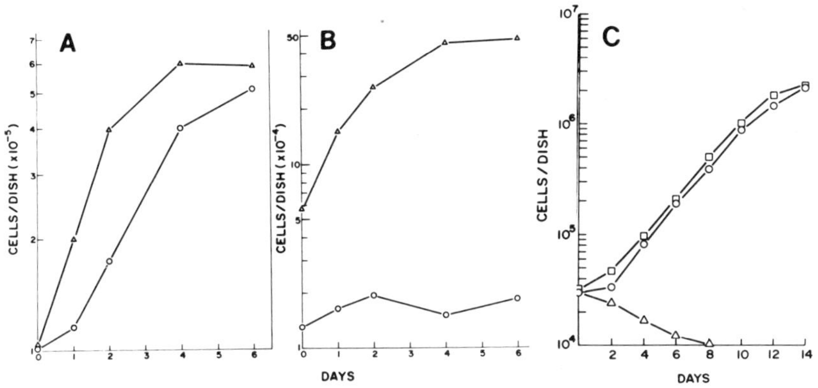

Fig. 4. Proliferation of Ewing's sarcoma cells when maintained on plastic versus basement lamina-coated dishes.

(A, B) 10^5 cells in 2 ml DMEM containing 0.5% calf serum were seeded into each plastic (o) or ECM-coated (▲) 35 mm dishes. Duplicate cultures were counted every day to determine the number of floating cells (present in the tissue culture medium) and of cells that are firmly attached (dissociated with STV). (A) Total cell number (floating plus attached). (B) Firmly attached cells. The number of firmly attached cells was higher than 80% of the total cell number found in dishes coated with ECM and lower than 10% of the total cell number obtained on plastic.

(C) Ewing sarcoma cells (4 X 10^4 cells) were seeded in total absence of serum on 35 mm ECM-coated dishes and exposed to DME alone (△) or to DME-supplemented with transferrin (10 µg/ml) and HDL (750 µg/ml, o) or 10% fetal calf serum (□).

The observation that tumor cells will divide actively when maintained on an ECM triggered our interest in their growth requirements. In most cases examined thus far (Table I), we found that tumor cells show a unique requirement for HDL alone in order to proliferate actively (Gospodarowicz et al 1982b). Two mammary carcinoma cell lines (MCF-7 and ZR-75-1) were exceptions to this rule in that they required insulin in addition to HDL in order to proliferate actively (Gospodarowicz et al 1982b). Since it would be expected that most of the tissues from which these tumor cells are derived would have a sophisticated growth requirement, it is possible that when cells become transformed they can revert to a primitive type of growth control in which hormones play a minor part and in which HDL becomes the main plasma factor involved in their proliferation. This was examined by looking at the growth control of normal rat fibroblasts (Rat-1) before and after transformation (B31 cells) by an avian sarcoma virus. While the Rat-1 cells do require HDL, insulin, and EGF in order to proliferate at an optimal rate, in the process of transformation their requirement for insulin and EGF was nearly lost and HDL alone was able to support their proliferation at an optimal rate (Giguere, Gospodarowicz 1983) (Table I). The substrate upon which cells were maintained was also an important factor to consider if tumor cells were to respond to HDL. This was best seen in the case of Ewing cells, which when maintained on ECM-coated dishes responded to HDL by proliferating as actively as when exposed to serum (Fig. 4C). Yet, when the same cell type was maintained on plastic and exposed to serum, the cells which adhered loosely to plastic did not proliferate actively (Fig. 4). This suggests that in that configuration they no longer responded to the stimuli provided by serum HDL.

TABLE I. Growth factors requirements for the proliferation of normal diploid and transformed cells maintained on ECM-coated dishes and exposed to defined medium

	HDL (μg protein/ ml)	Insulin or somato C (ng/ml)		FGF or EGF (ng/ml)		Transferrin (μg/ml)
Normal diploid cells:						
Vascular endothelial cells	500	--	--	--	--	10
Corneal endothelial cells	250	2500	100	10	50	10
Vascular smooth-muscle cells	250	2500	100	10	50	10
Granulosa cells	30	1000	100	10	50	10
Adrenal cortex cells	30	50	10	10	--	5
Lens epithelial cells	250	2500	100	10	--	10
Kidney tubule cells	800	--	--	--	--	50
Embryo fibroblasts (Rat-1)	500	5000	--		25	25
Transformed cells (Tumor):						
A-431 Carcinoma	500	--	--	--	Toxic	10
Colon carcinoma cells	500	--	--	--	--	10
Ewing sarcoma cells	500	--	--	--	--	10
Rhabdomyosarcoma	500	--	--	--	--	10
MDCK (kidney-derived)	500	--	--	--	--	10
B-31 cell line	1000	--	--	--	--	25

IV. Effect of ECM on the attachment, migration, proliferation, and differentiation of nerve cells

Studies on the role of cell-substrate adhesion in the initiation, elongation, and branching of axons have led to the conclusion that adhesive interaction between nerve cells and their microenvironment could be a crucial part of the initiation and elongation of neurons. Regulation of neuronal morphogenesis may therefore be expressed in part through the physicochemical properties of the interacting cell surface and its extracellular environment (Johnston, Wessels 1980). However, in most cases the substrates considered have been artificial in nature, consisting of plastic, chemically modified surfaces (palladium, polyornithine or polylysine-coated surface), collagen gels, as well as the remains of killed non-neuronal cells and the substrate-associated material produced by them. The ability of cultured corneal endothelial cells to produce a matrix similar to those found in vivo provides an opportunity to study the properties of a natural substrate with regard to nerve cell adhesion and the subsequent neurite initiation and outgrowth. It also allows study of how nerve cells respond to a trophic and chemotactic agent such as nerve growth factor (NGF) may differ from the response previously observed when cells were maintained on various artificial substrates.

The rat pheochromocytoma cell line PC12, which shares many properties with cultured sympathetic ganglion cells, was selected to study the role of cell-substrate interaction in regulating nerve cell attachment and neurite outgrowth. The advantage of using PC12 cells instead of normal sympathetic cells is that, although these cells do not require NGF in order to survive, they depend on it in order to initiate neurite outgrowth. When the attachment of PC12 cells to ECM-coated dishes and plastic or collagen-coated dishes was compared, it was observed that, in contrast to collagen-coated or plastic dishes, cells attach rapidly and tenaciously to ECM-coated dishes. Following cell attachment, cell spreading was observed, reflecting the functional association of the cells with their substratum (Gospodarowicz, Fujii 1981; Fujii et al 1982). After this initial cell spreading, neurite outgrowth occurred within 24 hours. Even in the absence of NGF, cells were capable of extending neurites for 5 to 10 days. In contrast, no neurite outgrowth occurred on either plastic or collagen-coated dishes unless NGF was present. It is therefore likely that the cell-substratum interaction between PC12 cells and the ECM is solely responsible for this initial neurite outgrowth. However, the presence of NGF is still required for the long-term maintenance (over 10 days) and expression of new neurite outgrowth

(Gospodarowicz, Fujii 1981; Fujii et al 1982). This also suggests that NGF may be required not so much for initiating neurite outgrowth as for stabilizing it.

The morphological appearance of neurites from PC12 cells maintained on ECM-coated dishes in the presence or absence of NGF was similar, with varicosities, branching, some fascicles, and growth cones (Fig. 5). Even after 1 or 2 days, some neurites in cultures not exposed to NGF could have a length greater than 100μ. Particularly interesting was the disposition on both sides of some neurites of microspikes, which extended from the neurite at regular intervals and appeared to staple it to the substrate. A similar configuration of microspikes or branchlets has been observed by Roberts (1976) for actively growing axons in vivo that move along the inner surface of an epidermal basement lamina.

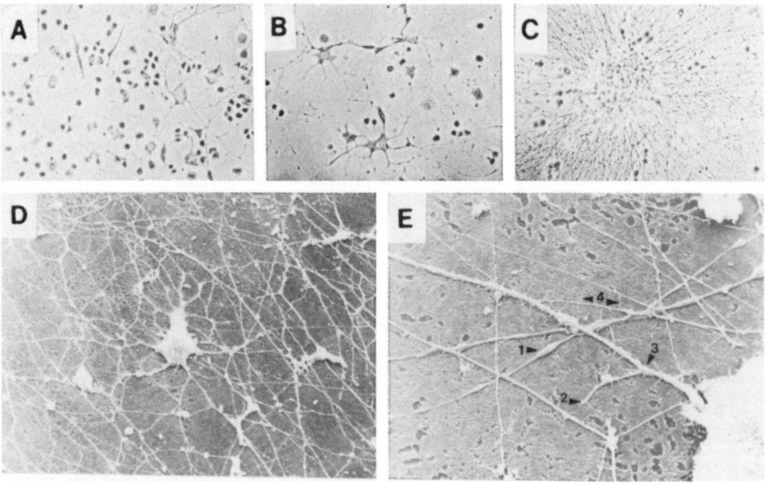

Fig. 5. Morphological appearance of PC12 cells maintained on ECM in the presence or absence of NGF. (A-C) Phase-contrast micrographs of unfixed PC12 cells cultured on ECM-coated dishes in the absence of NGF for 3 days (A) and in the presence of NGF for 3 days (B) and 13 days (C). (D, E) Scanning electron micrographs of PC12 cells on ECM in the presence of NGF for 12 days. (E) Arrows point to (1) a varicosity in a neurite, (2) the

end of a neurite, (3) a branching point, and (4) fine projections extending from a neurite.

Adhesion and differentiation of PC-12 cells to ECM-coated dishes also strongly affected their metabolic activity. This was best observed when one compared the pattern of proteins synthesized by PC12 cells maintained on collagen gel versus ECM. A reduction in the labeling by (^{35}S)methionine of high molecular weight proteins could be observed readily with cultures maintained on ECM. In the presence of nerve growth factor (NGF), qualitative changes in cellular protein synthesis also took place which were the same regardless of the substratum (either collagen or ECM) upon which cells were maintained. Particularly interesting was the observation of the induction of synthesis of a new protein with a molecular weight of 55,000 to 56,000 and an isoelectric point of 5.6. Cultures on ECM exhibiting neurites (e.g., day 2) in the absence of NGF also contain the protein, which is apparently associated with the cellular cytoskeleton (Fujii et al 1982).

Therefore, the adhesive interaction of nerve cells with the ECM produced by cultured corneal endothelial cells may not only provide a model with which to study the trophic and chemotactic effects of NGF on neurites developing on a natural substrate, but may also prove to be useful for the development in culture of neurons from the central nervous sytem which require intimate contact with glial cells for survival and growth. Although the role of glial cells may be to provide trophic factor(s), it is equally possible that they could provide a suitable surface (such as extracellular material) for neuronal cell adhesion and axon outgrowth.

V. Proliferation and differentiation of normal diploid epithelial cells on HR-9-ECM

As reviewed above, BCE-ECM provides an adequate substrate for the growth and differentiation of a variety of cell types derived from the primary or secondary mesenchyme or from the neural crest. These cell types *in vitro* grow in multiple cell layers (vascular smooth muscle cell) or adopt at confluence the morphology of a monolayer composed of small, flattened, and highly contact inhibited cells (vascular and corneal endothelial cells). The growth and differentiation of true epithelial cells, which are cuboidal or tall and columnar, are extremely poor when they are maintained on BCE-ECM, however. This can be seen particularly well in the case of bovine kidney epithelial cells derived from the distal part of the kidney nephron. This could be due in part, or *in toto*, to the composition of the BCE-ECM, which is produced by highly flattened cells and would therefore be inappropriate for supporting the proliferation and differentiation of epithelial cells which are cuboidal or tall and columnar. Since both the growth and differentiation of these cells *in vivo* correlate with the appearance of a basement membrane composed of collagen type IV, heparin sulfate proteoglycan and laminin (review in Ekblom 1981), we have analyzed the effect of such a substratum produced by PF-HR-9 teratocarcinoma cells on kidney tubule epithelial cell growth, proliferation, and differentiation (Gospodarowicz et al 1983a).

Distal kidney tubule microdissected from the medullary region of an adult bovine kidney yield two distinct cell populations (Fig. 6) based on their morphological appearance. These behave differently when maintained on plastic, BCE-ECM, or HR-9-ECM-coated dishes. The cell population which has a fibroblastic appearance does not grow on plastic but will grow actively when maintained on dishes coated with either BCE-ECM or HR-9-ECM (Fig. 7A). Its growth-rate and final cell density will be higher on dishes coated with BCE-ECM than on dishes coated with HR-9-ECM. In contrast, the other cell population, which is typically epithelioid in appearance, will grow very poorly on BCE-ECM-coated dishes. The growth-rate is improved when cells are maintained on plastic, but cells grow in islands composed of large cells and do not reach confluence (Fig. 7B). The best growth-rate and final cell density is observed when cells are maintained on HR-9-ECM-coated dishes. Under these conditions, cells grow rapidly and form a monolayer composed of extremely small cells. The differences appear in even higher relief when the growth-promoting abilities of the different substrates are analyzed as a function of initial cell density at which the epithelioid cell population were seeded (Fig. 8C). Also remarkable is the stage of differentiation that the epithelioid cell population derived from kidney tubule cells can achieve when maintained on HR-9-ECM-coated matrix. While dome formation, reflecting vectorial transport of fluid, can be observed, cells also form extensive tubules (Figs. 6 & 8). This type of morphological differentiation, similar to that seen *in vivo*, has not been reported previously for kidney tubule cells maintained *in vitro*. Histological section of such tubules indicates that they form true tubules (Fig. 8) with a lumen containing amorphous material, as has been described in the case of tubules formed by human capillary cells (Folkman,

Haudenschild 1980). The cell organization around the lumen is reminiscent of that observed in distal nephron tubule or collecting tubule (Fig. 9).

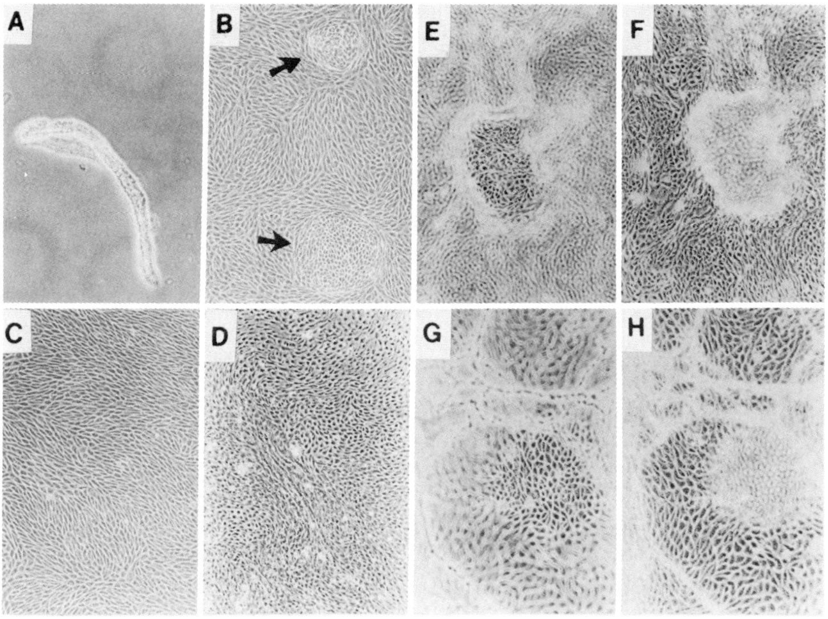

Fig. 6. Cell types growing out of a distal kidney tubule dissected from the medullary region of an adult bovine kidney.

(A) Kidney tubule explant maintained in the presence of serum-supplemented medium on BCE-ECM-coated dishes. After three weeks, two distinct cell populations have migrated from the kidney tubule explant (B), one cell type forming a uniform monolayer composed of cells with a fibroblastic appearance in which a few islands (arrows) of epithelioid cells growing in isolated colonies can be seen. (C) Kidney tubule cells with a fibroblastic appearance has been passaged on BCE-ECM and grown to form a monolayer from which islands of epithelioid cells are absent. (D) An island of kidney tubule cells with an epithelioid appearance passaged on HR-9-ECM matrix. A monolayer of small epithelioid cells has formed within 3 weeks. After one week at confluence, dome formation can be observed in the monolayer, indicating that cells have retained their ability to transport fluid. (E) Phase-contrast micrograph with focus on the apical part of the dome, (F) with focus on the monolayer. G and H show a region where dome and tubule formation coexist. Pictures were taken when the apical part of the dome was in focus (G) or when the monolayer was in focus (H).

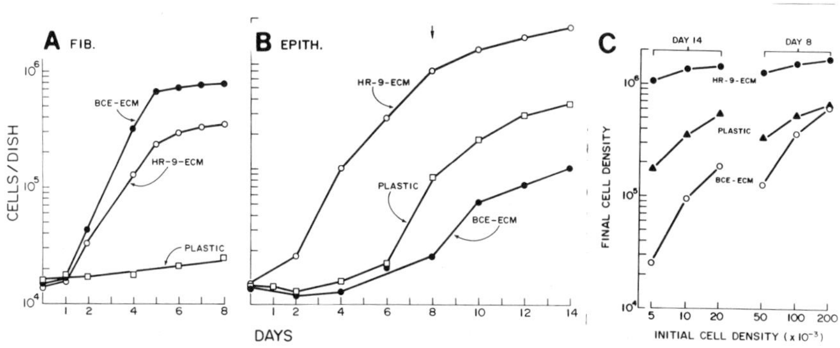

Fig. 7. Proliferation of kidney tubule epithelial cells on BCE-ECM versus HR-9-ECM-coated dishes.

(A) 2 X 10^4 kidney tubule cells (fibroblastic morphology) or (B) 4 X 10^4 kidney tubule cells (epithelioid morphology) were seeded on 35 mm plastic tissue culture dishes or on either BCE-ECM- or HR-9-ECM-coated dishes. The medium was DME-H21/F12 at a ratio of 1 to 1 supplemented with 10% fetal calf serum. Triplicate plates were trypsinized at regular intervals and cells were counted with a Coulter counter.

(C) Proliferation of kidney tubule cells (epithelioid morphology) on HR-9-ECM-coated dishes as a function of their initial cell density. Cells in serum-supplemented medium were seeded at an initial cell density ranging from 2 X 10^3 to 2 X 10^5 cells per 35 mm dish on plastic dishes ( ) or dishes coated with BCE-ECM (o) or HR-9-ECM (o). After 8 days in culture for cells seeded at an initial cell density of 50, 100, or 200 X 10^3 cells per 35 mm dish, or after 14 days for cells seeded at an initial cell density of 5, 10, or 20 X 10^3 cells per 35 mm dish, cultures were trypsinized and cells were counted in a Coulter counter.

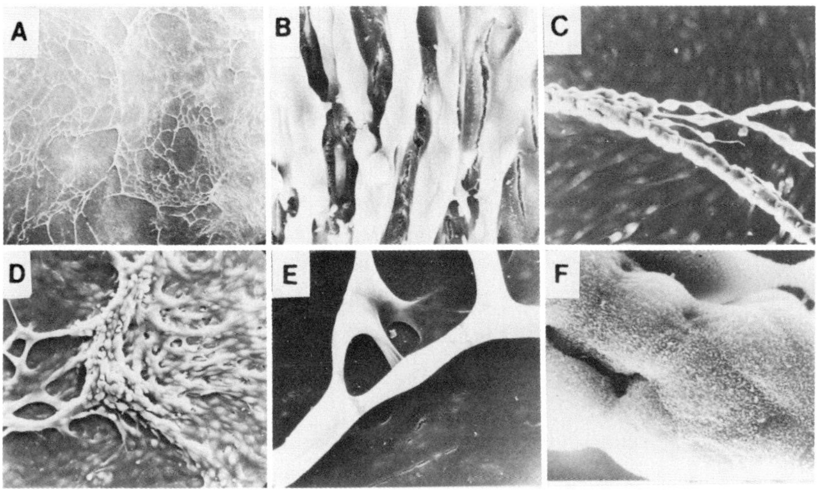

Fig. 8. Scanning electron micrograph of kidney tubules forming *in vitro*.

(A) Confluent monolayer of kidney tubule cells maintained on HR-9-ECM in the presence of serum-supplemented media and showing an extensive network of tubules. (B) An area from which the tubules originate. Numerous rounded cells are in the process of forming tubules. (C) The tubules still attached to the cell monolayer run, as *in vivo*, in parallel. (D) Point of attachment of tubules floating *free in* the medium to the cell monolayer. (E) Three floating tubules have formed and start to intertwine, (F) Intertwined tubules with numerous villi present on their abluminal surface.

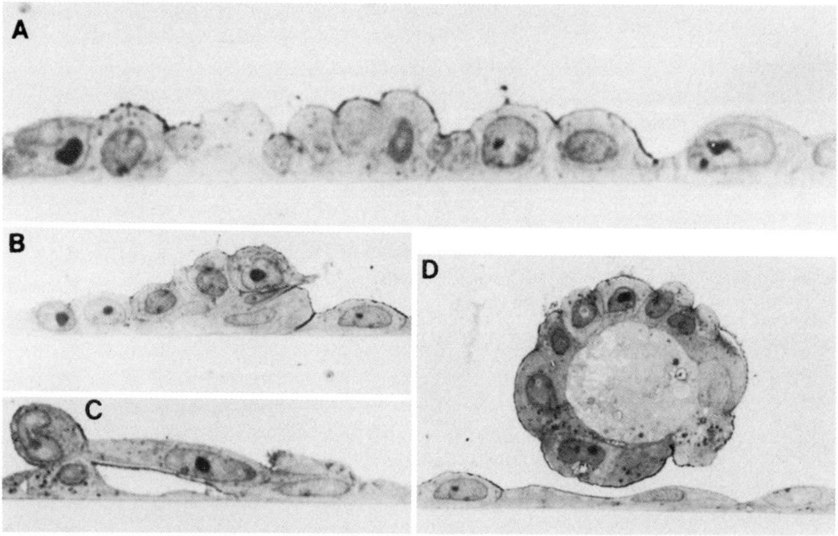

Fig. 9. Cross-section of kidney tubule epithelial cells maintained on HR-9-ECM.

(A) Cross-section of a monolayer of closely apposed cuboidal cells. (B) First step in the formation of a tubule. Cells start overgrowing each other. (C) A lumen has appeared between the cells. (D) Cross-section of a fully differentiated tubule. The inside of the lumen is filled with amorphous material.

Since kidney epithelial cells grown in the presence of serum-supplemented medium can differentiate on HR-9-ECM, we have attempted to identify the plasma component(s) responsible for their proliferation. As in the case of vascular endothelial cells (Gospodarowicz, Ill 1980b), only HDL and transferrin were required in order to promote their growth (Gospodarowicz et al 1983a) (Fig. 10), and cells maintained on HR-9-ECM and exposed to serum-free conditions differentiate as well as did cells maintained in the presence of serum, forming an extensive network of tubules. One major difference, however, was that differentiation of kidney cells in forming tubules could be observed even in sparse cultures exposed to HDL and transferrin-supplemented medium. When cells were exposed to serum-supplemented medium, such differentiation could only be observed when cells formed a monolayer. A similar growth requirement for HDL and transferrin was also observed when MDCK cells, a cell line derived from the distal part of the kidney tubule, were studied (Gospodarowicz et al 1983b). As in the case of vascular endothelial cells (Gospodarowicz et al 1982a), this mitogenic effect of HDL was closely associated with its ability to induce the enzyme HMG CoA reductase, whose catalytic product, mevalonic acid, is a precursor of both sterol and non-sterol compounds (Brown, Goldstein 1980).

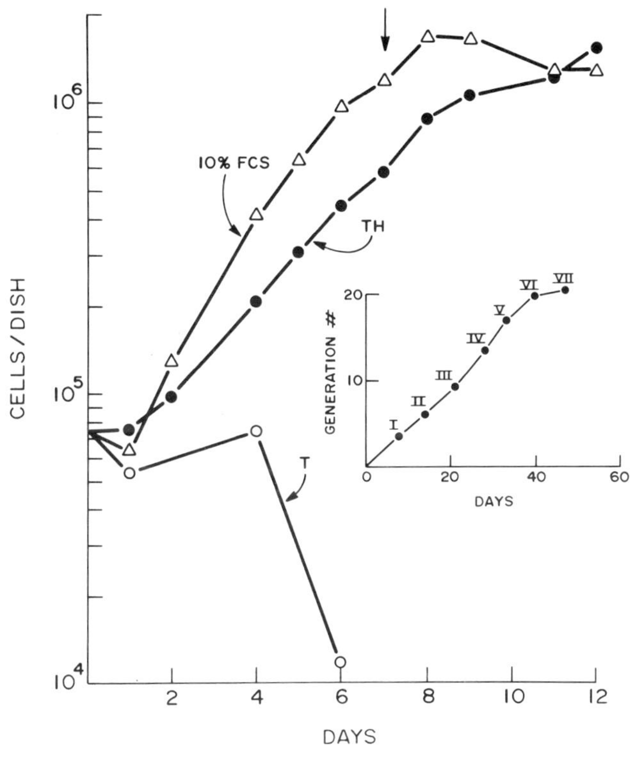

Fig. 10. Proliferation of kidney epithelial cells with an epithelioid morphology in serum-supplemented medium versus serum-free medium.

Kidney epithelial cells were seeded at an initial cell density of 7 X 10^4 cells per 35 mm HR-9-ECM-coated dish in the presence of 10% fetal calf serum (10% FCS,▲); transferrin (50 μg/ml) and HDL (750 μg protein/ml) (TH); or transferrin (50 μg/ml) alone (T). Triplicate plates were trypsinized and counted at regular intervals. The insert shows the lifespan of kidney epithelial cells maintained in HDL and transferrin supplemented medium and passaged at weekly intervals.

VII. Conclusion

Because the various cell types studied thus far respond to plasma factor(s) when maintained on a natural substrate and no longer require growth factors such as FGF in vitro, it is clear that the proliferative response of cells to plasma factors can be modified dramatically by the substrate upon which the cells are maintained. It is possible that the lack of response of different cell types in vitro to agents responsible for their proliferation and differentiation in vivo could be attributed to the artificial substrate (whether plastic or glass) upon which the cells rest. Maintenance on such a surface could limit both the cells' response to mitogenic factors and their ability to produce an ECM, either of the correct composition or in adequate amounts.

It also helps to explain why cells which in vivo rest in close association with their natural substrate respond differently to various growth-promoting agents than the same cells when they rest on plastic. A better understanding of the role that the ECM plays in cell proliferation and differentiation could affect the way in which we view various problems of cell biology currently being explored using in vitro techniques. For example, it is likely that, if one starts with a primary culture, cells are selected which in the subsequent passages retain their ability to produce an ECM. Alteration in their phenotypic expression could be the direct result of an alteration in the type of ECM produced. It is therefore possible that the widely acknowledged instability of the phenotypic expression of cultured cells could be due to their inability, when maintained on plastic, to continue to produce a normal ECM. If this should be the case, providing the cells with an artificial substrate closely resembling that produced in vivo should stabilize their phenotypic expression.

In the field of tumor cell biology, the growing recognition that the substrate upon which cells are maintained could modify their phenotypic expression is also important. One of the main characteristics of tumor cells grown in tissue culture is their loss of anchorage-dependence. This is reflected in their ability to grow either in soft agar or in suspension. Yet tumor cells from solid tumors, which can adhere loosely to one another in vitro, in an in vivo site can adhere tenaciously to the substrate which is provided by the host tissue or which they themselves produce. This is best reflected in the phenomenon of metastasis, in which tumor cells carried through the bloodstream attach tenaciously to basement membrane, infiltrate through it, and form secondary tumors at sites located far from the original tumor. It is therefore likely that, if tumor cells in culture are provided with an adequate substrate, they could shift their pattern of growth from anchorage-independence to anchorage-dependence. This could in turn result in an increased responsiveness to factors to which cells growing in suspension are not sensitive.

The ways in which the ECM exerts its permissive effect on the proliferation of normal diploid cells can only be the object of speculation. One possible effect is to modify the cell shape in order to make it responsive to factor(s) to which the cells do not respond unless they adopt an appropriate shape.

ACKNOWLEDGMENTS

This work was supported by grants from the National Institutes of Health (HL-20197, HL-23678, and EY-02186).

REFERENCES

Brown M, Goldstein J (1980). Multivalent feedback regulation of HMG CoA reductase, a control mechanism coordinating isoprenoid synthesis on cell growth. J Lipid Res 21:505.

Cohen DC, Massoglia SL, Gospodarowicz D (1982a). Correlation between two effects of high density lipoproteins on vascular endothelial cells: the induction of 3-hydroxy-3-methylglutaryl Coenzyme A reductase activity and the support of cellular proliferation. J Biol Chem 257:9429.

Cohen DC, Massoglia S, Gospodarowicz D (1982b). Feedback Regulation of 3-hydroxy-3-methylglutaryl Coenzyme A reductase in vascular endothelial cells: separate sterol and non-sterol components. J Biol Chem 257:11106.

Ekblom P (1981). Formation of basement membranes in the embryonic kidney. An immunohistological study. J Cell Biol 91:1.

Folkman J, Greenspan HP (1975). Influence of geometry on control of cell growth. Biochim Biophys Acta 417:211.

Folkman J, Moscona A (1978). Role of cell shape in growth control. Nature 273:345.

Folkman J, Haudenschild D (1980). Angiogenesis in vitro. Nature (Lond) 288:551.

Fujii DK, Massoglia SL, Savion N, Gospodarowicz D (1982). Neurite outgrowth and protein synthesis by PC12 cells as a function of substratum and nerve growth factor. J Neurosci 2:1157.

Giguere L, Gospodarowicz D (1983). Effect of RSV transformation of Rat-1 fibroblasts upon their growth factor and anchorage requirements in serum-free medium. Cancer Research 43:2121.

Gospodarowicz D, Greenburg G, Birdwell CR (1978). Determination of cellular shape by the extracellular matrix and its correlation with the control of cellular growth. Cancer Research 38:4155.

Gospodarowicz D, Vlodavsky I, Greenburg G, Johnson LK (1979). Cellular shape is determined by the extracellular matrix and is responsible for the control of cellular growth and function. In Ross R, Sato G (eds): "Hormones and cell culture", Vol 6, Cold Spring Harbor, N.Y.: Cold Spring Harbor Conferences on Cell Proliferation, p 561.

Gospodarowicz D, Ill CR (1980a). The extracellular matrix and the control of proliferation of vascular endothelial cells. J Clin Inv 65:1351.

Gospodarowicz D, Ill CR (1980b). The extracellular matrix and the control of proliferation of corneal endothelial and lens epithelial cells. Exptl Eye Res 31:181.

Gospodarowicz D, Tauber J-P (1980). Growth factors and extracellular matrix. Endocrine Reviews 1:201.

Gospodarowicz D, Vlodavsky I, Savion N (1980). The extracellular matrix and the control of proliferation of vascular endothelial and vascular smooth muscle cells. J Supramolec Struct 13:339.

Gospodarowicz D, Fujii DK (1981). The extracellular matrix and the control of cell proliferation and differentiation. Miami Winter Symposium 18:113.

Gospodarowicz D, Vlodavsky I, Savion N (1981). The role of fibroblast growth factor and the extracellular matrix in the control of proliferation and differentiation of corneal endothelial cells. Vision Res 21:87.

Gospodarowicz D, Cohen DC, Fujii DK (1982a). Regulation of cell growth by the basal lamina and plasma factors: relevance to embryonic control of cell proliferation and differentiation. In "Hormones and cell culture," Vol 9, Cold Spring Harbor, New York: Cold Spring Harbor Conferences on Cell Proliferation: Growth of Cells in Hormonally Defined Media, 295.

Gospodarowicz D, Lui G-M, Gonzalez R (1982b). High density lipoproteins and the proliferation of human tumor cells maintained on extracellular matrix-coated dishes and exposed to defined medium. Cancer Research 42:3704.

Gospodarowicz D (1983). The control of mammalian cell proliferation by growth factors, extracellular matrix, and lipoproteins. J Invest Dermatol 815:41.

Gospodarowicz D, Lepine J, Massoglia S (1983a). Ability of various basement membranes to support differentiation in vitro of normal diploid bovine kidney tubule cells. J Cell Biol submitted.

Gospodarowicz D, Massoglia S, Cohen DC (1983b). Effect of high density lipoprotein on the proliferative ability of MDCK Cells and HMG CoA reductase activity. J Cell Biol submitted.

Hay ED (1981). Extracellular matrix. J Cell Biol 91:205.

Johnston RN, Wessels NK (1980). Regulation of the elongating nerve fiber. Curr Top Dev Biol 16:165.

Kleinman HK, Klebe FJ, Martin GR (1981). Role of collagenous matrices in the adhesion and growth of cells. J Cell Biol 88:473.

Quesney-Huneeus V, Wiley HH, Siperstein HD (1980). Isopentenyladenine as a mediator of mevalonate-regulated DNA replication. Proc Natl Acad Sci USA 77:5842.

Roberts A (1976). Neuronal growth cones in an amphibian embryo. Brain Res 118:526.

Sugrue, SP, and Hay ED (1981). Response of basal epithelial cell surface and cytoskeleton to solubilized extracellular matrix molecules. J Cell Biol 91:45.

Vlodavsky, I, Lui GM, and Gospodarowicz D (1980). Morphological appearance, growth behavior and migratory activity of human tumor cells maintained on extracellular matrix versus plastic. Cell 19:607.

Vlodavsky I, Gospodarowicz D (1980). Respective involvement of laminin and fibronectin in the adhesion of human carcinoma and sarcoma cells. Nature 289:304.

Discussion

Wicha: Can you comment on specificity, especially in inducing differentiation? You have in a very general kind of way two different types of basement membrane like materials that do different things to cells, but they're still not organ specific as are the kinds of mesenchymal epithelial interactions that we've heard about before. Is it possible that the differentiation that you see relates to extracellular material as specifically laid down by the types of differentiating cells in culture? The fact that you have a time delay before you see expression of differentiation may not be just a manifestation of the density in cell culture or the confluence but the time required for extracellular matrix synthesis by the cells themselves. I wonder if you could comment whether you think the cells themselves are making more extracellular matrix.

Gospodarowicz: That's one way the cell can react to the substrate, by making its own matrix in response to the appropriate substrate. That's also one way to explain the extensive cell migration taking place. As long as the cell is on appropriate substrate it can start moving, going to the place where it will feel confident to be able to build up its own nest. It is evident that final cell density is very important for cell differentiation. Most cell differentiation we see in vitro simply shows that the cells don't proliferate as they should. Final cell density will be below the level of 2000 cells per square milliliter will not differentiate properly.

Story: In those cases where fibroblast growth factor (FGF) fulfilled the role of the extracellular matrix, do you know what FGF is turning on to provide the material that is found in the extracellular matrix? Does FGF stimulate collagen production, fibronectin, etc.?

Gospodarowicz: Those studies done were done by Plank. What the fibroblast growth factor does is to more or less promote the formation of a collagen type extracellular matrix component. If you maintain the cardiovascular or arterial cell in the absence of FGF they will mostly make collagen type I and type III, and a little bit of collagen type IV and none of type V. If you on the other hand get a shift in the type of collagen being produced in such a way that synthesis of collagen type I is completely blocked, that of collagen type III is greatly increased and collagen types IV and V are also being made. This will also greatly reduce the synthesis of fibronectin. Quite the opposite, if you remove FGF, fibronectin synthesis is increased by a factor of 10-50 fold. So, as far as basement membrane components are concerned, FGF can moderate their synthesis. We made a correlation between the production of basement membrane component and the ability of FGF to produce or induce cell growth. But its only a correlation, there is no probability yet.

Story: Some investigators have shown with epidermal growth factor that there is a decrease in collagen production. I suspect you would maintain that one needs to look at collagen types rather than total collagen production.

Gospodarowicz: When you alter the mitogen there is a decrease in the total quantity of basement membrane component being produced and an increase in quality. What you would like to do is to increase the synthesis of basement membrane collagen and decrease the synthesis of interstitial collagen, if possible. That's more or less what you achieve when you add the mitogen. Production of fibronectin also should go to a rather low level. Fibronectin is not really what you would like to have when you deal with various mesothelial cells or atypical cells in particular. Fibronectin also has been shown to increase cell migration and to promote dedifferentiation of the cell rather than differentiation. Those basement membrane components are the ones specifically affected by the mitogen. If you keep cells in the presence of mitogen they can express their specific expression for longer periods of time.

Cunha: What is the specificity of cell attachment to basement membranes? In your system using the corneal endothelial basement membrane, do corneal endothelial cells attach faster or more tightly than cells from other organs?

Gospodarowicz: I don't know. The problem is that to study cell attachment we ordinarily use tumor cells which make an attachment factor. Since normal diploid cells can make their own attachment factor they could attach to the substrate even if it did not contain those molecules. If you do the experiment with normal cells you would have to use cyclohexamide to block the synthesis by the cell of those attachment factor to study only a part of the basement membrane. We did not do that.

W. Isaacs: When you see tubule and hemicyst formations by the kidney cells, the cells are actually coming out of contact with your basement membrane. Do you think that these cells are triggered to differentiate, and can they continue to differentiate even though they've come out of contact with the basement membrane?

Gospodarowicz: They've not really come out of contact with the basement membrane. If you look at the section of the tubule you will see it's full of amorphous material. As a matter of fact, I even closed the contact from the tubules and they don't form this material. It's a problem that people working on capillary formation did not realize. It's apparent that the cell secretes a strand of basement membrane and uses it as a lumen. The second step is to hydrolyze what is inside the lumen and empty it. But first it will organize around that amorphous material which is the basement membrane itself. It's a reverse polarity to that which occurs *in vivo*.

New Approaches to the Study
of Benign Prostatic Hyperplasia, pages 129–142

INTERACTION OF RAT MAMMARY EPITHELIUM WITH EXTRACELLULAR MATRIX COMPONENTS

Max S. Wicha
Division of Hematology/Oncology
Department of Internal Medicine
Simpson Memorial Research Institute Univ. of Michigan
Ann Arbor, MI 48109

It is now clear that mesenchymal-epithelial interactions play a crucial role in tissue differentiation. There is increasing evidence that some of these interactions may be mediated by extracellular matrix components. Using the rat mammary gland as a model system, we have been investigating the role that extracellular matrix plays in cell growth and differentiation. The mammary gland is an ideal system to study these processes since *in vivo* mammary epithelium undergoes hormonally mediated growth, differentiation, and involution (15). We have studied the interaction of primary cultures of rat mammary epithelial cells with both defined extracellular matrix components and complex extracellular matrices extracted from mammary glands.

It has been appreciated for some time that cell behavior *in vitro* may be influenced by placing cells on matrices of stromal (type I, III collagen). The fusion of myoblasts into myotubes is facilitated by a substratum of denatured stromal collagen (9). More recently, Michalopoulos and Pitot described a system for the culture of hepatacytes on floating membranes of stromal collagen which promoted cellular diffferentiation (16). Based on this report, Emerman and Pitelka succeeded in culturing mouse mammary cells on floating collagen gels (5,4,2). Mammary epithelial cells isolated from pregnant mice were able to synthesize casein when cultured on these gels but not on standard tissue culture plastic dishes. Yang, et al. reported that if mammary epithelial cells from rodents or humans were imbedded within, rather than on top of stromal collagen gels, there was extensive cell growth but little differentiation (27,28), a finding recently confirmed with rabbit mammary cells (20). It has been suggested from these studies and others (8,7) that cell shape changes imposed by collagen gel systems may be important in controlling cell growth and differentiation. Although stromal collagen gel substrata clearly influence the behavior of mammary epithelial cells _in vitro_, no system using this matrix alone has been described which can duplicate the _in vivo_ sequence of mammary growth and differentiation.

I. Interaction of rat mammary cells with defined basement membrane components.

Although previous studies have utilized stromal collagen types I and III as substrata for mammary cell culture, _in vivo_ these cells are associated with the genetically and biochemically distinct type IV collagen. In addition, basement membranes contain laminin, entactin, heparin sulfate proteoglycans, and other glycoproteins (See 10 for Review).

A. Interaction of mammary cells with type IV collagen

We demonstrated that primary cultures of rat mammary cells produce collagen exclusively of the type IV variety in a process which is under hormonal control (13). Furthermore, these cells preferentially attach to and proliferate on a substratum of purified type IV collagen compared to stromal collagen (24). This matrix can reduce the cell requirements for hydrocortisone and epidermal growth factor (19). If mammary epithelial cell deposition of basement membrane collagen is blocked with the proline analogue cis-hydroxyproline (22), epithelial cells degenerate if they are growing on a matrix of stromal but not type IV collagen (24). We have extended this observation _in vivo_ by administering cis-hydroxyproline to rats whose mammary glands were hormonally stimulated with perphenazine. Although cis-hydroxyproline had no effect on unstimulated mammary glands, in hormonally stimulated glands, this compound caused defective basement membrane collagen deposition. This was followed by epithelial cell degeneration which histologically was identical to that seen in mammary involution (25). On the basis of these experiments, we proposed a model in which the formation and turnover of basement membrane components play a key role in the regulation of mammary growth and involution.

B. Interaction of mammary cells with laminin.

Laminin in a glycoprotein of approximately 800,000 M W found in the lamina lucida of all basement membranes. It is interposed between the cell surface and the lamina densa of the basement membrane which contains type IV collagen (6). The laminin molecule has distinct binding domains for type IV collagen and for the cell surface, and thus, can serve as an attachment protein (21). We postulated that the selective attachment of mammary epithelial cells to type IV collagen might be laminin mediated. Using both immunofluorescence and immunoprecipitation techniques, we have found that primary rat mammary cultures synthesize intact laminin which they deposit in an extracellular matrix. By inhibiting endogenous laminin synthesis with cyclohexamide, we were able to study the effects of exogenous laminin on mammary cell attachment to type IV collagen. As can be seen in Fig. 1, the addition of

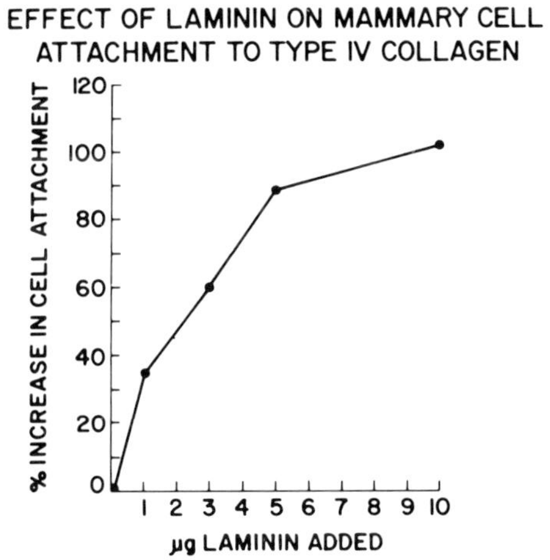

Fig. 1. Mammary epithelial organoids were prepared from perphenazine stimulated virgin rats as previously described. Attachments were to type IV collagen substrata (14) and done in medium 199 + 5% fetal calf serum + 25 µg/ml cyclohexamide to prevent endogenous protein synthesis. Attachment performed over 18 hours.

exogenous laminin stimulated mammary cell attachment to a purified type IV collagen subtratum in a dose dependent manner. Pretreatment of either the type IV collagen matrix with laminin or the addition of soluble laminin to freshly isolated mammary epithelial cells resulted in enhanced cell attachment. This attachment could be blocked with affinity purified antilaminin antibodies.

The observation that mammary cells pretreated with laminin showed enhanced binding to type IV collagen suggested that these cells had the ability to directly bind exogenous laminin to their surface. We found that [^{125}-I] laminin bound to mammary epithelial cells and that this binding could be partially displaced with an excess of cold laminin (Table 1). We have recently

Table 1.

SPECIFIC BINDING OF ^{125}-I LAMININ TO RAT MAMMARY EPITHELIUM

+	^{125}-I -Laminin Bound CPM x 10^2 /μ DNA
- Cold Laminin	49.6 ± 3
+ Cold Laminin	21.2 ± 2

Laminin binding was performed on freshly isolated cells as we have previously described (20). ^{125}-I laminin was incubated with approximately 2 x 10^5 cells for 90 minutes at 20° C ± 100 fold excess of unlabeled laminin.

described the isolation of a cell surface laminin receptor protein from murine fibrosarcoma cells that retains the ability to bind laminin with specificity and high affinity (Kd laminin 2 x 10^{-9} M) (14). Similar laminin receptors have now been isolated from B16 melanoma cells (18) and smooth muscle cells (12). We have found that the isolated laminin receptor protein also has the ability to bind directly to cellular actin (1). Based on the ability of this protein to bind both extracellular laminin and intracellular actin, we have name the protein "connectin". We postulate that connectin may be an example of a transmembrane protein capable of mediating the interaction of cells with the extracellular matrix (1). Using techniques similar to those described above, we are currently attempting to isolate laminin receptors from rat mammary epithelium and determine the role of these receptors in mediating cell shape changes and cytoskeletal rearrangements by extracellular matrix.

Part II. Interaction of rat mammary cells with complex extracellular matrices.

A. Matrix preparation.

Although the purified basement membrane components type IV collagen and laminin can interact with mammary epithelial cells and promote their attachment and growth, we found that these matrix proteins alone were unable to support long term mammary growth or differentiation *in vitro*. In order to more closely simulate the *in vivo* environment, we developed a system for the primary culture of rat mammary epithelium on an acellular matrix derived from pregnant rat mammary glands (26). This technique involved a modification of the procedure of Rojkind, et al, for the isolation of liver biomatrix (17). We have recently introduced several modifications which allow for more efficient matrix production and its deposition on culture dishes. Briefly, pregnant rat mammary glands are homogenized in 3.4 M NaCl with protease inhibitors (26). Insoluble matrix material is collected on 140 μ nitex filters. Lipids are removed with butanol-diisopropyl ether and nucleic acids with DNase and RNase (26). The matrix is pulverized under liquid nitrogen in a freezer mill (Spex Industries, Metachusen, New Jersey) and the resulting matrix powder is suspended in water and aliquoted on culture dishes. The material is then allowed to dry and sterilized with cobalt radiation. This matrix which is firmly attached to the dish provides an excellent substratum for cell growth studies. In the mammary system, cell differentiation is facilitated by plating cells on free floating matrix which is flexible, permitting cell shape changes (See Below).

B. Cell behavior on mammary extracellular matrix.

Primary cultures of rat mammary cells rapidly attach to mammary extracellular matrix and spread over the surface (Fig. 2). Unlike cells on tissue culture

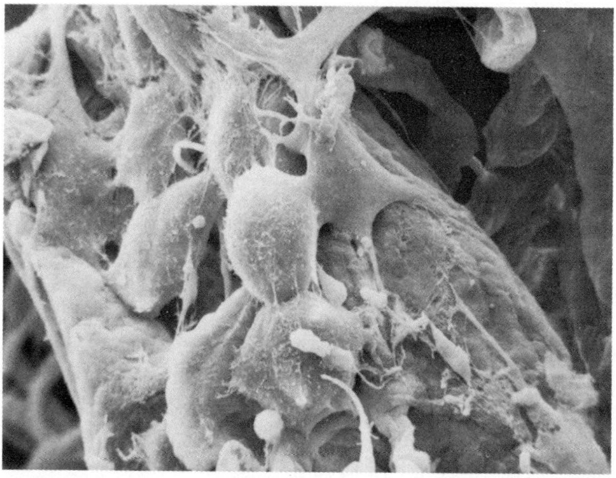

Fig. 2. Scanning electron micrograph of a primary culture of rat mammary epithelium. Conditions were as previously described (24). 2 month culture x 2,200.

plastic, these cells retain a more rounded shape (Fig 2). These cultures remain viable for at least four months.

1. Differentiated function.

Mammary cells plated on mammary extracellular matrix express considerably more differentiated function than cells on tissue culture plastic. Cultures plated on this substratum produce 40 x the α lactalbumin of those on tissue culture plastic. This enzyme is a marker of mammary differentiation (26). We have also found that cultures of mammary cells on mammary extracellular matrix continue to secrete lactose into the medium while those on tissue culture plastic or on floating collagen gels rapidly lose this ability. The confirmation of mammary gland extracellular matrix as well as its composition appear to be important in the induction of differentiated function. Cells on floating mammary matrix produce more α lactalbumin than those on extracellular matrix attached to culture dishes (23). As has been suggested for floating collagen gels, the ability of cells to undergo shape changes may play a role in their differentiation.

We compared the time course of α lactalbumin secretion for cultures on floating collagen gels to those on floating mammary gland extracellular matrix. Mammary cells on floating collagen gels gradually differentiate with increasing time in culture. αlactalbumin is maximal after approximately 3 to 4 weeks. On mammary extracellular matrix, differentiation proceeds more rapidly although there is still an increase in αlactalbumin production with time in culture (Fig 3).

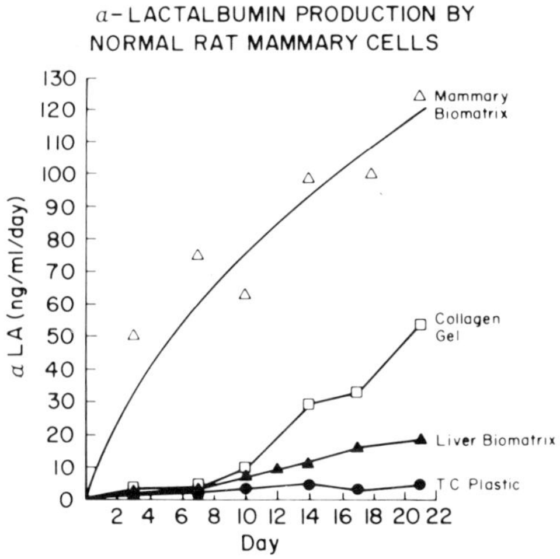

Fig. 3. Cultures were plated on tissue culture plastic, collagen gel, or extracellular matrix prepared from rat mammary glands or liver. After 24 hours in culture, the matrices were released to float.

The organ specificity of mammary gland extracellular matrix is indicated by the lower level of differentiation of cells plated on matrix prepared from rat liver (Fig 3). Although there appears to be organ specificity in induction of differentiation, we have recent evidence that extracellular matrix prepared from the EHS tumor which contains large amounts of basement membrane material (11), is also efficient in inducing mammary differentiation. These results may indicate that there are both organ specific and more general effects of extracellular matrix components on mammary cell differentiation.

We have been able to sustain long term survival and differentiation of mammry cultures under serum-free conditions. With added insulin hydrocortisone, transferrin, epidermal growth factor, and prolactin, and Pederson fetuin (19), these cultures continue to produce αlactalbumin for at least four months. The expression of this differentiated function is dependent on the continued presence of prolactin in the medium. αlactalbumin secretion rapidly falls when prolactin is removed.

2. Cell growth.

DNA synthesis and cell growth is rapid over the surface of mammary gland extracellular matrix as indicated by cell counts, ^{3}H-thymidine incorporation and autoradiography (26, 23). ^{3}-H-thymidine incorporation is greater for cells on mammary gland extracellular matrix than for those on tissue culture plastic or on extracellular matrix prepared from rat liver (Table 2).

Table 2.

^{3}-H-Thymidine Incorporation by Rat Mammary Cells on Various Substrata

MATRIX	CPM/μg DNA x 10^2
TISSUE CULTURE PLASTIC	42 ± 7
LIVER BIOMATRIX	28 ± 12
MAMMARY BIOMATRIX	82 ± 16

Cells were plated in medium 199 + 5% fetal calf serum (24). They were labeled with ^{3}H-thymidine from 48-72 hours in culture.

Furthermore, we find that mammary biomatrix promotes the mitogenic effect of estrogens and the inhibitory effect of antiestrogens on mammary cells when compared to cells on tissue culture plastic (23). Although the mechanism of this potentiation of steroid hormone effects by matrix is currently unknown, we have preliminary evidence that cells on mammary extracellular matrix have significantly higher levels of estrogen receptors than those on tissue culture plastic.

3. Role of synthesized extracellular matrix components in expression of differentiated function.

It is unclear at this time whether mammary cells respond directly to components in mammary extracellular matrix or whether it is necessary for them to synthesize other molecules which are then stabilized by the mammary extracellular matrix. Others have shown that there are interactions between extracellular matrix components (11). For instance, is has been demonstrated that stromal collagen can potentiate the accumulation of glycosaminoglycans into an extracellular matrix by reducing their turnover (3). We find that mammary epithelial cells rapidly deposit the basement membrane components type IV collagen, laminin, and fibronectin when cultured on mammary extracellular matrix (Fig 4).

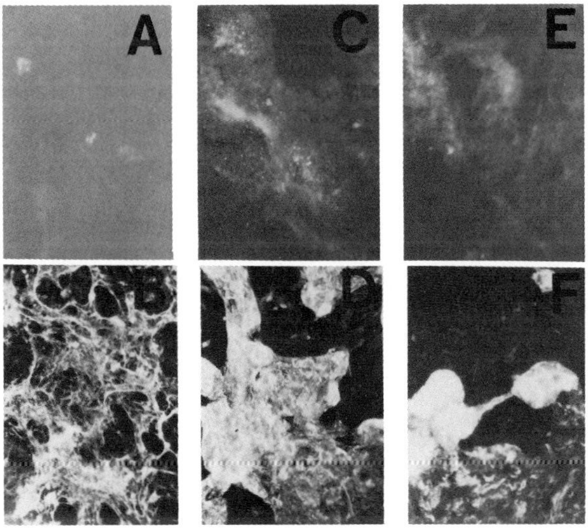

Fig. 4. Immunofluoresence detection of fibronectin, laminin, and type IV collagen in mammary gland extracellular matrix before and after cell culture. Rat mammary cells were cultured on mammary gland extracellular matrix (24) for 3 weeks and then cells removed with 1% Np-40 in phosphate buffered saline. Indirect immunofluresence was performed on resulting matrix or on freshly isolated extracellular matrix. Antibodies and immunofluoresence techniques have been described previously (24). A,C, E fresh matrix, B,D,F after cell culture, AB-fibronectin, C,D, laminin, E,F type IV collagen x 100.

Although the deposition of these components by mammary epithelium on mammary extracellular matrix or on collagen gels correlates temporally with αlactalbumin production, we do no know whether this de novo extracellular matrix deposition is required for the expression of differentiated function.

Summary.

Primary cultures of rat mammary epithelium synthesize the basement membrane components type IV collagen and laminin and utilize these components for attachment and growth. These cells may interact with matrix componetns via specific cell surface receptors. However, neither laminin nore type IV collagen alone can sustain mammary differentiation or promote culture longevity _in vitro_. We have developed a system for the culture of mammary cells on matrices derived from rat mammary glands. This complex matrix promotes cell growth, differentiation, and hormonal responsiveness. Although the mechanisms responsible for these effects are still unknown, one possibility is that cell surface matrix receptors interact with cytoskeletal components leading to alterations in cell shape and hormone receptor configurations. The mammary gland provides an excellent model system to study the interaction of extracellular matrix components with soluble signals, e.g. hormones and growth factors, in the control of cell growth and differentiation. The way these components may interact to influence cell behavior is depicted schematically in Fig. 5.

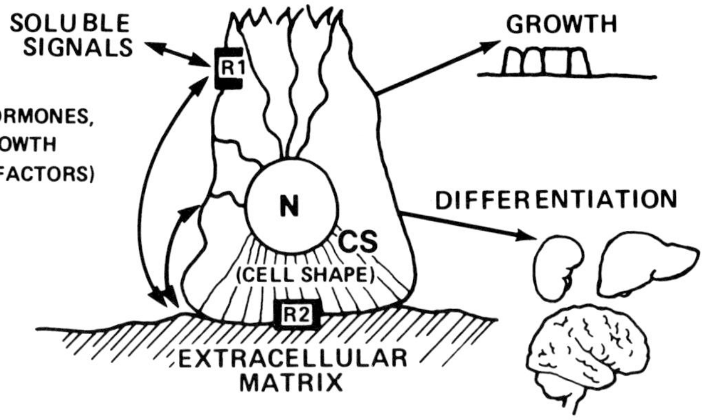

Fig. 5. Schematic representation of the interaction of soluble signals and growth factors in the control of growth and differentiation. Cells have receptors for both soluble signals (hormones and and growth factors) and for extracellular matrix components. These receptors may interact with each other and with the cellular cytoskeleton to produce cell shape changes and to influence both cytoplasmic and nuclear events.

ACKNOWLEDGEMENTS: Thanks to George Lowrie for excellent research assistance and Barbara Gorenflo for help in preparing the manuscript. This work was supported by grants BC-357-A from the American Cancer Society and HD 16721 from the National Institutes of Health.

REFERENCES

1. Brown SS, Malinoff HL, Wicha, MS (1983). Proc Natl Acad Sci USA In Press.
2. Burwen SJ, Pitelka DR (1980). Exp Cell Res 126:249.28.
3. David G, Bernfield M (1981). J Cell Biol 91:281.5.
4. Emerman JT, Enami J, Pitelka DR, Nandi S (1977). Proc Natl Acad Sci USA 74:4466.
5. Emerman JT, Pitelka Dr (1977). In Vitro 13:316.

6. Foidart JM, Bege EP, Yaar M, Rennard S, Gullino M, Martin J, Katz SI (1980). Lab Invest 42:336.
7. Folkman J, Moscona A (1978). Nature 273:345.
8. Gospodarowicz D, Greenberg G, Birdwell Cr (1978). Cancer Res 38:4155.
9. Hauschka SD, Konigsberg IR (1966). Proc Natl Acad Sci USA 55:119.
10. Hay ED (1982). Cell Biol Extracellular Matrix New York, Plenum Press
11. Kleinman HK, Woodley DT, MCGarvey ML, Robey PG, Hassell, Martin GR (op cit p 45.
12. Lescot H, Kuhl U, Vonder Mark K (1983). Embo Journal G:861.
13. Liotta LA, Wicha MS, Fodart JM, Rennard SI, Garbisa S, Kidwell WR (1979). Lab Invest 41:511.
14. Malinoff HL, Wicha MS (1983). J Cell Biol 96:1475.
15. Martinez-Hernandez, Fink LM, Pierce (1976). Lab Invest 34:455.
16. Michaelopoulos G, Pitot HC (1975). Exp Cell Res 94:70.
17. Rao NC, Barsky SH, Terranova VP, Liotta LA (1983). Biochem Biophys Res Commun 111:804.
18. Rojkind M, Gatmatan A, Mackensen S, Giambrone M, Ponce P, Reid LM (1980). J Cell Biol 87:255.
19. Solomon DS, Liotta LA, Kidwell WR (1981). Proc Natl Acad Sci USA 78:382.
20. Suaro YM, Haeuptle MT, Farinon E, Kraehenbuhl, K (1983). J Cell Biol 96:1435.
21. Terranova VP, Rao CN, Kalebic T, Liotta LA (1983). Proc Natl Acad Sci USA 80:444.
22. Uitto J, Prockop D (1977). Arch Biochem Biophys 181:293.
23. Wicha MS. In Extracellular Matrix. Hawks S, Wang J (ed) p 309 Academic Press.
24. Wicha MS, Liotta LA, Garbisa S, Kidwell WR (1979). Exp Cell Res 124:181.
25. Wicha MS, Lowrie G, Kohn E, Bagavandoss P, Jahn T (1982). Proc Natl Acad Sci USA 79:3213.
26. Wicha MS, Liotta LA, Vonderhaar BK, Kidwell WR (1980). Develop Biol 80:253.
27. Yang J, Richards J, Bowman P, Guzman R, Enami J, McCormic K, Hamamoto S, Pitelka D, Nandi S (1979). Proc Natl Acad Sci 76:3401.
28. Yang J, Richards J, Guzman R, Imagawa W, Nandi S (1980). Proc Natl Acad Sci USA 77:2088.

Discussion

Katzenellenbogen: When you look at alpha-lactalbumin production on different matrices, do you have hormones in the media during that time, or is the stimulation in the animal adequate to continue the alpha-lactalbumin in vitro?

Wicha: I didn't show that, but it is necessary to add hormones. In serum free medium it is necessary to add hydrocortisone and prolactin. When prolactin is removed alpha-lactalbumin production rapidly falls.

Katzenellenbogen: Also, I was interested in another point concerning the normal mammary cells and DMBA tumor cells. There seemed to be no modulation of the thymidine incorporation in the tumor cells by the matrix, but there was modulation in the case of normal mammary cells. Would you comment on this?

Wicha: I wasn't going to talk about the tumors today, but it does appear to be interesting. DMBA is a carcinogen which induces well differentiated mammary adenocarcinomas. There seems to be several fundamental differences between these cells and normal mammary cells; although, morphologically they look identical in culture. DMBA induced mammary tumor cells express only limited differentiated function on any substratum. Unlike normal mammary cells, the growth and differentiation of these cells is similar on tissue culture plastic, floating collagen gels or mammary extracellular matrix (ECM). This supports the concept that tumors lose the ability to recognize signals in the ECM, or at least react to them in abnormal ways.

W. Isaacs: Oftentimes when you put epithelial cells in culture, they undergo a massive shift in their protein synthetic patterns. Have you looked at methionine labeling of proteins synthesized by cells on plastic versus cells on the matrix, and compared overall protein patterns?

Wicha: We are beginning such studies, but we have not compared labeling patterns of cells plated on different substrata.

Cunha: There are many reports in the literature indicating that epithelial cells can produce a basal membrane. That isn't to say that that basal membrane is the same basal membrane that develops in vivo when you have mesenchymal cells on the other side. Aside from fibronectin, is there any evidence that mesenchymal cells contribute substances to the basal membrane?

Wicha: Not really, but there is an indication that components produced by stromal cells may produce may affect the accumulation of components in the basement membrane. At the simplest level, Merton Bernfield has shown that stromal collagen will cause epithelial cells to accumulate glycosaminoglycans and proteoglycans in a layer under the cells. What it seems to do is stabilize the turnover of the glycosaminoglycans. There is certainly the possibility that the ECM that we are putting in culture acts as a stabilizing factor for other ECM components synthesized *in vitro*. *In vivo* it may be that the mesenchyme is making these critical elements that interact with the ECM made by the epithelial cells.

Chung: Have you tried to culture your epithelium and stroma together, and then add the hormone? In this confronting culture condition what is the real effect of hormone and antihormone?

Wicha: We haven't done that yet. It certainly would be interesting, in light of the hormone receptors described in the stromal tissue. We now have good systems, because we can separate stroma, mesenchyme and ECM components and combine them systematically.

New Approaches to the Study
of Benign Prostatic Hyperplasia, pages 143–158

PRELIMINARY STUDIES ON THE RELATIONSHIP BETWEEN COLLAGEN AND THE GROWTH OF MALE ACCESSORY SEX ORGAN EPITHELIAL CELLS

Mark O. Thornton, Richard Frederickson,
Lucinda Mata† and Michael Mawhinney

Departments of Urology, Pharmacology and Anatomy
West Virginia University Medical Center
Morgantown, WV 26506
† Present address: Cell Biology
Glubenkian Institute of
Science ,Oeiras, Portugal

Introduction

Evidence has accrued in a variety of adult organ systems indicating that collagenous matrices support epithelial cell proliferation and differentiation. Elucidating the significance of these cell-extracellular collagen matrix relationships has often involved use of inhibitors of collagen metabolism such as cis-hydroxyproline (CHP). For example, *in vitro* CHP effectively inhibited mammary gland proliferation of type I collagen (Wicha et al., 1979) and blocked the *in vivo* proliferation of normal (Wicha et al., 1980) and neoplastic (Vembu et al., 1979; Wicha et al., 1981 and Lewko et al., 1980) mammary epithelial cells. Such effects of CHP on cellular proliferation in various organ systems have been attributed to its ability to cause a reduction in the accumulation of collagen in the extracellular matrix by being incorporated into newly formed collagenous peptides in place of proline, and preventing the molecule from forming its normal helical structure (Uitto and Prockop, 1974). Consequently, the CHP containing collagens were secreted at a reduced rate (Rosenbloom and Prockop, 1971; Kao et al., 1979) and were susceptible to degradation by relatively non-specific proteases (Uitto and Prockop, 1974). However, there has been disagreement about whether CHP selectively perturbs collagenous proteins. The reports that CHP had little effect on non-collagenous protein synthesis (Wicha et al., 1975; Uitto and Prockop, 1974) could have resulted from the use of ^{14}C-leucine or

C^{14}-lysine instead of C^{14}-proline to quantify protein synthesis, but Uitto and colleagues (1975) have used C^{14}-proline as a probe and found no effect of CHP on non-collagenous protein. It must also be considered that the apparent specificity of CHP action on mammary gland collagenous proteins (Wicha et al., 1980; Uitto et al., 1975) may have been due to endogenous collagenases degrading CHP containing non-helical collagens without comparable endogenous mechanisms to degrade CHP containing non-collagenous proteins. In contrast Kao et al.,(1979) and Rosenbloom and Prockop, (1971) showed that CHP could inhibit total protein synthesis in tendon regardless of whether ^{14}C-leucine or ^{14}C-proline was used as the probe, but effects on collagenous vs. non-collagenous proteins were not discriminated. Therefore the specificity of CHP action on collagenous and non-collagenous proteins has not been entirely resolved. Nevertheless, it has been shown that only those cells which require an interaction with collagenous matrices for proliferation were susceptible to inhibition by CHP (Lewko et al,, 1981), indicating that the effects of the drug on cellular proliferation were due only to its inhibition of collagen accumulation.

In view of the theories which have been offered since the early 1900's, that the epithelial cell proliferation in human BPH may occur in response to stimulation from the fibromuscular stroma (Deming and Wolfe, 1939; LeDuc, 1939; Pradham and Chandra, 1975; McNeal, 1978; Neubauer, 1983), we sought to determine if a cause and effect relationship does exist between production of the extracellular collagenous matrix and epithelial cell proliferation and differentiation in the normal prostate. The problem was approached by analyzing the temporal relationships between androgen-induced changes in collagen and DNA and by determining if cis-hydroxyproline (CHP), an inhibitor of collagen accumulation, perturbed epithelial cell growth. The rat ventral prostate was used in these studies since the androgenic regulation of its cell cycle has been well defined (Coffey et al., 1968) and the organ contains an overwhelming predominance of acinar epithelial cells (DeKlerk and Coffey, 1978).

Materials and Methods

All rats used in this study were purchased from Hilltop Labs, Scotdale, PA, and ranged in body weight between 275-350 gms. Dihydrotestosterone (DHT) (Sigma Chemical) was prepared in peanut oil, and subcutaneously injected each day (10 mg/kg) in a volume of 0.1-0.2 mls. Castrate controls for DHT-treated groups received injections of peanut oil. CHP (Cal Biochem.) and β-amino-proprionitrile fumarate (BAPN) (Sigma), were disolved in saline and injected subcutaneously twice daily with 1/2 the total daily dose. The 200 mg/kg dose was previously shown to effectively inhibit normal mammary gland growth without overt systemic toxicity (Wicha et al., 1980). The dose of BAPN chosen was 600 mg/kg which represented approximately 1/2 the LD_{50} in rats (Keiser et al., 1967). Controls for drug treated animals received the saline vehicle. Unless otherwise stated, all rats were maintained on a standard rat chow purchased from Purina. In those experimental designs in which a proline-free diet (PFD) was used, it was purchased from U.S. Biochemical Corp. with control rats being fed the balanced synthetic rat chow from the same company.

Endogenous collagen levels were quantified using the colorimetric hydroxyproline method of Kivirikko et al., (1962). Specific discription of this procedure used to quantify hydroxyproline in rat accessory sex organs have been previously described (Mariotti et al., 1981). To measure prostate collagen synthesis, prostates were excised, blotted free of secretions, and chopped into 1.0 mm squares. Samples were incubated in a proline free Eagles minimum essential medium containing 0.5 Ci/ml ^{14}C-proline (New England Nuclear, Boston, Massachusetts), and 0.35 mg/ml $NaHCO_3$, 50 μg/ml BAPN fumarate, 50 μg/ml ascorbate and 0.8 mM ferrous ammonium sulfate. At the end of incubation, tissue samples were rinsed, blotted, and homogenized in 2.0 ml ice-cold 10% TCA, centrifuged (1,000 x g for 10 minutes) and pellets were rinsed once in 10% TCA. The pellets were either directly assessed for radioactivity or assayed for radioactive ^{14}C-proline and ^{14}C-hydroxyproline as outlined below.

The method to determine ^{14}C-hydroxyproline and ^{14}C-proline incorporated into newly synthesized protein utilized the procedure of Juva and Prockop (1966) and Berg (1982) with slight modification. In particular, after the initial toluene extraction for ^{14}C-proline, the remaining aqueous phase was, in order to remove ^{14}C-proline contamination, further extracted with toluene (for a total of eight extractions) in the following manner: 5 ml of toluene was added to each tube, the tube was secured, and the tubes were inverted manually ten times. After separation of the phases, the organic phase was removed by suction and the process was repeated with 5 ml of tolune. After the eighth extraction, the samples were boiled, cooled, and another 5 ml of tolune added. The tubes were shaken and centrifuged as mentioned and 4.5 ml of the tolune phase was eluted through a silicic acid column prepared exactly as described by Berg (1982). The eluted fraction, representing 94% of the total ^{14}C-hydroxyproline, was mixed with 1 ml of counting solution (.3 g POPOP and 24 g PPO in 300 ml tolune) and counted for 1 minute in a scintillation counter. ^{14}C-proline contamination of this fraction was 0.2% and all ^{14}C-hydroxyproline values were corrected for this contamination.

RNA and DNA were measured by the procedures of Hutchinson and Monroe (1961) and Schneider (1957) respectively, while prostatic DNA synthesis was quantified as described by Coffey et al, (1968).

Results

Two weeks after castration of adult male rats the temporal relationship between DHT (2-10 mg/kg)-induced changes in rat ventral prostate wet weight, DNA content and collagen content and synthesis were analyzed. DNA content increased on day 3 of daily DHT treatment, while collagen content did not increase until day 7 (Figure 1). From day 7 until day 14 for the 10 mg/kg DHT group, and from day 7 until day 22 for the 2 mg/kg group, there were close correlations between the androgen-induced accumulations in ventral prostate weight, DNA content and collagen content as the parameters approached and exceeded normal levels (Figure 1). Focusing on the first 7 days of androgen treatment of castrate adult rats, and analyzing the VP for collagen and DNA synthesis it was found that the relationship between increases in newly synthesized DNA and collagen were different than for total endogenous levels of the two parameters. On day 1 of DHT treatment, the concentration of collagen synthesized in the VP increased 101% above castrate and continued to increase until plateauing between days 5 and 7 (Table 1). DNA synthesis also increased significantly on day 1, but rose dramatically by day 2, peaked on day 3 and declined thereafter to relatively low levels by day 7 (not shown).

Figure 1. Temporal Relationship Between Androgen Induced Increases In Total DNA and Collagen In Rat Ventral Prostate.

Rats were castrated and two weeks later androgen (DHT) was given at a maximally stimulating (10 mg/kg/day) dose for 2,3,5,7,10 or 14 days or a sub-maximally stimulating dose (2 mg/kg/day) for 1,3,7,10, 15, or 23 days. Twenty-four hours after the final hormone injection, rats were sacrificed and the VP was removed and analyzed for either DNA or collagen content. Each group contained from 5 to 20 animals and the points on the time course were presented as a percentage of sham controls (which were sacrificed with the longest treated group). The asterisk (*) represented the first significant increase compared to castrate controls.

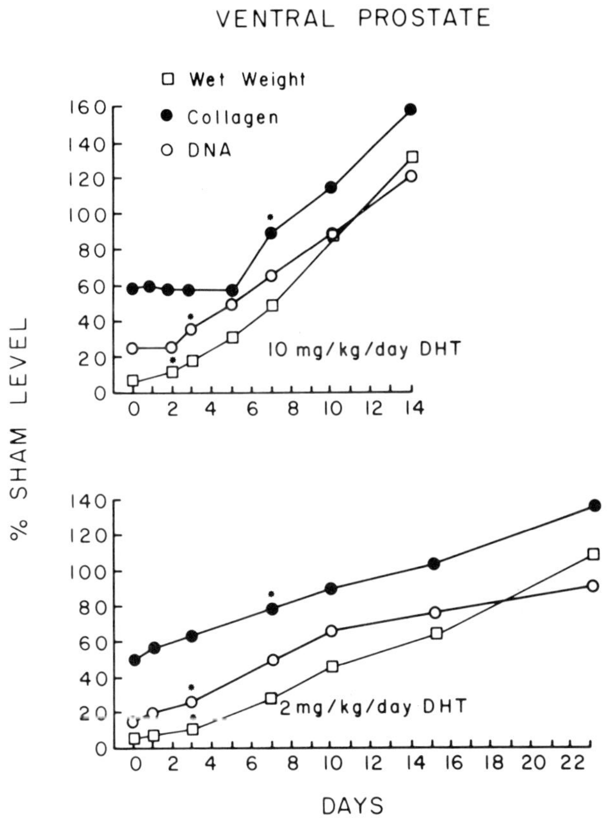

Days DHT treatment following two-week castration-induced regression

Table 1: COMPARISON OF VP ORGAN CONTENT AND CONCENTRATION OF SYNTHESIZED AND ENDOGENOUS HYDROXYPROLINE

	Endogenous Hydroxyproline	
	Content, ug/organ	Concentration, ug/mg
Normal	(11) 280 ± 23	(5) 0.61 ± 0.03
Castrate	(13) 165 ± 8	(6) 6.70 ± 0.60
Castrate + DHT (days)		
+ 1	(5) 165 ± 17	(5) 3.80 ± 0.17
+ 2	(16) 163 ± 14	(6) 4.20 ± 0.60
+ 3	(11) 162 ± 10	(6) 1.60 ± 0.12
+ 5	(13) 163 ± 15	(5) 1.38 ± 0.08
+ 7	(7) 255 ± 10	(5) 1.37 ± 0.18

	Synthesized ^{14}C-Hydroxyproline	
	Content, dpm/organ	Concentration, dpm/mg
Normal	(5)341.4 ± 51.7	(5) 0.77 ± 0.10
Castrate	(6) 45.0 ± 9.5	(6) 0.94 ± 0.11
Castrate + DHT (days)		
+ 1	(4)116.0 ± 14.9	(4) 1.89 ± 0.14
+ 2	(6)140.0 ± 12.2	(6) 2.18 ± 0.21
+ 3	(4)250.0 ± 12.1	(4) 2.54 ± 0.17
+ 5	(3)560.0 ± 173.2	(3) 2.97 ± 0.37

Synthesis of ^{14}C-hydroxyproline or accumulation of endogenous hydroxyproline was determined in sham operated rats or two-week castrate rats and two week castrates treated for 1,2,3,5, and 7 days with DHT (10 mg/kg/day). Data was presented as content of synthesized or endogenous hydroxyproline per organ or concentration of synthesized or endogenous hydroxyproline per milligram VP organ weight.

Figure 2. Effect of CHP and BAPN Fumerate on DHT-Induced Growth of Adult Rat Accessory Sex Organs.

Adult animals were castrated and two weeks later were treated daily with DHT (10 mg/kg) or oil for 7 days. In addition, groups of DHT treated castrates were also subjected to twice daily injections with either BAPN (600 mg/kg/day) or CHP (200 mg/kg per day). Drug injections were initiated 3 days prior to the onset of DHT treatment and continued throughout the course of DHT treatment. The asterick (*) denoted statistical significance from DHT controls.

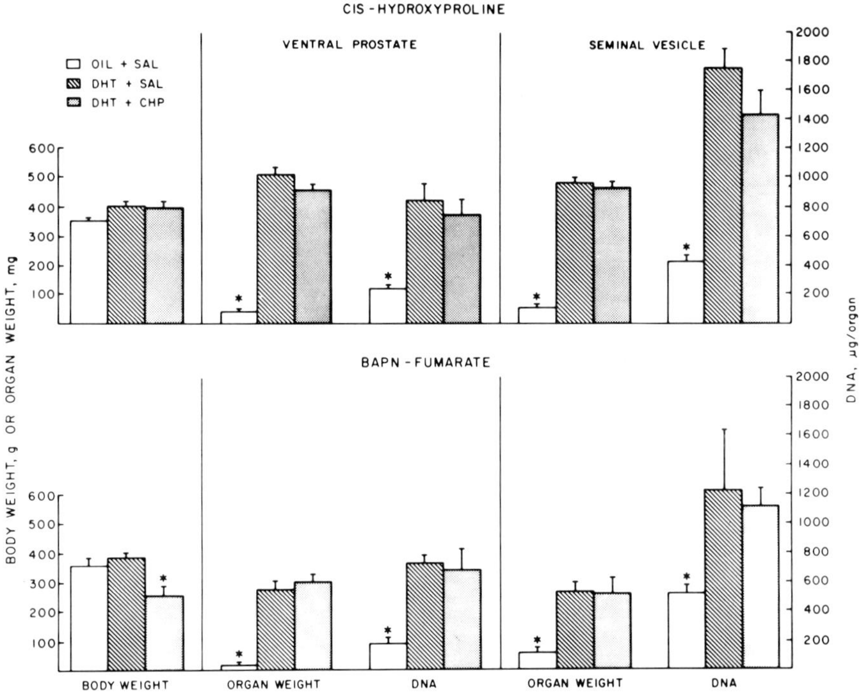

Table 2: EFFECT OF CIS-HYDROXYPROLINE ON DHT INDUCED GROWTH OF ADULT RAT ACCESSORY SEX ORGANS FED A PROLINE-FREE DIET

	VENTRAL PROSTATE			SEMINAL VESICLE			HEART	KIDNEY
Group	OW mg	DNA ug/Organ	RNA ug/Organ	OW mg	DNA ug/Organ	RNA ug/Organ	OW g	OW g
Oil + Saline	49* ± 5 (4)	435* ± 81 (4)	88* ± 28 (4)	92* ± 7 (4)	869* ± 20 (4)	265* ± 34 (4)	---	---
DHT + Saline	294 ± 9 (8)	997 ± 47 (8)	2054 ± 100 (8)	470 ± 13 (8)	2432 ± 169 (6)	4499 ± 39 (6)	1.432 ± .050 (5)	1.556 ± .042 (5)
DHT + CHP	204* ± 13 (6)	738* ± 16 (5)	1430* ± 118 (5)	379* ± 12 (6)	1731* ± 49 (6)	3747* ± 114 (3)	1.229 ± .028 (3)	1.688 ± .087 (3)
Oil + CHP	35 (2)	--- ---	--- ---	74 (2)	--- ---	--- ---	1.186 (2)	1.340 (2)

Adult animals were castrated and two weeks later were treated daily with DHT 10 mg/kg or oil for 7 days. In addition, castrate controls or DHT treated groups were treated twice daily with CHP (200 mg/kg/day). CHP-injections were started 3 days prior to and continued throughout the course of DHT treatment. Proline free diets were given to all animals 10 days prior to and during drug treatment, but during the last 3 days of the experiment when food consumption declined dramatically in the CHP + DHT group, the diet was fed to all animals in amounts equal to that consumed by the DHT + CHP treated group. The asterisk (*) denoted statistical difference from the DHT + saline group. The lack of a standard error on the oil + CHP group was due to the fact that N = 2. The average number of observations in all other groups was 5.

Considering that the DHT-induced changes in the collagenous component of the prostate might be an essential component in supporting the normal androgenic restoration of cell number, we determined the effects of BAPN and CHP on DHT-induced growth of the ventral prostate of adult rats. BAPN, an inhibitor of collagen cross-linking proved to have significant systemic toxicity in that it caused body weight to decrease approximately 30% relative to DHT controls (Figure 2) and animals appeared to be emaciated with skeletal anomalies. Since DHT-induced growth of ventral prostate in the emaciated BAPN animals was not altered from normal (Figure 2), we discontinued any further studies with the drug. CHP was free of any overt systemic toxicity, but also had no affect on DHT-induced growth of the adult accessory sex organ, as measured by changes in organ weight or DNA content (Figure 2).

In view of the fact that CHP-induced perturbations in collagen accumulation are dependent upon its incorporation into collagen in place of proline, we repeated the previously described experimental designs of CHP action on androgen-induced ventral prostate growth in rats which were subjected to a proline-free diet. In combination with the PFD, CHP proved to be a most effective inhibitor of androgen-induced hyperplasia in the prostate (Table 2). The PFD alone had no significant effect on DHT-induced growth.

Discussion

Androgen-induced changes in ^{14}C-hydroxyproline formation and incorporation into the TCA precipitable protein fraction may involve several processes including changes in the net synthesis of collagen chains, accumulation of free ^{14}C-proline by the organ, degree of proline hydroxylation per collagen chain and shifts in the production of collagen types. Direct measurements of free ^{14}C-proline by ventral prostate in two week castrates and castrates treated with androgen for 1 day (the first increase in synthesis of ^{14}C-hydroxyproline), indicated that the concentration of free ^{14}C-proline did not differ between the castrate and androgen treated group (not shown). Therefore, the androgenic effect on the increased rate of ^{14}C-hydroxyproline formation was not likely due to an increased accumulation of the free ^{14}C-proline substrate. Changes in proline-hydroxyproline ratios were not directly measured in these experiments and could have been at least partially involved in the androgen-induced increased in ^{14}C-hydroxyproline formation. However, in view of the magnitude of the change involved, as much as a 400% increase in ^{14}C-hydroxyproline formation, it was not possible that an increased proline hydroxylation per collagen chain could account for this increase. For example, given the same number of collagen molecules in the control and treated groups, hydroxylation of all ^{14}C-proline residues in the collagen from the androgen treated group would have accounted for only a 100% increase in ^{14}C-hydroxyproline. With respect to alterations in the synthesis of individual collagen types, this effect could only have contributed to an approximate 15% increase in synthesized ^{14}C-hydroxy-proline. This calculation was based on the fact that differences in hydroxyproline residues in type IV vs. I collagen was 116 vs. 103 (Miller and Bay, 1982) and assumed a complete shift in collagen production from I to IV without any change in the number of chains. Thus, it appears that the measurements of C^{14}-hydroxyproline formation primarily reflected synthesis of new collagen chains.

Focusing on androgen action on new collagen synthesis vs. endogenous hydroxyproline levels, it was apparent that collagen synthesis rates (per mg prostate weight) were similar in the normal and 2 week castrate, yet endogenous hydroxyproline concentrations were increased above normal in the castrate. Expressing the same parameters on a total organ basis also indicated that castration caused a much greater decline in collagen synthesis than endogenous collagen. These comparisons indicate that the castration-induced regression of the endogenous collagen content involved not only a decline in collagen synthesis but a decrease in collagenolytic activity as well. Similarly, analyzing the effects of androgen replacement on collagen synthesis and endogenous collagen indicated that the collagenous activity in castrate rat VP was restored by androgen treatment. This conclusion was based on the observations that androgen-induced increases in total prostate collagen synthesis were of much greater magnitude than changes in total endogenous collagen and that as the concentration of synthesized collagen increased with androgen treatment, the endogenous collagen concentration decreased. A recent report by Kneifel _et al._ (1982) examining the effect of estrogen action on uterine plasminogen activator can be considered consistent with these conclusions. Estrogen treatment of immature rat uterus increased plasminogen activator, which may be ultimately important in activating collagenase and enhancing collagen turnover. Further studies directly quantifying androgen-induced changes in collagenase activity may provide greater insight into factors regulating collagen accumulation during cell proliferation and differentiation in the prostate. At the present time, it appears that androgen-induced accumulation of collagen in the ventral prostate involved both the increased synthesis and degradation of collagen chains; hydroxyproline accumulated in response to androgen because the increases in synthesis were of a greater magnitude than that in degradation.

Should a cause and effect relationship exist between androgen-induced changes in collagenous matrices and epithelial cell proliferation, increased endogenous collagen accumulation should occur prior to or at the same time as the onset of DNA synthesis and/or accumulation of endogenous DNA. However, the first significant increase in endogenous total collagen did not take place until 4 days after the first increase in DNA. Androgen-induced changes in collagen synthesis did occur on day 1 of hormone treatment without a detectable change in total hydroxyproline levels. Possibly there was an increased net accumulation of basement membrane collagens during the wave of new DNA synthesis and cell proliferation which represented a very small percentage of the total collagen pool and was not detectable with the methodologies employed.

Use of CHP provided support for the idea that androgen-induced changes in collagen synthesis and possible accumulation during the first 7 days of hormone replacement represented essential components in the normal proliferation and differentiation of rat prostate epithelial cells. Although (Uke et al, 1983) reported that CHP inhibited prostatic in a dose of 0.1 mg/kg cell proliferation, our initial experiments with CHP indicated that it was ineffective in perturbing androgen-induced cell proliferation in the adult castrate. Considering that the basal lamina or other collagenous components of the extracellular matrix might not be sufficiently altered to perturb epithelial growth and that granuloma collagen incorporated very little CHP unless animals were fed a proline-free diet (Dr. Sergio Jimenez; personal communications), endogenous proline pools were depleted by feeding rats a proline-free diet in order to enhance CHP incorporation into collagen molecules and its effects on collagen accumulation. Indeed, use of the proline-free diet proved the essential component in causing an inhibitory action of CHP on epithelial cell proliferation.

Conclusion

This study was designed to determine if a cause and effect relationship exists between androgen-induced changes in collagen and epithelial cell proliferation and/or differentiation in rat ventral prostate. Analyses of the temporal relationship between dihydrotestosterone (DHT)-induced changes in the synthesis and levels of collagen in the regressed ventral prostates of adult castrates demonstrated that the collagen synthesis first increased as early as 24 hours after initiating DHT treatment, while total prostate collagen levels did not increase significantly until day 7 of DHT treatment. Such findings indicated that during the first 7 days of androgen-induced restoration of prostatic growth there was both enhanced synthesis and degradation of collagen. Since CHP treatment (200 mg/kg) during the first 7 days of androgen-stimulated prostate growth combined with maintenance of animals in a proline free diet, produced a 50% reduction in ventral prostate weight and DNA content, it is concluded that the collagenous components of the male accessory sex organs may be important in supporting the normal androgen dependent proliferation of epithelial cells.

References

Berg RA (1982). Determination of 3- and 4-hydroxyproline. In Cunningham LW, Frederickson, DW (eds.),: "Methods in Enzymology" New York; Academic Press, Vol. 82, p. 372.

Coffey DS, Shimizaki J, Williams-Ashman HG (1968). Polymeryation of deoxyribonucleotides in relation to androgen-induced prostatic growth. Arch. Biochem. Biophys. 124: 184.

DeKlerk DP, Coffey DS (1978). Quantitative determination of prostatic epithelial and stromal hyperplasia by a new technique: biomorphometrics. Invest. Urol. 16: 240.

Deming CL, Wolf JS (1939). The anatomical origin of benign prostatic enlargement. J. Urol. 42: 566.

Hutchinson WC, Munro HN (1961). The determination of nucleic acids in biological materials. Analyst 86: 1961.

Juva K, Prockop DJ (1966). Modified procedure for the assay of ^{3}H or ^{14}C labelled hydroxyproline. Anal. Biochem. 15: 77.

Keiser HR, Harris ED, Sjoerdsma A (1967). Studies on beta-aminoproprionitrile in animals. Clin. Pharm. and Ther. 8: 587.

Kivirikko KI, Laitinen O, Prockop DJ (1967). Modifications of a specific assay for hydroxyproline in urine. Anal. Biochem. 19: 249.

Kneifel MA, Leytus SP, Fletcher E, Weber T, Mangel WF, Katzenbellenbogen BS (1982). Uterine plasminogen activator activity: Modulation by steroid hormones. Endocrinology 111: 493.

Lewko W, Liotta L, Wicha MS, Vonderhaar BK, Kidwell WR (1981). Sensitivity of n-nitro-somethylurea-induced rat mammary tumors to cis-hydroxyproline, an inhibitor of collagen production. Cancer Res. 41: 2855.

LeDuc IE (1939). The anatomy of the prostate and the pathology of early benign hypertrophy. J. Urol. 42: 1217.

Mariotti A, Thornton MO, Mawhinney MG (1981). Actions of androgen and estrogen on collagen levels in male accessory sex organs. Endocrinology 109: 837.

McNeal J (1978). Origin and evalution of benign prostatic enlargement. Invest. Urol. 15: 340.

Miller EJ, Gay S (1982). Collagen: An Overview. In Cunningham LW, Fredericksen DW (eds.): "Methods in Enzymology", New York: Academic Press, Vol. 82, p.3.

Neubauer BL (1983). Endocrine and cellular inductive factors in the development of human benign prostatic hypertrophy. In Hinman F Jr (ed): "Benign Prostatic Hypertrophy", New York: Springer-Verlaz, Chapter 17, p. 179.

Pradhan BK, Chandra K (1975). Morphogenesis of nodular hyperplasia of the prostate. J. Urol. 113: 210.

Schneider WC (1957). Determination of nucleic acids in tissues by pentose analysis. In Coldwich, S.P. and Kaplan, N.O. (eds.): "Methods in Enzymology", New York: Academic Press, Vol. 3, p. 384.

Uitto J, Prockop DJ (1974). Incorporation of proline analogues into collagen polypeptides. Biochim. Biophys. Acta. 336: 234.

Uke E, Lee C, Grayhack J (1983). Effect of cis-hydroxyproline on ventral prostatic growth in rats. J. Urol. 129: 171.

Vembu D, Liotta L, Paranjpe M, Boone CW (1979). Correlation of tumorigenicity with resistance to growth inhibition by cis-hydroxyproline. Expl. Cell. Res. 124: 247.

Wicha MS, Liotta LA, Vonderhaar BK, Kidwell WR (1980). Effects of inhibition of basement membrane collagen disposition on rat mammary gland development. Dev. Biol. 80: 253.

Wicha MS, Liotta LA, Garbisa S, Kidwell WR (1979). Basement membrane collagen requirements for attachment and growth of mammary epithelium. Expl. Cell. Res. 124: 1981.

Wicha MS, Liotta LA, Lewko WM, Kidwell WR (1981A). Blocking basement membrane collagen deposition inhibits the growth of 7,12-dimethylbenzanthracene induced rat mammary tumors. Cancer Letters 12: 9.

Discussion

J. Isaacs: Mike, when you make a rat vitamin A deficient, you induce squamous metaplasia in the prostate. In the mouse, estrogen treatment also induces squamous metaplasia. However, the rat prostate doesn't develop squamous metaplasia following estrogen treatment. Would you comment on this difference?

Mawhinney: It depends on the specific tissue. For example, the rat seminal vesicle and anterior prostate exhibit squamous epithelial metaplasia, while the ventral prostate does not.

J. Isaacs: When you reduce dietary proline and also give cis-hydroxyproline, are you absolutely sure that what you observed wasn't a type of squamous metaplasia due to some dietary complication in the animals? From what you showed of the morphologic disorganization, it looked a little bit like the early beginnings of squamous metaplasia.

Mawhinney: The cells do not appear to be squamous to me.

J. Isaacs: What does cis-hydroxyproline do to the liver? Some of the diets that make an animal deficient in proline affect multiple organs.

Mawhinney: I don't know. I know under these conditions cis-hydroxyproline doesn't affect the heart, kidneys or body weight. I don't know about the liver. I believe that it requires a depletion of dietary proline to get the effect. Whether this effect will progress to frank squamous metaplasia, I don't know. The cells at the light level don't look squamous.

I think retinoids may be important in prostatic growth. One experiment we want to try is to see if retinoic acid can prevent this effect of cis-hydroxyproline.

Wicha: I wonder if you could answer that type of question using very short term organ culture? Then you could directly examine the effects of cis-hydroxyproline on cell growth. Have you tried this approach?

Mawhinney: No.

Cunha: Mike, if an organ culture system could be established to study this fascinating problem, there's a study in the literature on the development of the tooth that I think is very appropriate to what you're doing. It's a study by Galbraith and Kollar in which they found that a variety of substances that affected collagen synthesis, azetidine, 2-carboxylic acid, alpha-alpha dipyridyl, would disrupt tooth development reversibly. One criticism of that work as it was originally published, was that you could wonder what azetidine is doing other than disrupting collagen synthesis. Perhaps the same thing could be said for cis-hydroxyproline in your experiment as well. But what Galbraith and Kollar showed was that if they kept the drug present continuously, exogenous procollagen completely overode the effect of the drug. This might be a neat way to go if the organ culture could be adapted to your system.

Mawhinney: The specificity of cis-hydroxyproline is a serious question. Dr. Wicha's group and others have indicated that it acts primarily on collagen synthesis, but there are some alternative interpretations to that data. Collagenases will degrade cis-hydroxyproline containing collagens. But if there are cis-hydroxyproline containing proteins and there's no endogenous mechanisms to immediately degrade them, it may not look as if the non-collagenous proteins are altered, although they may be nonfunctional. If I can quote data from Wicha's work, I think some of the best evidence that cis-hydroxyproline acts on collagen to inhibit proliferation is that those cells which require production of collagen for proliferation are susceptible to inhibition by cis-hydroxyproline. Tumor cells that don't require an interaction with collagen to proliferate are resistant. So, if the drug was nonspecific in its action, it should theoretically inhibit all cells.

New Approaches to the Study
of Benign Prostatic Hyperplasia, pages 159–179

THE IMPORTANCE OF STROMAL TISSUE IN BENIGN PROSTATIC HYPERPLASIA: MORPHOLOGICAL, IMMUNOFLUORESCENCE AND ENDOCRINOLOGICAL INVESTIGATIONS

G. Bartsch[*], A. Brüngger[+], U. Schweikert[o], H. Hintner[**], U. Stanzl[***], Ch. Marth[***], G. Daxenbichler and H.P. Rohr[+]

Department of Urology[*], Dermatology[**] and Gynecology[***], University of Innsbruck, Austria; Department of Internal Medicine[o], Bonn, FRG; Department of Pathology[+], University of Basel, Switzerland

MORPHOLOGICAL APPROACH:

The histology of the normal human prostate and the histo-pathology of benign prostatic hyperplasia have been well documented (Franks, 1954; Franks, 1975; Mao et al, 1965; Moore, 1943; Brandes et al, 1964; Brandes, 1974; Narbaitz, 1974; McNeal, 1975). The possible role of stromal tissue in the pathogenesis of benign prostatic hyperplasia was for the first time suggested in 1925 (Reischauer, 1925); the initial lesions of benign prostatic hyperplasia were apparently fibromyomatous nodules into which penetration of glandular elements occured. In order to be able to establish a structure-function relationship, these morphological methods were complimented by quantitative techniques which yield objective and reproducible values for any morphological structure thus allowing statistical comparisons. This can be achieved by stereological methods.

Supported by the Fonds zur Förderung der wissenschaftlichen Forschung (P 4020) Austria and the Swiss National Foundation No. 3190-0.82.

Stereology, a term coined by the International Society in 1961, is based on geometric probability and makes it possible to quantitate three-dimensional structures by extrapolation from measurements of two-dimensional cross-sections thereof. Further methodological details (calculations, multistage sampling were described by Weibel and Rohr (Weibel, 1969; Rohr et al, 1976).

LIGHT MICROSCOPIC FINDINGS:

To evaluate the prostatic gland and its components in stereological terms a morphometric model of the human prostate was developed (Rohr et al, 1976; Bartsch et al, 1975; Bartsch and Rohr, 1977). Figure 1 shows how the human prostate was divided into morphologically defined compartments. Essentially the model has two major divisions - the stromal part (ST) including connective tissue, blood vessels, nerves and smooth muscle fibres and the glandular part (EP) including the lumina of the acini and the glandular epithelial cells.

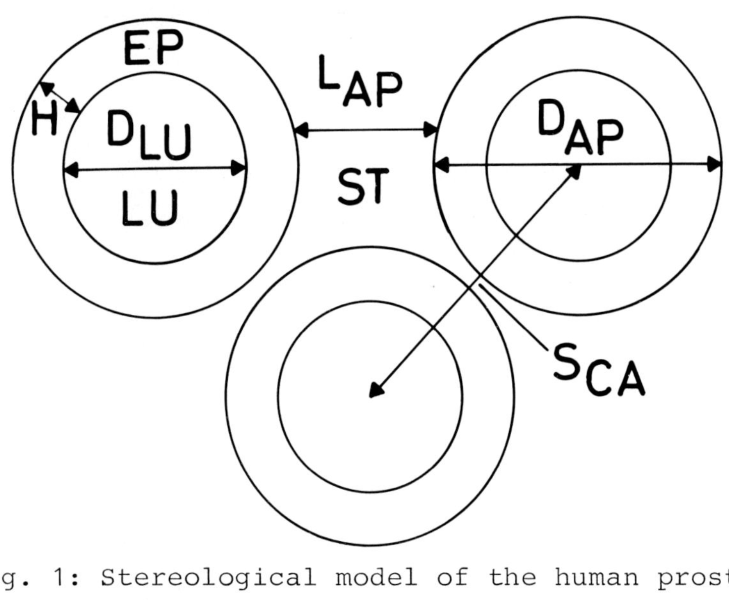

Fig. 1: Stereological model of the human prostate.

Whereas the stromal part of the normal human prostate accounts for 45 % of the tissue, the glandular cells represent 21 % (tab. 1). Compared to the normal human prostate in benign prostatic hyperplasia a statistically significant increase in the stromal tissue can be observed.

		V_{VST}	V_{VEP}	V_{VLU}
Normal human prostate	m	0.45	0.21	0.34
(N = g)	SE	0.02	0.01	0.02
Benign prostatic hyperplasia	m	0.60	0.12	0.28
(N = 7)	SE	0.04	0.01	0.05
Analysis of significance		s	s	ns

m = Mean, SE = Standard error, Differences are only significant (s) if the error of probability 2P was < 0.05.

Table 1: Volume densities of the stromal tissue (VVST), the glandular cells (VVEP) and the acinar lumina (VVLU) in the normal human prostate and in benign prostatic hyperplasia.

The following absolute stereologic parameters were determined:
Surface density of the glandular epithelium (S)
Volume density of the stromal part (V_{ST})
Volume density of the epithelial part (V_{EP})
Volume density of the glandular lumen (V_{LU})
Length density of the glandular tubules (L)
Height of the glandular epithelium (H)
Diameter of the glandular lumen (D_{LU})
Diameter of the glandular tubules (D_{AP})
Mean free distance between the glandular tubules (L_{AP})

Mean distance between the centers of the glandular tubules (S_{CA}).

As can be seen from the absolute data (tab.2) in benign prostatic hyperplasia in comparison to normal prostatic tissue there is a statistically significant increase in the volumetric amount of stromal tissue and the glandular lumina; contrary, regarding the volumetric amount of glandular epithelium no difference between normal and hyperplastic tissue can be found; there is also no difference regarding the surface density and the height of epithelial cells; as a consequence of the highly significant increase in stroml tissue

a significant increase in the mean free distance between the glandular tubules (= L_{AP}) and the mean distance between the centers of the glandular tubules (= S_{CA}) was found in hyperplastic tissue.

	case	age	weight (gm)	S $x10^5 mm^2$	V_{LU} $x10^3 mm^3$	V_{EP} $x10^3 mm^3$	V_{ST} $x10^3 mm^3$	L $x10^5 mm$	H μ	D_{LU} μ	D_{AP} μ	L_{AP} μ	S_{CA} μ
HYPERPLASTIC	1	80	87	7.63	43.2	12.9	31.4	18.3	17	226	260	199	459
	2	72	42	2.58	8.7	4.9	28.4	8.1	19	134	173	479	652
	3	63	36	2.98	8.9	4.9	22.3	7.4	16	120	153	332	485
	4	52	79	5.96	14.5	11.7	52.6	15.0	20	97	137	392	529
	5	73	62	3.32	7.0	7.9	46.9	13.9	24	84	132	613	745
	6	76	204	17.90	78.6	29.1	97.0	50.0	16	176	208	249	457
	7	72	42	34.60	13.5	6.4	22.6	11.4	19	156	193	298	492
	8	79	56	3.92	16.7	6.4	33.8	13.2	16	170	203	378	581
	9	71	50	3.49	13.9	7.5	28.6	12.1	22	159	202	371	574
	10	62	84	1.94	10.9	3.4	16.1	5.6	18	225	261	368	629
	m±SD	71±9	74±49	8.4±10.3	21.5±22.5	9.5±7.4	37.9±23.5	15.5±12.7	18.7±2.7	154.7±47.9	192.2±45.1	367.9±116.4	560.3±94.3
NORMAL	1	24	19	2.30	5.32	4.23	6.7	7.9	18	93	129	152	382
	2	26	24	3.17	6.78	7.38	10.2	5.1	23	85	132	176	308
	3	21	22	2.49	5.57	4.55	9.6	5.5	18	89	126	190	316
	m±SD	23±2	21.6±2.5	2.6±0.4	5.8±0.7	5.3±1.7	8.8±1.8	6.1±1.5	19.6±2.8	89.0±4.0	129.0±3.0	172.6±19.2	335.3±40.6

Table 2: Absolute data of normal and hyperplastic prostatic tissue.

ULTRASTRUCTURAL FINDINGS:

The smooth muscle cells in the normal human prostate are spindle-shaped. Most of the organelles are located near the nucleus or in small clusters in the cell periphery. Most of the cytoplasm is occupied by myofilaments. The rough endoplasmic reticulum consists of a few profiles of membranes, a great part of which is often devoid of ribosomes; sometimes a small Golgi apparatus and few mitochondria can be observed. Contrary to these findings, in benign prostatic hyperplasia the perinuclear zone is markedly increased. The abundant rough endoplasmic reticulum shows enlarged cisternae studded with ribosomes. The Golgi apparatus is also enlarged and contains more vesical than cisternal elements (Bartsch et al, 1979; Rohr and Bartsch, 1980).

Data for the various smooth muscle cell compartments are given in tab. 3. In benign prostatic hyperplasia there is a statistically significant increase in the volume fractions of rough endoplasmic reticulum, mitochondria and Golgi apparatus.

	Golgi apparatus*	Organelles*	Myofilaments*
Normal human prostate, 5 pts.			
Mean	0.002	0.048	0.950
Standard error	0.001	0.005	0.026
Benign prostatic hyperplasia, 5 pts.			
Mean	0.013	0.134	0.853
Standard error	0.001	0.006	0.032

* Analysis of variance-significant.

Table 3: Volume densities of smooth muscle cells in the normal human prostate and benign prostatic hyperplasia.

These light and electron microscopic measurements show that tissue overgrowth in human benign prostatic hyperplasia is mostly due to an increase in stromal tissue; as shown by the electron microscopic measurements, in the benign prostatic hyperplasia-changed prostatic tissue activated smooth muscle cells are observed, which possibly play a key role in the pathogenesis of human benign prostatic hyperplasia.

CORRELATION OF STEREOLOGICAL AND BIOCHEMICAL RESULTS:

Since the initial studies of Siiteri and Wilson in 1970 it has become apparent that alterations in androgen metabolism are responsible for the spontaneous development of human benign prostatic hyperplasia. At present there are strong indications that it is above all androgens which control the function of the stromal part of the human prostate; therefore, an attempt was made to correlate the quantitative morphologic and biochemical values of normal and hyperplastic prostatic tissue to find out, if this altered steroid metabolism in benign prostatic hyperplasia is reflected in the morphologic architecture.

Using the Spearman rank correlation coefficient a statistical analysis was performed for age, weight and the prostate, absolute stereological and the following biochemical data: endogenous prostatic hormones (5α-dihydrotestosterone, testosterone, progesterone, estradiol, estrone and estriol), receptors (androgens, estrogens and progesterone). Benign prostatic hyperplastic tissue specimens were obtained by open prostatectomy; normal prostatic tissue was obtained from kidney donors.

As can be seen from the statistical analysis (tab. 4) the endogenous 5α-dihydrotestosterone concentration and the age of the patient as well as the weight of the prostate show statistically significant correlation coefficients; a statistically significant correlation could also be found for the following stereologic parameters: volumetric amounts of stromal and glandular tissue, surface density of glandular epithelium, length density of glandular tubules and diameter of glandular tubules; estriol, estradiol, estrone and endogenous progesterone steroid levels, however, did not correlate significantly with the morphometric data investigated; regarding the receptor levels a statistically significant correlation was found between the nuclear androgen receptor and the volumetric amount of stromal tissue and as a consequence of stromal overgrowth to the mean free distance between the glandular tubules (L_{AP}); regarding the cytoplasmic progesterone receptor the diameters of the glandular lumina (D_{LU}) and the diameters of the glandular tubules (D_{AP}) were found to correlate significantly.

	AGE	WEIGHT	V_{LU}	V_{EP}	V_{ST}	S	L	H	D_{LU}	D_{AP}	L_{AP}	S_{CA}
Testosterone										o		o
5α-dihydrotestosterone	o	●	o	o	o	o	●			o		o
Estradiol												
Estrone												
Estriol												
Progesterone												
Androgen Receptor (N)					o						o	
Androgen Receptor (C)												
Estrogen Receptor (N)												
Estrogen Receptor (C)												
Progesterone Receptor (C)			o						o	o		

● $p < 0.01$ N: Nucleus

o $p < 0.05$ C: Cytoplasm

All other values do not show a statistically significant correlation

Table 4: Correlation of age, weight of the prostate, biochemical and absolute stereological data.

These data show that stromal overgrowth in benign prostatic hyperplasia correlates with high 5α-dihydrotestosterone and nuclear androgen receptor levels; therefore, quantitative biochemical differences of androgen metabolism are reflected in the morphological architecture of human benign prostatic hyperplasia.

HORMONE SENSITIVITY OF STROMAL TISSUE:

There is some evidence that interactions between stromal and epithelial cells play a crucial role in the regulation of the coordinated growth of the prostatic gland. Since the separation of prostatic acinar parenchyma and stroma is difficult or even impossible and in common biochemical practice prostatic tissue is homogenized prior to biochemical assays, most biochemists overlooked the cellular elements of the stromal tissue. Therefore the stromal function regarding hormonal response is virtually not understood. Despite the fact that receptor proteins have been found for estrogens, testosterone and 5 -dihydrotestosterone the action site of these steroids in the different glandular and stromal cell components has not been demonstrated. Thus the role of glandular and stromal elements of the prostate in steroid metabolism is still unclear.

It was shown that the endogenous concentration of 17ß-estradiol in the stromal part of the prostate of guinea pigs exceeded those of blood plasma and prostatic epithelium; this fact supports the assumption that endogenous estrogen may play a role in the regulation of male accessory sex tissue and smooth muscle cell function (Blume and Mawhinney, 1978); an activation of the smooth muscle cells of the uterus of prepubertal rats was demonstrated after injection of 17ß-estradiol (Ross and Klebanoff, 1967). In young female virgin mice estrogen injections for 3 days led to an increase in the cell organelles of the smooth muscle cells of the uterus (Rohr and Jurukova, 1978). These autoradiographic findings show that under definite experimental conditions the smooth muscle cells can participate in the synthesis of ground substance of connective tissue. In strong A/J strain mice enlargement of the prostate and the periurethral gland can be produced by estrogens (Fingerhut and Veenema, 1966). Similar results of smooth muscle cell activation were obtained in beagle dogs following estrogen administration, which indicates that possibly estrogens play a role in the induction of stromal growth by smooth muscle cell activation (Rohr et al, 1981). In relation to the unit volume of smooth muscle cell cytoplasm, in castrated dogs treated with estrogens (2.5 mg of estradiol-benzoate twice a week over a period of 3 weeks) a statistically significant increase in the volume of rough endoplasmic reticulum, vacuolesand vesicles can be seen compared to the control group (Rohr et al, 1981). These stereological results are very similar to those obtained for smooth muscle cells in human benign prostatic hyperplasia. These data possibly reemphasize the fact that estrogens play a role in the development of human benign prostatic hyperplasia.

A precise understanding of the estrogenic action at the cellular level of human benign prostatic hyperplasia and in particular on the stroma is still lacking. An important supposition for discussing specific estrogenic action is the demonstration of estrogens in human benign prostatic hyperplastic tissue. When comparing stroma to the epithelium in human benign prostatic hyperplasia Krieg et al. found an accumulation of estrogens in the nuclei of stromal cells (Krieg et al, 1983). Krieg et al. furthermore showed in the stromal cells more estrogen receptor positive cases than in the epithelial cells (Krieg et al, 1983). These data possibly support the hypothesis that 17-ß-estradiol plays a special role in stimulating the growth of the stromal part of the human prostate.

At present there are strong indications that it is above all androgens which control the function of the stromal part of the human prostate. In 1977 Cowan and coworkers for the first time reported that 5α-reductase activity, which regulates 5α-dihydrotestosterone formation, was found predominantly in the stromal tissue of the prostate (Cowan et al, 1977). Using a mechanical technique for separating the glandular and stromal parts Krieg (Krieg et al, 1981), Romijn (Romijn et al, 1980) and Bruchovsky (Bruchovsky et al, 1980) found that 5α-reductase activity in the stromal fraction of the prostate was considerably higher than in the glandular fraction; by comparing the stromal fractions of the normal human prostate and benign prostatic hyperplasia it was shown that the mean specific activity of 5α-reductase in benign prostatic hyperplasia is three times greater (Bruchovsky et al, 1980).

The 5α-reductase and 3α(ß)hydroxysteroid oxidoreductase activity of the stromal and glandular parts in the normal human prostate and in benign prostatic hyperplasia were analyzed without the use of these separation techniques which possibly destroy the cell architecture and the stromal/glandular interrelationships. In a correlative biochemical and light microscopic stereological study testosterone metabolite formation was measured in small biopsy specimens; afterwards a stereological analysis was performed to determine the amounts of glandular and stromal tissue (Schweikert et al, 1983).

As can be seen from the correlation coefficient there is no difference between 5α-dihydrotestosterone and 5α-androstane 3α(ß)17ß-diol formation when the testosterone metabolism of the stromal part is compared to that of the glandular part (fig. 2 and 3). These data on intact tissue show that 5α-reductase and 3α(ß)-hydroxysteroid oxidoreductase activity is found in benign prostatic hyperplasia in the stromal part as well as in the glandular part.

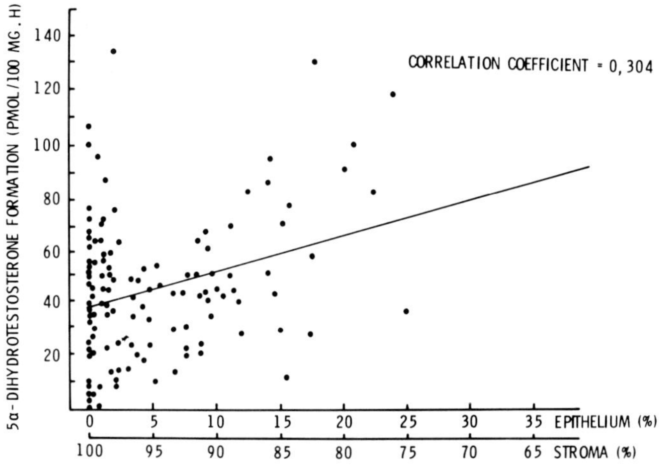

Fig.2 : Correlative biochemical and morphometric study on human biopsy specimens, 5α reductase activity is correlated to the amount for stromal and glandular tissue of the biopsy specimen (= 100 %), hyperplastic prostatic tissue.

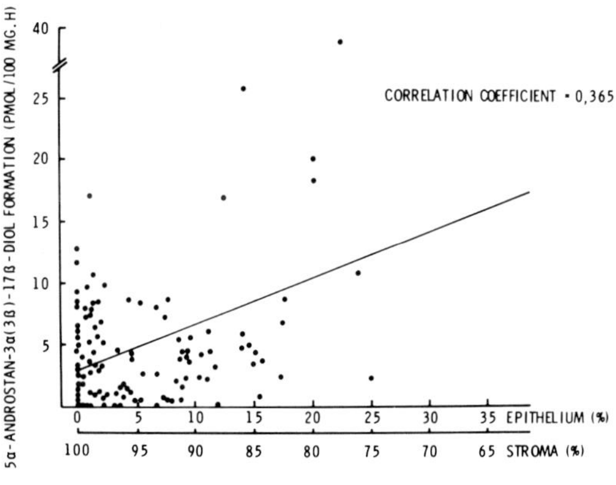

Fig.3: Correlative biochemical and morphometric study on human biopsy specimens, 3α (β) hydroxysteroid-oxidoreductase activity is correlated to the amount of stromal and glandular tissue of the biopsy specimen (=100 %), hyperplastic prostatic tissue.

The discrepancy of these values may be due to the methods employed. It is understandable that mechanical separation disturbs the integrity of the cells, in particular of the more vulnerable epithelial cells, which in turn may affect the cellular metabolism. The advantage of the method employed in this study over the methods in which the stromal and glandular parts are separated mechanically is that the tissue used for assessing the metabolic rates is left intact.

Summarizing the results of these biochemical and morphological investigations on the hormone responsiveness of prostatic stromal tissue one can say that stromal tissue is possibly sensitive to both estrogens and androgens: regarding androgen metabolism these investigations also show that stroma is not only a target tissue but also an active metabolizing component in the prostate.

EXTRACELLULAR MATRIX

There is strong evidence that the extracellular matrix acts as an interface between epithelial and stromal cell elements, such as smooth muscle cells and fibroblasts; although the exact nature and composition of the extracellular matrix in the prostate, is not known at present, in most tissues it is composed of collagen, glycosaminoglycans and glycoproteins. Glycosaminoglycans were shown to play an important role in the development and growth of normal and neoplastic tissue. As compared to the normal human prostate, increased levels of chondroitin sulphate were shown in benign prostatic hyperplasia (DeKlerk, 1982). It was shown that this interface plays an important role in glandular-stromal interactions as well as in the development of the normal prostate and in benign prostatic hyperplasia. The biochemical mechanism of these interactions remains obscure; however, the understanding of the mechanism of the interface and the influence of ageing and hormonal alterations on this factor will be of great help in the understanding of the pathogenesis of benign prostatic hyperplasia.

Numerous studies performed over the past decade support the concept that smooth muscle cells are multifunctional cells capable of synthesizing collagen, elastin, myosin and glycosaminglycans. It was demonstrated in cultures that in vitro these smooth muscle cells can synthesize type I and III collagens (Lajman et al, 1977). On the other hand smooth muscle cells were shown to be involved also in the process of collagen phagocytosis and degradation (Jurukova and Milenkov, 1981).

Previous studies have shown that type I and III collagens comprise the major fibrillar protein components found in the connective tissue of skin, blood vessels and stromal tissue of visceral organs. Other types of collagen are restricted to hyaline cartilage (type II) and basement membrane (type IV). The purpose of the present study was to investigate the presence and distribution of various types of collagen (type I, III and V) and laminin, a non-collagenous basement membrane glycoprotein found in the normal human prostate and in benign prostatic hyperplasia.

Cryostat sections of normal human (n=3) or benign hyperplastic prostates (n=5) were first incubated, for thirty minutes with rabbit anti-type I, III and IV collagen serum (concentration: 1:80) or with rabbit anti-laminin serum (concentration: 1:40). All sera were kindly provided by Dr. S.J. Katz, National Institutes of Health, Bethesda, Maryland. After extensive washes in phosphate-buffered saline (PBS), the specimens were exposed in a second incubation period of thirty minutes to a fluorescin isothiocyanate-(FITC) labelled swine anti-rabbit serum of a dilution of 1:20.

In a control group these specific antisera were substituted by PBS or by a non-immune rabbit serum during the first incubation period. A cryostat section of a normal human prostate, which was incubated with PBS and afterwards with FITC-labelled swine anti-rabbit serum served as a negative control; beside the very faint background there was no specific staining, neither in the epithelium nor in the stromal part of the specimen.

Specific immunofluorescence staining of sections of normal human and hyperplastic prostates with rabbit antibodies against type I collagen was observed only within the stromal tissue, whereas the glandular cells remaind completely unstained. Note that antibodies against type I collagen in the normal human prostate (fig. 4) stain strongly and appears as bundles around a group of smooth muscle cells, whereas among the individual smooth muscle cells only faint staining can be observed.

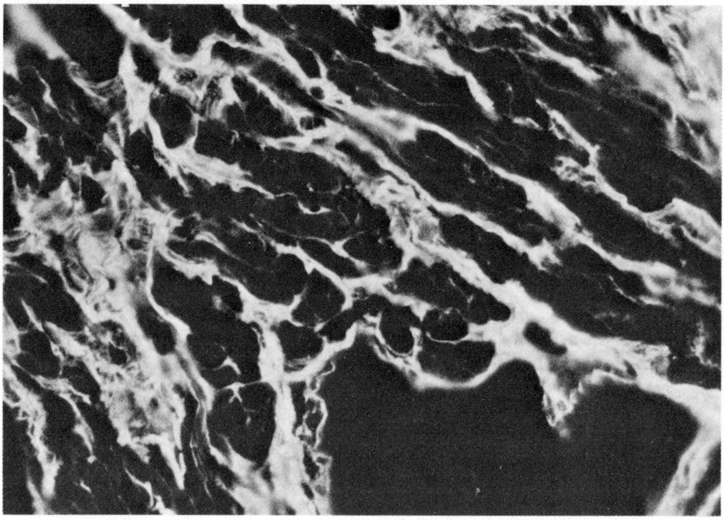

Fig. 4: Collagen type I: specific immunofluorescence staining of sections of normal human prostatic tissue.

In benign prostatic hyperplasia, due to the stromal overgrowth, this typical scaffold pattern is replaced by a strong, diffuse distribution of the antibody reactivity (fig. 5).

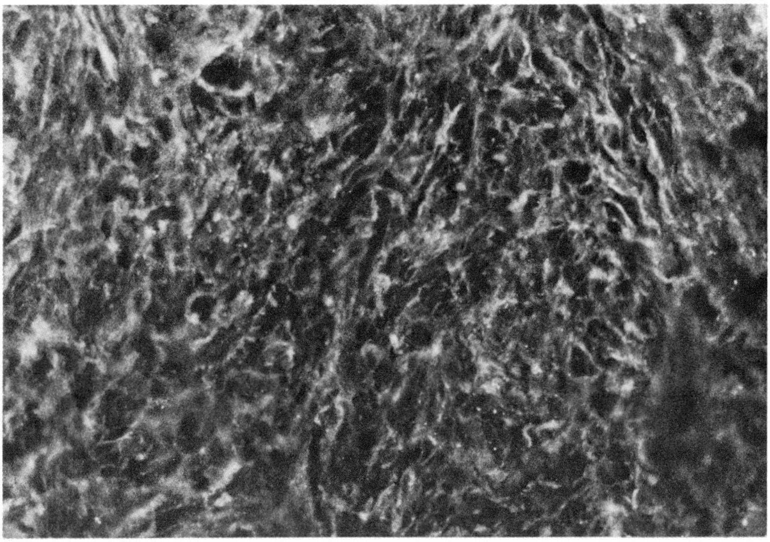

Fig. 5: Collagen type III: specific immunofluorescence staining of sections of hyperplastic prostatic tissue.

Very similar to type I collagen, the antibody reactivity of collagen type III was present only within the stromal tissue, whereas the glandular cells remained unstained. Individual or grouped smooth muscle cells are interwoven with delicate type III positive fibres originating from a scaffold of thick, coarse collagen bundles in normal prostatic tissue. In benign prostatic hyperplasia this subtle architecture is replaced by a dense array of irregularly interlaced wavy type III collagen fibers between the stromal cells (=fibroblasts, smooth muscle cells).

Contrary to type I and III collagen the fluorescence staining of type IV collagen in normal as well as in benign prostatic hyperplasia tissue was found to outline smooth muscle cells in a regular honey-comb pattern; due to the increase in stromal tissue in benign prostatic hyperplasia a more irregular pattern of type IV collagen immunofluorescence was observed in benign prostatic hyperplasia; nevertheless, the antibody reactivity was found to outline only the stromal cells in a regular honey-comb pattern; as regards the immunofluorescence staining with antilaminin serum the same picture as with type IV collagen antiserum was observed.

These studies suggest a considerable overproduction of type I and III collagens in benign prostatic hyperplasia, which demonstrates that these two collagens are principal factors in the stromal character of human benign prostatic hyperplasia; whether the overproduction of collagen observed is the cause of the result of the stromal function has to be elucidated in future studies.

Further studies will have to find out whether collagen synthesis is hormone-sensitive; we furthermore will have to study collagen degradation and find out whether type I or III collagen synthesis in hyperplastic tissue is reversible by hormonal manipulation.

References:

Bartsch G, Fischer E and Rohr HP (1975). Ultrastructural morphometric analysis of the rat prostate (ventral lobe). Urol.Res.3, 11, 1.

Bartsch G and Rohr HP (1977). Ultrastructural stereology: a new approach to the study of prostatic function. Invest.Urol. 14, 301-306.

Bartsch G, Frick J, Ruegg I, Bucher M, Holliger O, Oberholzer M and Rohr HP (1979). Electron microscopic stereological analysis of the normal human prostate and of benign prostatic hyperplasia. J. Urol. 122, 481-486.

Bartsch G, Müller HR, Oberholzer M and Rohr HP (1979). Light microscopic stereological analysis of the normal human prostate and of benign prostate hyperplasia. J. Urol. 122, 487-491.

Blume DCh and Mawhinney MG (1978). Estrophilic Molecules in the male guniea-pig. J.Steroid Biochem.9, 515-529.

Brandes D (1974). Fine structure and cytochemistry of male sex accessory organs. In: Male Accessory Sex Organs: Structure and Function in Mammals. Edited by D Brandes, New York: Academic Press, pp. 18-44.

Brandes D, Kirchheim D and Scott WW (1964). Ultrastructure of the human prostate: normal and neoplastic. Lab.Invest.13, 1541.

Bruchovsky N, Callaway T, Lieskovsky G and Rennie PS (1980). Markers of androgen action in human prostate: potential use in the clinical assessment of prostatic carcinoma. In Steroid Receptors and Hormone Dependent Neoplasia (Edited by JL Witliff and O Dapunt) Masson, USA, 121-132.

Cowan RA, Cowan SK, Grant JK and Elder HY (1977). Biochemical investigations of separated epithelium and stroma from benign prostatic hyperplastic tissue. J. Endocr. 74, 111-116.

Fingerhut B and Veenema RJ (1966). Histology and radioautography of induced benign enlargement of the mouse prostate. Invest.Urol. 4, 112-124.

Franks LM (1954). Benign nodular hyperplasia of the prostate: a review. Ann. Roy.Coll.Surg., Engl.14 92.

Franks LM (1975). Benign prostatic hyperplasia: gross and microscopic anatomy. In: Benign Prostatic Hyperplasia. National Institute of Arthritis, Metabolism and Digesive Disease Workshop Proceedings. Edited by JT Grayhack, JD Wilson and MJ Scherbenske, Bethesda: National Institutes of Health, pp.63-89.

Jurukova Z and Milenkov Ch (1981). Involvement of smooth muscle cells in Collagen Degradation in the postpartum uterus. Virchows Arch.37, 237-244.

DeKlerk DP (1982). Glycosaminoglycans of benign prostatic hyperplasia. American Urological Association, Kansas City.

Krieg M, Klötzl G, Kaufmann J and Voigt KD (1981). Stroma of human benign prostatic hyperplasia: perferential tissue for androgen metabolism and estrogen binding. Acta Endocr., Copenh.96, 422-432.

Krieg M, Bartsch W, Thomsen M and Voigt KD (1983) Androgens and Estrogens: Their interaction with stroma and epithelium of human benign prostatic hyperplasia and normal prostate. J.Steroid. Biochem., Vol. 19, 1, 155-161.

Layman DL, Epstein Jr. EH, Dodson RF and Titus JL (1977). Biosynthesis of type 1 and 3 collagens by cultured smooth muscle cells from human aorta. Proc.Natl.Acad.Sci., Vol. 74, 671-675.

Mao P, Nakao K, Bora R and Geller J (1965). Human benign prostatic hyperplasia. Arch.Path. 79, 270.

McNeal JE (1975). Development and comparative anatomy of the prostate. In: Benign Prostatic Hyperplasia. National Institute of Arthritis, Metabolism and Digestive Disease Workshop Proceedings. Edited by JT Grayhack, JD Wilson and MJ Scherbenske. Bethesda: National Institutes of Health, pp. 1-9.

Moore RA (1943). Benign hypertrophy of the prostate. A morphological study. J.Urol. 50, 680.

Narbaitz R (1974). Embryology, anatomy and histology of the male sex accessory glands. In: Male Accessory Sex Organs: Structure and Function in Mammals. Edited by D Brandes, New York: Academic Press, pp.3-15.

Reischauer F (1925). Die Entstehung der sogenannten Prostatahypertrophie. Virch.Archiv 256, 357-389.

Rohr HP, Obholzer M, Bartsch G and Keller M (1976) Morphometry in experimental pathology (Methods, baseline, data and applications) Int.Rev.exp. Pathol. 15, 233-325.

Rohr HP and Bartsch G (1980). Human benign prostatic hyperplasia: a stromal disease. New perspectives by quantitative morphology. Urology, 625-633.

Rohr HP and Jurukova Z (1978). Beiträge zur Bildung bindegewebiger Matrix in glatten Muskelzellen. Path.Eur. 3, 571-592.

Rohr HP, Naef HF, Holliger O, Oberholzer M, Ibach B, Weissbach L and Bartsch G (1981). The effect of estrogen and stromal growth of the dog prostate. Urol.Res. 9, 201-207.

Romijn JC, Oishi K, Belt de Vries J, Schweikert U, Mulder E and Schröder FH (1980). Androgen metabolism and androgen receptors in separated epithelium and stroma of the human prostate. On Steroid Receptors, Metabolism and Prostatic Cancer (Edited by FH Schröder and HJ de Voogt), Exerpta Medica, Amsterdam, pp 134-139.

Ross R and Klebanoff SJ (1967). Fine structural changes in uterine smooth muscle and fibroblasts in response to estrogen. J.Cell.Biol. 32, 155-159.

Schweikert HU, Bartsch G, Totzauer P and Rohr HP (1983). Testosterone metabolism in the epithelium and stroma of normal human prostate in benign prostatic hyperplasia. In press.

Siiteri PK and Wilson JD (1970). Dihydrotestosterone in Prostatic Hypertrophy. I. The formation and Content of Dihydrotestosterone in the Hypertrophie Prostate of Man. J.Clin.Invest. 49, 1737-1745.

Discussion

J. Isaacs: Georg, could you show that slide again where you determined the actual weight of the various components of the normal versus BPH prostate. The reason I bring it up is that in several places you state that there is no increase in the glandular components of the gland in BPH. If Dr. McNeal is right, the transition zone gives rise to BPH and this zone only represents 5% of the gland. Thus, if the total amount of glandular tissue in the entire BPH gland increased by only 4 gm (i.e. going from 5 to 9 grams) that would mean the epithelium of the transition zone would have to increase by more than 4-fold. Therefore, a substantial amount of glandular overgrowth does appear to occur in human BPH.

Bartsch: You see here the absolute data for lumen, epithelium, and stroma. If you look at the stroma you find a significant increase in BPH, but you don't find a significant increase of the epithelial cells, if you compare normal prostatic tissue to BPH. This normal prostatic tissue is from kidney donor patients where we made a morphometric analysis of the whole normal prostate.

McNeal: Dr. Bartsch, in reference to what Dr. Isaacs was saying, you're not measuring absolute volumes -- but proportionate zones?

Bartsch: No, these data don't mean grams proportions; these represent grams of stroma, or grams of epithelium as these are absolute data. These are not our old slides where we always gave the relative volumetric amount; these are absolute data. That means, for instance, that you have this amount of grams of stromal and this amount of epithelial cells in the normal human prostate; and this amount in BPH.

McNeal: All right, in that case, you do show an absolute increase in the amount of gland cell mass. The blue area is twice as large on the right as it is on the left.

Bartsch: These differences are not statistically significant. If you analyze the glandular portion, we have a big increase of the lumina, but the glandular cells themselves don't show an absolute increase.

McNeal: There is a discrepancy here, at which Dr. Isaac hinted. In the nodules that I see at autopsies, transurethral resections, and suprapubic prostatectomy, frequently I see nodules in which the packing of glands is much closer than it is in the normal prostate with a tremendous overgrowth of epithelium and only narrow bands of stroma between the nodules. In addition, in looking at autopsy material many glands show a tremendous variability in the histological appearance of BPH nodules. This includes nodules where there appears to be a greatly increased proportion of epithelial cells. Some nodules are in between and some show a greater proportionate increase in stromal cells. I don't know how to explain this discrepancy. In early nodules, it is almost universal that there is at first a tremendous proliferation of the glandular component with a relative proportionate decrease in stroma. I recognize that I haven't got stereologic analyses to support these assertions, but the differences are so striking, I think they ought to be apparent to the eye.

Bartsch: That is right, in the sense that we are comparing the whole normal prostatic tissue to benign prostatic hyperplasia, but, if you look to the single values of normal prostatic tissue, and you have to know that we have taken for one assay for one prostate about 140,000 points; there is no big difference. I think this sum of the so-called normal transitional zone would not have another tissue distribution.

This was the slide we had in 1979. When we saw these data, we did not want to publish it because the pathologist told us that this was not possible because they found a lot nodules which are more glandular than stroma. We have now measured 37 prostates, 3 times, by different people with the morphometric procedures and we have not found one BPH above 60 grams of tissue which has more glandular elements than stromal elements. There may be one nodule that is more glandular, and one nodule that is more stromal. If you look at the objective data of the whole disease, it is a stromal disease.

Walsh: You measured the content of dihydrotestosterone in three normal and eight BPH patients and found that dihydrotestosterone content was increased in BPH. My question is, what was the content in normal tissue, how old were the patients and how was the tissue obtained in those three cases?

Bartsch: The patients were 20-30 years old. They were kidney donor patients, and we obtained the tissue about 1-2 hours after the kidney was taken out.

Walsh: What was the level of dihydrotestosterone?

Bartsch: It was about .05 ng/gm.

Walsh: Is that after 1-2 hours of ischemia?

Bartsch: Yes. But I can tell you, we were recently allowed to take out a prostate within a half an hour after the kidney had been taken. The DHT level was 4.5 ng/gm, but this was the first patient like this we have had.

New Approaches to the Study
of Benign Prostatic Hyperplasia, pages 181–195

PROSTATE-DERIVED GROWTH FACTORS

Richard F. Parrish, Warren D.W. Heston, L. Susan Pletscher, Russell Tackett and William R. Fair

Department of Surgery/Division of Urology
Washington University School of Medicine
St. Louis, Mo. 63110

Polypeptide growth factors have been isolated and characterized from a wide variety of tissues (Bradshaw, Rubin 1980; Baserga 1981). Several years ago the observation was made that extracts of human prostatic tissue contained a material or materials capable of stimulating new cell growth in tissue culture (Jacobs, 1979). In this communication we present our own preliminary studies on growth factor activity in human prostatic tissue and expressed prostatic secretions.

Prostatic tissue samples were obtained at either open or transurethral surgery and stored frozen at -20^{0} C or immediately homogenized in two volumes of cold phosphate buffered saline utilizing a Polytron homogenizer. Samples stored frozen were allowed to slowly thaw and then homogenized in two volumes of cold phosphate buffered saline. The tissue homogenate was centrifuged for two hours at 48,000 x g at 4^{0} C. The clear supernatant that was not immediately used was stored frozen at -20^{0} C. Prostatic secretions were collected by rectal massage of the prostate into sterile plastic containers and stored at -20^{0} C. A diagnosis of benign prostatic hyperplasia (BPH) was made at the time of rectal examination of the prostate in patients with symptoms and physical findings compatible with BPH and the prostatic fluid obtained from that gland was so designated. Patients with no clinical symptoms of prostatic enlargement and no enlargement of the prostate, as judged by rectal examination, were designated as non-BPH patients and the prostatic fluid obtained from that gland was so designated.

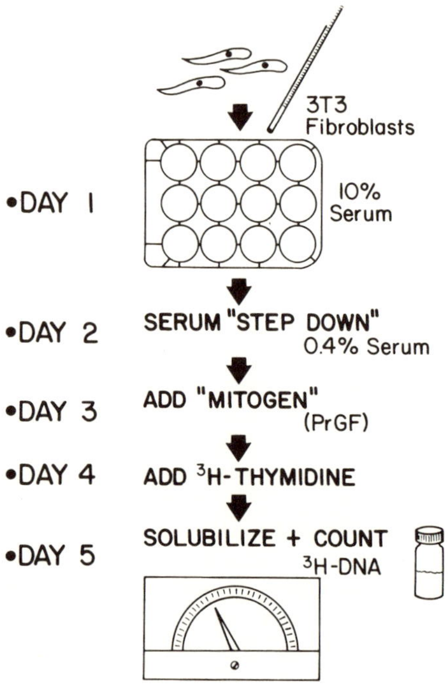

Figure 1. Schematic representation of the assay system employed to measure growth factor activity.

Growth factor activity was measured according to an established procedure (Thomas, 1980) which is schematically represented in Figure 1. Molecular weight estimates were obtained by gel filtration chromatography over a calibrated Sephadex G-200 column (Andrews, 1964). Molecular weight standards used for calibration were catalase (250,000), aldolase (150,000), bovine serum albumin (68,000), ovalbumin (45,000), chymotrypsinogen (25,000) and myoglobin (17,300). Protein profiles were monitored by absorbance at

280 nm (Layne, 1957).

When serial dilutions of human prostatic tissue extracts were examined for growth factor activity, a biphasic relationship between growth factor activity and increasing dilution was observed. A typical example of this is shown in Figure 2. Growth factor activity in the homogenate (indicated by the open circles) was highest at a 1:9 fold dilution and at a 1:243 fold dilution was still higher than at a 1:3 fold dilution. In contrast, when the

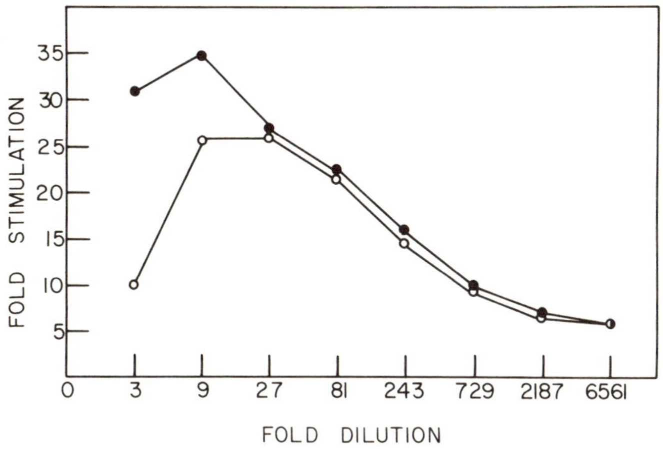

Figure 2. Serial dilution of a non-dialyzed prostatic homogenate (O) and a dialyzed prostatic homogenate (●). Fold stimulation was calculated by dividing the observed radioactivity present in those samples containing an aliquot of prostatic homogenate by the radioactivity present in samples that had received no prostatic homogenate (controls). Each point represents the mean of triplicate determinations.

same tissue homogenate was dialyzed against phosphate buffered saline prior to testing for growth factor activity, a significant increase in growth factor activity was observed in the 1:3 fold dilution of the dialyzed material, relative to the undialyzed material. At a 1:27

fold dilution the growth factor activity was substantially less than at the 1:3 fold dilution. These results indicate that human prostatic tissue homogenates contain a low molecular weight material, or materials, capable of modulation of the endogenous growth factor activity in the tissue. The nature of this inhibition and the mechanism of inhibition are not currently understood.

The molecular weight distribution of growth factor activity in human hyperplastic tissue was next examined. Tissue samples obtained at open prostatectomy (Figure 3)

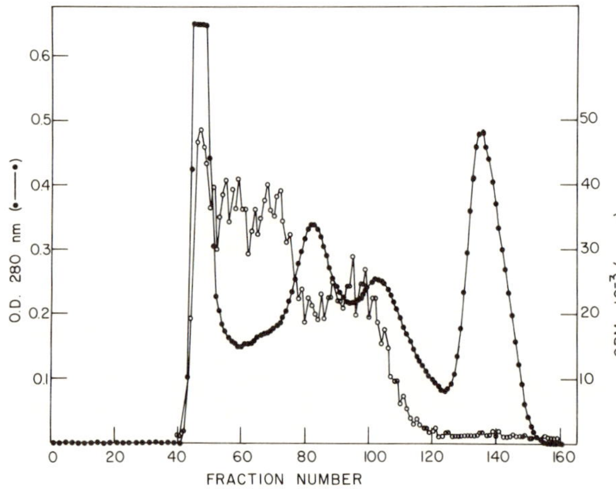

Figure 3. Protein profile (●) and tritiated thymidine incorporation (○) profile for a sample of prostatic tissue obtained at open prostatectomy, homogenized as previously described, and subjected to gel filtration chromatography over Sephadex G-200 equilibrated with phosphate buffered saline.

or transurethral resection (Figure 4) were homogenized, centrifuged and subjected to gel filtration chromatography over a Sephadex G-200 column. Several areas of growth factor activity were observed. A very high molecular weight material eluting in the void volume of the column and possibly three other areas of growth factor activity were observed. The estimated molecular weights of the non-void volume peaks were 300,000, 150,000 and 60,000. These must remain estimates of the molecular weight because of the overlapping nature of the three non-void volume

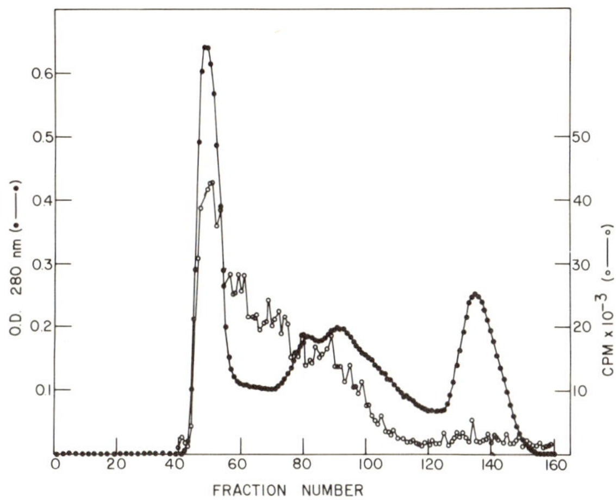

Figure 4. Protein profile (●) and tritiated thymidine incorporation (O) profile for a sample of prostatic tissue obtained during transurethral resection of the prostate. After homogenization as previously described, an aliquot was subjected to gel filtration chromatography over Sephadex G-200 equilibrated with phosphate buffered saline.

areas of growth factor activity. Both tissue sources, however, display qualitatitvely the same general number and position of peaks thus indicating that either surgical procedure should yield an acceptable source of tissue for isolation and characterization studies of prostate derived growth factor. Purification studies were then initiated. In a preliminary series of stability experiments it was observed that total growth factor activity was only moderately effected by acidification to pH 4.5. However, a significant precipitate was observed to form during the acidification. This acid treatment was therefore incorporated as a first purification step. The results shown in Figure 5 indicate that acidification followed by dialysis against phosphate buffered saline results in a

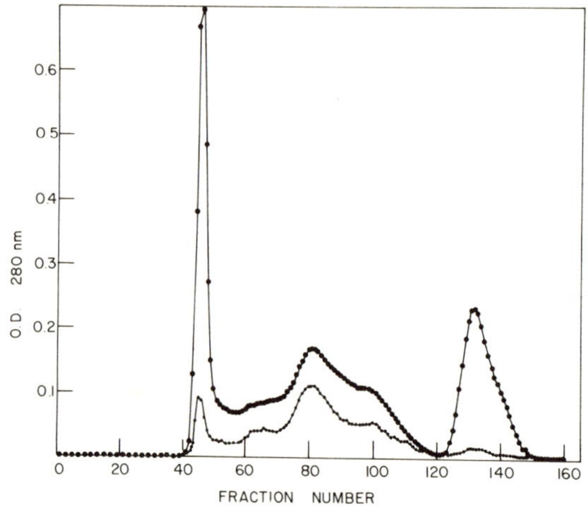

Figure 5. The effect of acidification and dialysis on the protein profile of a prostatic homogenate. The upper curve shows the 280 nm absorbance of the crude extract. The lower curve shows the 280 nm absorbance following acidification of the crude extract to pH 4.5, centrifugation to separate precipitated material, and readjustment of the pH of the supernatant to pH 7.3.

significant reduction in void volume protein and loss of the low molecular weight 280 nm absorbing material. Dilutional assays for growth factor activity before and after acidification and dialysis indicated that 80% of the growth factor activity was retained. The acid treated material was subjected to ammonium sulfate fractionation. Sufficient solid ammonium sulfate was added to the supernatant of the acid treated prostatic homogenate to bring the solution to 25% of saturation. After refrigeration for 1 hour the precipitate was separated by centrifugation and the supernatant brought to 50% of saturation by a second addition of solid ammonium sulfate. After refrigeration for one hour, the precipitate was separated by centrifugation and the supernatant brought to 75% of saturation by the addition of a third portion of solid ammonium sulfate. After refrigeration for 1 hour, the precipitate was separated by centrifugation. Precipitates were dissolved in phosphate buffered saline and dialyzed against phosphate buffered saline to remove the ammonium sulfate. A portion of the solution that had achieved 75% saturation was also dialyzed against phosphate buffered saline. As shown in Table 1 the mitogenic activity was split between the materials that precipitated at 50% of saturation and 75% of ammonium sulfate saturation.

TABLE 1

Growth Factor Activity Obtained by Ammonium Sulfate Fractionation of Acid Treated Prostatic Tissue Extract

Per Cent of Ammonium Sulfate Saturation	Tritiated Thymidine Incorporated (CPM)
0-25 [a]	18,807 ± 3.892 [c]
25-50	96.762 ± 7,974
50-75	131,668 ± 9,120
>75 [b]	10.517 ± 803
control	8,842 ± 740

a. Material that precipitated at the indicated fraction ranges for ammonium sulfate saturation.
b. Material remaining in solution at 75% of ammonium sulfate fractionation.
c. Performed at 1:3 dilution of dialyzed material. Mean±SD for triplicate determinations.

The material precipitated between 50 and 75 per cent of ammonium sulfate saturation was then subjected to gel filtration chromatography over Sephadex G-200 (Figure 6). The major area of mitogenic activity occured at an extrapolated molecular weight of 300.000. Another area of lower molecular weight activity was also observed. This, however, was only a minor area and is well resolved from the high molecular weight form by the gel filtration chromatography. These initial purification studies have developed a method that apparently selectively concentrates one of the high molecular weight growth factor species present in prostatic tissue extracts.

There is experimental evidence which indicates that the biochemical composition of human expressed prostatic secretions reflects the physiological status of the prostate (Anderson, Fair, 1976; Grayhack,1977). It appeared possible, therefore, that prostatic fluid might serve as a nonsurgical source material for purification of one or more of the prostatic growth factors. However, initial attempts to demonstrate growth factor activity in prostatic secretions was hampered by the presence of one or more cytotoxic agents present in the secretions. The

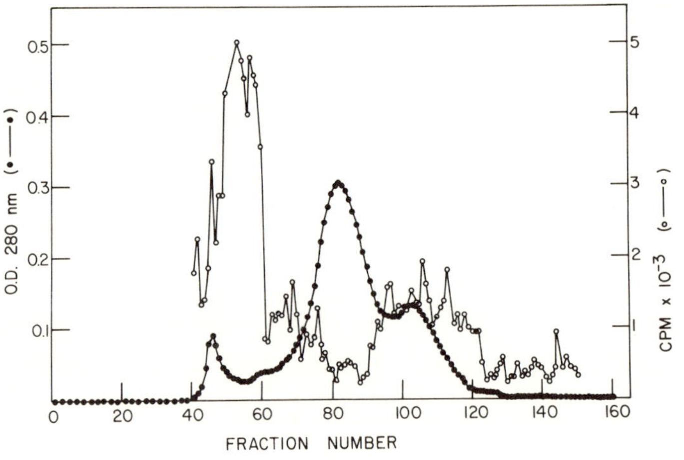

Figure 6. Protein profile (●) and tritiated thymidine incorporation (O) profile for the material present in the supernatant of acid treated prostatic tissue homogenate that precipitated between 50% and 75% of ammonium sulfate saturation. The precipitate was dissolved in phosphate buffered saline, dialyzed against phosphate buffered saline and subjected to gel filtration chromatography over Sephadex G-200 equilibrated with phosphate buffered saline.

TABLE 2

Effect of Dialysis on the Growth Factor Activity of Human Prostatic Fluid

Material Added	Tritiated Thymidine Incorporated (CPM)
No Prostatic Fluid	8,511 ± 896 [b]
Dialyzed Prostatic Fluid [a]	61.865 ± 6651
Nondialyzed Prostatic Fluid	39 ± 11

a. Approximate molecular weight cut off of the dialysis membrane was 3.500
b. Mean ± Standard error of the mean for triplicate determiations

TABLE 3

Comparison of Growth Factor Activity in Five Individual Samples of Prostatic Fluid Obtained from BPH Paients and from non-BPH Patients

Parameter	BPH	Non-BPH
Protein (mg/ml)	17.1 ± 2.3 [a]	28.4 ± 3.8 [a]
Growth Factor (Units/ml)	456 ± 110	737 ± 194
Growth Factor (Units/mg Protein)	27.8 ± 5	27 ± 4

a. Mean ± Standard error of the mean

results in Table 2, however, indicate that the cytotoxic agent(s) could easily be removed by dialysis, thus indicating the low molecular weight of the agent(s). Five individual samples of prostatic fluid obtained from BPH patients and non-BPH patients was then analyzed for total growth factor activity (Table 3). No quantitative difference in the growth factor activity was observed in prostatic fluid obtained from BPH patients or prostatic fluid obtained from non-BPH patients when results were expressed as units/mg of protein. Qualitative differences between growth factor activity in prostatic fluid obtained from BPH patients and from non-BPH patients was examined by gel filtration chromatography. This also allowed comparison of the number and molecular weight of species present in the secretions to be compared to those present in prostatic tissue homogenates. In Figures 7 and 8 are shown the elution profiles for prostatic fluid obtained from BPH patients and non-BPH patients. Since the fluid obtained from an individual patient is of limited amount, these profiles were established utilizing pools of fluids

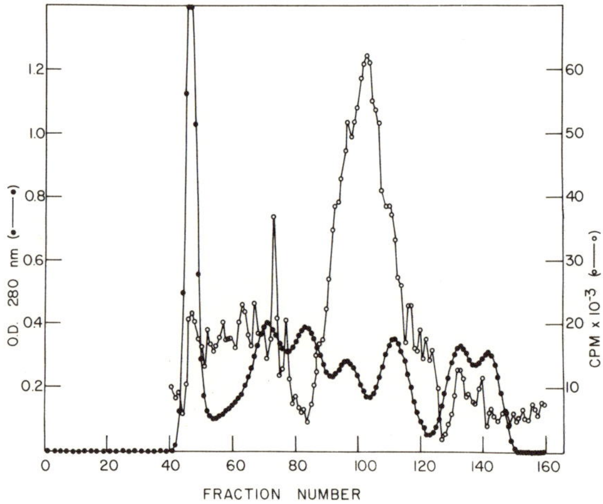

Figure 7. Protein profile (●) and tritiated thymidine incorporation profile (O) for a pooled sample of prostatic fluid obtained from BPH patients. The pooled prostatic fluid sample was centrifuged for 1 hr at 20,000 x g and subjected to gel filtration chromatography over Sephadex G-200 equilibrated with phosphate buffered saline.

obtained from patients with similar diagnoses. It is clear that there is a marked difference between the growth factors present in prostatic fluid and prostatic tissue. The major molecular weight species in prostatic fluid obtained from both BPH patients and non-BPH patients had an apparent molecular weight of 30,000. In the fluid obtained from non-BPH patients, this was the only significant form observed. However, in fluid obtained from BPH patients, additional areas of growth factor activity were seen in the void volume and in the area between the void volume and the major peak. These latter two areas of growth factor activity were significantly smaller than the main growth factor peak.

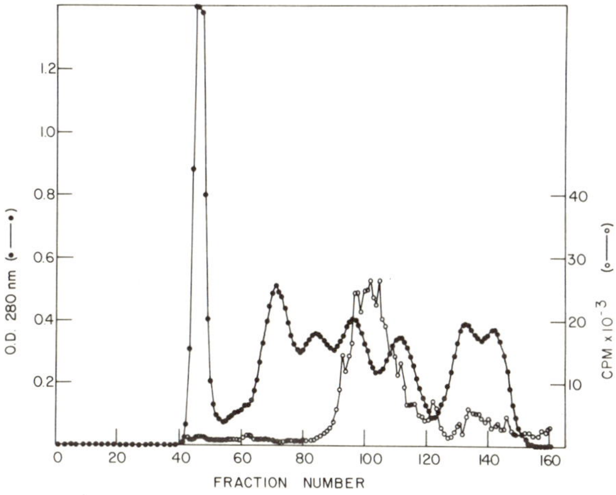

Figure 8. Protein profile (●) and tritiated thymidine incorporation profile (O) for a pooled sample of prostatic fluid obtained from non-BPH patients. The pooled prostatic fluid was centrifuged for 1 hr at 20,000 x g and subjected to gel filtration chromatography over Sephadex G-200 equilibrated with phosphate buffered saline.

These results offer the first confirmation of the results of Lawson and associates that human prostatic tissue extracts contain multiple molecular weight species of growth factors. In addition, we have extended these observations to now include the results that growth factor activity is also present in prostatic secretions obtained from BPH patients and from non-BPH patients. There are dramatic differences between the growth factor activity of prostatic tissue extracts and prostatic fluid. The majority of growth factor activity in tissue extracts exists as species with apparent molecular weights greater than 60,000. In prostatic fluid, however, the major portion of the growth factor activity appears to be associated with a material with a molecular weight of 30,000. Interestingly, there is little of the 30,000 molecular weight species present in the prostatic tissue extracts, even though this material was probably liberated during the extraction procedure. This suggests that some of the high molecular weight growth factor activity seen in prostatic tissue homogenates results from a complexation of lower molecular weight growth factors with specific binding proteins, or from nonspecific binding to materials liberated during the homogenization process. Alternately, the high molecular weight species may result from self-association of low molecular weight growth factors. At present there are insufficient data to discriminate between these different hypotheses. Purification studies of the high molecular weight species, coupled with treatment of the high molecular species with experimental conditions previously shown to disrupt protein complexes may provide a means to answer this question.

There are, in addition, apparently some subtle differences between the growth factors present in prostatic fluid obtained from BPH patients as opposed to the growth factors present in prostatic fluid obtained from non-BPH patients. In prostatic fluid obtained from BPH patients, the majority of the activity elutes from the column with an apparent molecular weight of 30.000. There are, however, additional areas of growth factor activity associated with the void volume material and with areas beween the void volume and the 30,000 molecular weight species. These areas comprise only a fraction of the total growth factor activity of the prostatic secretions. In contrast, no growth factor activity was observed in the area between the major growth factor activity and the void volume of the column when prostatic fluid obtained from non-BPH patients was chromatographed over the same column. Although this qualitative difference in growth factor activity present in prostatic fluid obtained from BPH and non-BPH patients is an intriging observation, it cannot yet be stated that it is diagnostic. When pooled samples are utilized, the possibilty of one grossly abnormal sample effecting the final results, out of proportion to its relative contribution to the final size of the pool, cannot be unequivocally eliminated. Examination of individual samples of prostatic fluid obtained from BPH patients and from non-BPH patients, for the presence of growth factors with molecular weights larger than 30,000 should allow the intriging possibility that there is a significant difference between these two groups of patients to be addressed.

Finally, the question of the relationship between prostate derived growth factors and benign prostatic hyperplasia must be addressed. At first glance, the presence of growth factors in normal, benign hyperplastic, and cancerous prostatic tissue, prostatic fluid from BPH patients and from non-BPH patients might lead one to conclude that there was no relationship. However, growth factors have not been purified from all the individual sources on normal and diseased tissues. There may be subtle differences between the growth factors produced by normal prostatic tissue and diseased prostatic tissue that simple gel filtration or total mitogenic activity measurements are not sensitive enough to detect but which have major biochemical and/or physiological consequences. It is, for example, a change in a single amino acid that distinguishes hemoglobin obtained from a normal patient and hemoglobin obtained from a patient with sickel cell anemia (Hunt, Ingram 1959). Alternately, a change in the biological regulation of the expression of growth factor activity present in prostatic tissue may be important. This could involve an altered response by the prostatic cell to endogenous prostatic growth factors; or an alteration in the synthesis, degradation or processing of endogenous growth factors. Thus, it is clear that unequivocal establishment of a realtionship between prostatic growth factors and benign prostatic hyperplasia requires purification of individual prostate derived growth factors; utilization of the purified growth factors for elucidation of the reaction mechanism by which growth factors stimulate cell growth and division; elucidation of the mechanism by which expression of growth factor activity is regulated; and demonstration that purified growth factors, alone or in conjunction with other modulators of tissue growth (i.e. hormones) can produce benign prostatic hyperplasia in an animal model system, organ culture, or tissue culture.

In summary, although at this time. no direct relationship can be demonstrated between benign prostatic hyperplasia and prostate derived growth factors. this is an area of research that has a significant potential for increasing the understanding of benign prostatic hyperplasia and merits further research.

REFERENCES

Anderson RU, Fair WR (1976). Physical and chemical determinations on prostatic secretion in benign hyperplasia, prostatitis and adenocarcinoma. Invest Urol 14:137.

Andrews P (1964). Estimation of the molecular weight of proteins by Sephadex gel filtration. Biochem J 91:222.

Baserga R (1981) "Tissue Growth Factors". New York: Springer-Verlag, p 57.

Bradshaw RA. Rubin JS (1980). Polypeptide growth factors: some structural and mechanistic considerations. J Supramol Structure 14:183.

Grayhack JT, Wendel EF, Lee C, Oliver L (1977). Analysis of prostatic fluid in prostatic disease. Cancer Treat Rep 61:205.

Hunt JA, Ingram VM (1959). A terminal peptide sequence of human heamoglobin. Nature 184 (Suppl 9):640.

Jacobs SC, Pikna D, Lawson RK (1979) Prostatic osteoblastic factor. Invest Urol 17:195.

Layne E (1957). Spectrophotometric and Turbidimetric methods for measuring proteins. Methods Enzymol 3:447.

Thomas KA. Riley MC, Lemmon SK, Baglan NC, Bradshaw RA (1980). Brain fibroblast growth factor. J Biol Chem 255:5517.

Discussion

Katzenellenbogen: I'm asking questions that you might not have addressed yet. The first is, why did you choose 3T3 cells as the test system?

Parrish: We happened to choose that particular system for two reasons; first, its easy to work with and second, when we got into this particular area, we went to people at the University who had done a lot of work on growth factors and they recommended it. Additionally, Dr. Story had previously shown that the mitogen worked both on 3T3 cells and human foreskin fibroblasts.

Katzenellenbogen: Do you assume that this growth factor is prostate-specific?

Parrish: We have not addressed that yet because we don't have it clean enough to answer that question.

Katzenellenbogen: Have you screened other cell lines?

Parrish: We have not. You might address that question to Dr. Story, they have done substantially more work in this area than we have.

Katzenellenbogen: The other two related questions are: is this a protein? Is it destroyed by proteinase?

Parrish: We believe at this time it is a protein. We haven't done the complete proteolytic digestion, but the growth factor is partially destroyed by proteinase so there may be non-proteolytic fragments which still retain activity.

Katzenellenbogen: It seems to me quite likely that you may, have some factor that is aggregated with other proteins so that you get it coming off at other points during column chromatography.

Parrish: That's true. That was our original working hypothesis. That has still not been eliminated.

Story: Do you notice the differences in the elution profile on G200 between expressed prostatic secretions and your tissue homogenates? Were your expressed prostatic secretions dialyzed prior to chromatography? How about your tissue extracts?

Parrish: No they weren't.

Story: When you dialyze the material from your secretions, what were they dialyzed against?

Parrish: They were dialyzed against PBS (phosphate buffered saline).

New Approaches to the Study
of Benign Prostatic Hyperplasia, pages 197–216

PRELIMINARY CHARACTERIZATION AND EVALUATION OF TECHNIQUES FOR THE ISOLATION OF PROSTATE-DERIVED GROWTH FACTOR

Michael T. Story, Ph.D., Stephen C. Jacobs, M.D., and Russell K. Lawson, M.D.

Department of Urology, Medical College of Wisconsin, 9200 W. Wisconsin Ave., Milwaukee, WI 53226

In 1979, Jacobs et al demonstrated the presence of a growth-promoting factor in crude extracts, of human prostatic tissue prepared from BPH, well-differentiated prostatic adenocarcinoma (pelvic lymph node), and normal post-pubertal prostate. This and subsequent work (Jacobs and Lawson 1980, Lawson et al 1981) led us to postulate that prostatic-derived growth factor (PrGF), perhaps acting in concert with androgens which are known to regulate the glandular content of growth factors (Bynny et al 1974), Ishii and Shooter 1975), might be involved in the fibrostromal proliferation characteristic of BPH (Bartsch et al 1979). A similar interaction of PrGF with osteoblasts might also explain the osteoblastic response to prostatic carcinoma. At this time we describe some of the properties of PrGF and our experience with various separation techniques that have been used in isolating the factor from BPH tissue.

MATERIALS AND METHODS

Cell Cultures and Assay for Growth Factor Activity

Human fibroblast cells were initiated in culture from explants of newborn foreskin by standard techniques (Hayflick 1973). Stock cultures, maintained in minimum essential medium, Eagle, with 10% newborn calf serum (NBS), 100 U/ml penicillin, 100 µg/ml steptomycin, and 0.25 µg/ml fungizone (MEM_{10}), were used between the 2nd and 8th passage in culture. All cell culture medium, serum, antibiotics, and enzymes were from Grand Island Biological Co.

Monolayer cultures were dispersed by Ø.25% trypsin, Ø.Ø1% ethylenediamine teteracetic acid, in Hank's balanced salt solution (HBSS) without Ca^{+2} and Mg^{+2}, counted by hemocytometer, and inoculated at 2x1Ø^5 cells per well in 24-well culture plates (Falcon). After 3 days incubation, 37°, in a humidified atmosphere of 5% CO^2 in air, cells were washed twice with HBSS and nutritionally down-shifted to Ø.8 ml of medium containing Ø.5% NBS ($MEM_{Ø.5}$). After 1 day, Ø.2 ml of sample to be tested for mitogenic activity or control material was added to cells. Additions included: (a) 5Ø% NBS, (b) sample buffer, and (c) test samples. After 23 hours incubation, ^{3}H-thymidine (Ø.1 uCi, 6.7 Ci/m mole, New England Nuclear (NEN), was added to all wells. After 1 hour the pulse medium was removed and cells were washed 3 times with cold Ø.1M sodium phosphate with Ø.15M sodium chloride, pH 7.4. Trypsin solution, Ø.3 ml, was added to each well. After 1Ø minutes incubation, 37°, cells were collected on glass fiber filters with the aid of a Multiple Sample Harvester (M.A. Bioproducts), fitted with a specially constructed suction-delivery head to accommodate the Falcon 24-well culture plate. Filters were air dried, and transferred to 7 ml vials and incubated, 6Ø°, 3Ø minutes, with Ø.25 ml Protosol (NEN), tissue solubolizer. Econofluor (NEN), scintillation cocktail, (5 ml) was added and the amount of radioactivity was determined with a liquid scintillation spectrometer (Packard). The mean of triplicate samples was determined and the relative mitogenic activity (RMA) calculated:

$$\text{RMA} = \frac{\text{CPM (test sample) - CPM (Sample buffer)}}{\text{CPM (10\% NBs) - CMP (Sample buffer)}}$$

One unit of growth factor activity was defined as a RMA equal to one determined by dose-response studies. Significance was assessed by student t-test. As published previously (Lawson et al 1981), ^{3}H-thymidine uptake correlated well with measurements of mitogenesis by autoradiography and cell number.

BPH EXTRACT

Human prostate tissue was from surgical specimens obtained at transurethral and open prostatectomy for BPH. Specimens were stored at -8Ø° prior to the preparation of extract. All steps in preparing BPH extract were at Ø° to

4°. The tissue was rinsed in HBSS and cut into small cubes. The pieces of tissue were weighed and placed in a sterile steel mortar and pistle and covered with liquid nitrogen. Immediately after boil-off of the liquid nitrogen, the tissue was pulverized. The powdered tissue was placed in Ø.Ø5M Tris with Ø.Ø5M sodium chloride, pH 7.6 at 25°, (Tris buffer), (1:1, wet weight: volume), and kept at 4° over night. The preparation was centrifuged 3,ØØØ rpm, 3Ø minutes, (Sorvall, RC-3) and the supernatant transferred to a clean tube. An equal volume of cold Tris buffer was added to the pellet. After suspending the pellet the centrifugation was repeated. The supernatant from the two centrifugation steps were pooled and centrifuged 14,ØØØ rpm, 4Ø minutes, (Sorvall, RC-2B). The supernatant was decanted through a funnel packed with glass wool to remove floating lipid and successively passed through 3.Ø, Ø.8, Ø.45 and Ø.22 μ filters (Millipore). To facilitate the extraction of larger quantities of tissue, specimens were pooled after cutting into small pieces and homogenized with a model PT 1Ø-35 "Polytron" homogenizer quipped with a PT 2Ø ST probe generator (Brinkmann instruments). Homgenization was performed at a setting of 8 for a total of 35 seconds. The volume of Tris buffer used to prepare extracts, the centrifugation proceudre, and filtration was as described for extract prepared from tissue pulverized after freezing in liquid nitrogen.

Ammonium Sulfate Precipitation of BPH Extract

The BPH extract was brought to 33% saturation by the slow addition of saturated ammonium sulfate, pH 7.6. After mixing for 2 hours the preparation was centrifuged 3,ØØØ rpm, 3Ø minutes, and the pellet was dissolved in Tris buffer (33% ammonium sulfate precipitate). The supernatant was brought to 67% saturation with ammonium sulfate. After centrifugation, the pellet was dissolved in Tris buffer (33-67% ammonium sulfate precipitate). The supernatant (67% ammonium sulfate supernatant) as well as the 33% and 33-67% ammonium sulfate precipitates were dialyzed extensively against Tris buffer.

Chromatography

Chromatographic separation of BPH extract precipitated between 33 and 67% saturation with ammonium sulfate was performed in columns (Pharmacia) at 4° with downward flow regulated by a peristaltic pump. The absorbance (206 nm) was recorded and column elutes were collected in fractions (LKB). Sephadex and Con-A-Sepharose were obtained from Pharmacia. DEAE Cellulose (Cellex D) was from Bio-Rad. Further details are given in RESULTS.

Concentration, Dialysis, Filtration, and Protein Determination

Samples were concentrated by ultrafiltration in a stirred cell apparatus with a type YM-10 membrane (Amicon). Dialysis was performed in bags prepared from membrane with a molecular weight (MW) cut-off of 3,500 (Spectrum Medical Industries). Concentration and dialysis was performed at 4°. Samples were sterilized by filtration (Gelman) before being tested for growth factor activity. Protein determination was as described by Lowry et al (1951) or by a Coomassie blue dye binding procedure (Bio-Rad) when dilute samples were assayed in Tris buffer. Both procedures used bovine serum albumin as standard.

RESULTS

Growth Factor Activity of BPH Extract

To date, extracts have been prepared from more than 100 glands obtained at open prostatectomy. An average of 420 units (range 300-890 units), of growth factor activity were recovered per gram wet weight of tissue. The extracts averaged 20 units/mg (range 10-47 units/mg). Tissue obtained by transurethral resection (TUR) has also been used as a source of growth factor. However, extracts prepared from individual TUR specimens or prepared from pooled specimens yielded fewer units of growth factor activity per gram wet weight of tissue (average 190 units, range 110-320 units) and the specific activity was lower (average 14.5 units/mg) than from extracts prepared from glands obtained by open prostatectomy.

pH vs. PrGF Activity

PrGF activity was unstable at acid pH (Figure 1). A 30% to 50% loss in activity was seen when the pH of BPH extracts was lowered from 7.3 to 6. The activity did not decrease further until the pH was lowered to 3 in one study, or to 1.5 in a second study, at which time only about 20% of the original activity was present. About a 20% loss in activity was also seen when the pH was raised from 7.3 to 8.8. At about pH 6, a precipitate formed in the preparation. The precipitate did not solubolize when the pH was readjusted to 7.3. When dialyzed against 0.1M acetic acid (pH 2.9) only 24% of the activity remained (Table 1). In addition, treatment with 6M urea or 6M guanidine-HCI at pH 7.6 inactivated more than 50% of the growth factor activity.

Figure 1: pH vs. PrGF Activity

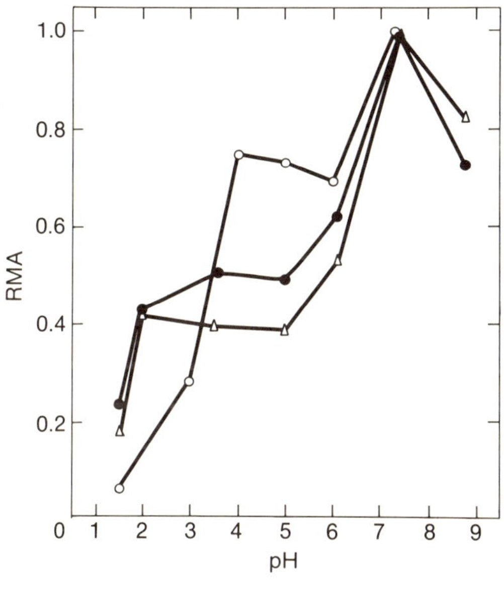

Crude BPH extract, pH 7.3, was titrated with 1N HCl or 1N NaOH to the pH indicated. A sample was removed, adjusted to pH 7.3, filtered (0.2μ), and assayed for growth factor activity. The different symbols show the results from three separate studies. The same BPH extract was used for two of the studies (●, △) and a second BPH extract was used for the third study, (O). Values are the mean of quadruplicate fibroblast cultures.

Table 1: Influence of dissociation agents on PrGF activity

Agent	Activity (% Control)
Urea (6M)	25, 46
Guanadine-HCl (6M)	12, 32
Acetic acid (Ø.1M)	24

Ammonium sulfate precipitated BPH extract was dialyzed against the agent prepared in Tris buffer, pH 7.6, or saline (acetic acid) for 1 day and then dialyzed against Tris buffer for 2 days. Values are expressed as the % of control extract dialyzed 3 days against Tris buffer.

Ether Extraction of BPH Extract

To determine if the growth factor activity in BPH extract was due to a component in the lipid fraction, a preparation was extracted with ether. All of the activity remained in the aqueous phase (data not shown).

Ammonium Sulfate Precipitation of BPH Extract

Table 2 shows the typical distribution of growth factor activity after precipitation of BPH extract with ammonium sulfate. The material that precipitated between 33 and 67% saturation with ammonium sulfate contained 36% (range 25-36%) of the protein and 58% (range 52-64%) of the growth factor activity in crude BPH extracts. Eighteen percent of the activity was recovered in the 33% ammonium sulfate pellet; whereas, 8% of the activity was not precipitated at 67% saturation with ammonium sulfate. The 33-67% ammoniun sulfate precipitated material was the only fraction that showed an increase in growth factor activity compared to the crude extract. Although the recovery of growth factor was higher in a 67% ammonium sulfate precipitate compared to the 33-67% precipitate, the material had a lower specific activity than material precipitated between 33-67% saturation (data not shown). Despite a 4Ø to 5Ø% loss in activity after ammonium sulfate precipitation between 33 and 67% saturation, the procedure provided a means of reducing the sample volume by 1Ø-fold and resulted in material that remained in solution after freeze-thawing and during subsequent fractionation steps.

Table 2: Distribution of Growth Factor Activity after Precipitation with Ammonium Sulfate

Preparation	Growth Factor Activity (units/mg)	% Recovery Protein	% Recovery Activity
Crude BPH Extract	15.5	100	100
Ammonium Sulfate Precipitate			
33%	12.0	23	18
33-67%	25.0	36	58
Ammonium Sulfate Supernatant			
67%	10.3	13	8
Ammonium Sulfate Precipitate 33-67%	45.9 *(25-67)	30.4 (25-36)	56.4 (52-64)

*Mean of five preparations, (Range).

Fractionation of Ammonium Sulfate Precipitated BPH Extract on a Column of Sephadex (G-200)

The typical elution profile of ammonium sulfate precipitated BPH extract from a column of Sephadex G-200 is shown in Figure 2. The growth factor activity was distributed in the MW region ranging from 17,000 to material that was excluded from the gel (>100,000). About 60% of the activity was found in fractions 44 to 61.

Fractionation of Ammonium Sulfate Precipitated BPH Extract on a Column of DEAE Cellulose

The typical elution profile of ammonium sulfate precipitated BPH extract from a column of DEAE-cellulose is shown in Figure 3. About 50% of the protein and 80% of the growth factor activity bound to the anion exchanger and was eluted from the column when the concentration of sodium chloride in the elution buffer was increased to 0.35M. The ionic strength of the elution buffer was previously optimized for recovery of growth factor by elution with a linear salt gradient (not shown). A small amount of protein, without growth factor activity was eluted from the column when the sodium chloride concentration was increased to 1.ØM. The growth factor activity that did not bind to DEAE also did not bind to a second column packed with the ion-exchanger (data not shown).

Figure 2: Elution profile of Ammonium Sulfate Precipitated BPH Extract from a Column of Sephadex (G-2ØØ)

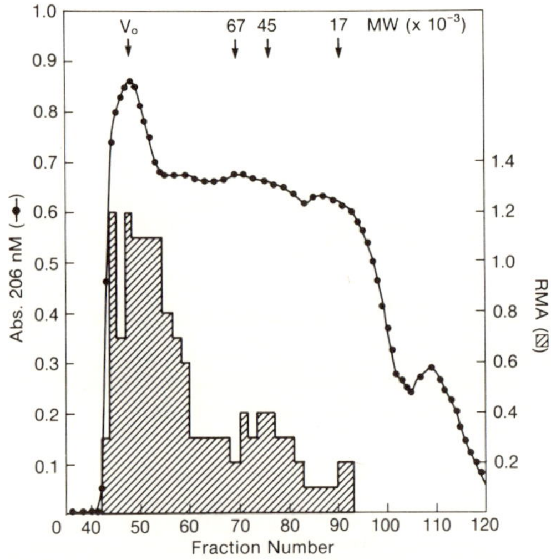

Ammonium sulfate precipitated BPH extract (175 mg, 21ØØ units) was applied to 2.6 x 95 cm column of Sephadex (G-2ØØ) equilibrated with Tris buffer. The sample was eluted with the same buffer at 22 ml/hr. Fractions (4.5 ml) were diluted 1:5 in HBSS and assayed for growth factor activity. The elution positions of blue dextran (Vo), bovine serum albumin (67,ØØØ), ovalbumin (45,ØØØ), and myoglobin (17,ØØØ) are indicated.

Figure 3: Elution Profile of Ammonium Sulfate Precipitated BPH Extract from a Column of DEAE Cellulose

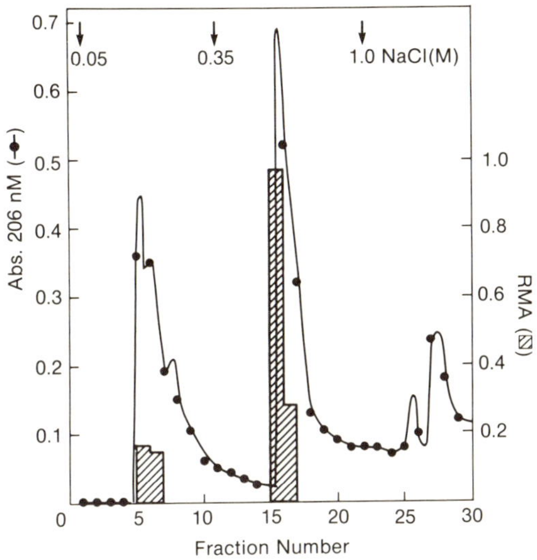

Ammonium sulfate precipitated BPH extract (17.5 mg, 214 units) was applied to a 1.6 x 36 cm column of DEAE cellulose equilibrated with Tris buffer. The material that did not bind to the anion exchanger was eluted with Tris buffer at 2Ø ml/hr. At the indicated time, the ionic strength of the buffer was increased to Ø.35M and 1.ØM NaCl. Fractions (14.1 ml) were assayed for growth factor activity.

Electrofocusing of Ammonium Sulfate Precipitated BPH Extract.

The predominate growth factor activity in an ammonium sulfate precipitate of BPH extract was found between pH 4.7 and 5.3 after flat-bed electrofocusing in a granulated gel (Figure 4). Only 15% of the applied growth factor was recovered from the gel.

Figure 4: Preparative Flat-bed Electrofocusing of **Ammonium** Sulfate Precipitated BPH Extract in a Granulated Gel.

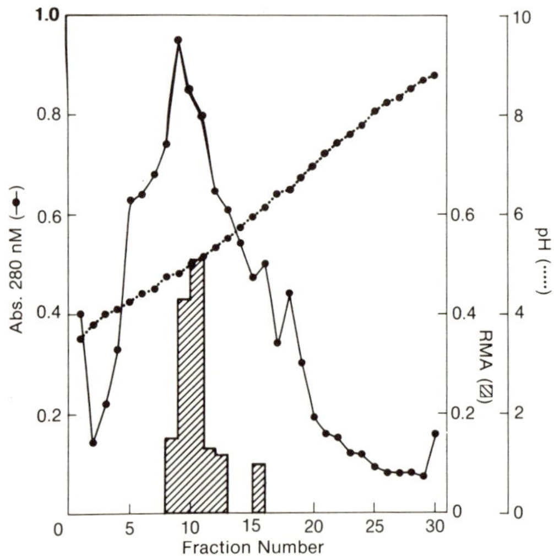

Ammonium sulfate precipitated BPH extract (1Ø5 mg, 1355 units) was dialyzed against a 1% solution of Ampholine, pH 3.5 - 9.5 (LKB). The sample was applied to a granulated gel with a formed Ampholine pH gradient on a LKB Multiphor unit as described by Winter et al (1975). After focusing, the gel was cut into 3Ø equal slices and the material was eluted from the gel with saline. The pH, absorbance (28Ø nm), and growth factor activity (following dialysis and dilution) of the eluted material was determined.

Fractionation of Ammonium Sulfate Precipitated BPH Extract on a Column of Con A-Sepharose

Ammonium sulfate precipitated BPH extract was fractionated on a column of Con A-Sepharose (Table 3). Fifty three percent of the protein and 65% of the growth factor activity was recovered in the material that did not bind to the immobilized lectin. No activity was found in the material that bound to the column and was eluted with 1-Ø-Methyl α-D-glucopyanoside.

Table 3: Fractionation of Ammonium Sulfate Precipitated BPH Extract on a Column of Con A-Sepharose

Sample	Protein (mg)	Growth Factor Activity units	units/mg	% Recovery Protein	% Recovery Activity
BPH Extract	16.9	324	19.2	100	100
Con A					
Unbound	9.0	210	23.3	53	65
Bound	6.4	0	0	38	0

Ammonium sulfate precipitated BPH-extract was applied to 1.6 x 16 cm column of Con-A Sepharose 4B equilibrated with Tris buffer continaing 1 mM $MgCl_2$ and 1 mM $CaCl_2$. The column was eluted with the same buffer until the absorbance reached zero (unbound). The buffer was changed to Tris containing 1 M 1-0-Methyl α-D-glucopyranoside (sigma) and the column was eluted until the absorbance reached zero (bound). The fractions were dialyzed against Tris buffer, concentrated, and assayed for growth factor activity.

Fractionation of Ammonium Sulfate Precipipated BPH Extract on a Column of Sephadex G-75 with Low and High Salt-containing Buffer

To facilitate the recovery of the apparent large MW growth factor seen on G-200 fractionation (Figure 2), ammonium sulfate precipitated BPH extract was fractionated on a column of Sephadex G-75 (Figure 5A). As expected, most of the growth factor activity was excluded from the gel (MW >67,000). The mean recovery of growth factor activity in concentrates of fractions 13-15 (determined from 5 separate columns) was 57 + 7%. Fractions 13-15 were concentrated and brought to 1.55 M NaCl. Figure 5B illustrates the elution profile of this material from a G-75 column with the high salt-containing buffer. Three peaks of growth factor activity were found. Peak I eluted in the same position as the major peak of activity from the G-75 column with the low salt-containing buffer (i.e., >67,000). Peak II eluted one fraction below the BSA standard (<67,000), and a third peak of activity eluted between the position of the 30,000 and 17,000 MW standards. Only a trace of growth factor activity was seen in the region of Peak III on G-75 frationation with the low salt-containing buffer. The distribution of growth factor activity after G-75 fractionation with the low and high salt-containing buffers is shown in Table 4. About 50% of the growth factor activity, recovered in concentrates of elutes after G-75 fractionation with the high salt-containing buffer was in Peak III (apparent MW 17,000 to 30,000). The specific activity of the growth factor in Peak III was 667 units/mg compared to 43.9 units/mg in the ammonium sulfate precipitated BPH extract. About 30% of the growth factor activity was recovered in each of Peaks I and II, but the specific activity of this material was lower than the starting sample.

Table 4: Distribution of Growth Factor Activity After G-75 Fractionation with Low and High Salt-containing Buffer.

Sample[a]	Protein (mg)	Growth Factor Activity units	Growth Factor Activity units/mg
Ammonium Sulfate Precipitated BPH Extract	47.4	2081	43.9
G-75 - Low Salt (fractions 13-15)	27.0	1234	45.7
G-75 - High Salt[b]			
Peak I	5.5	25	4.5
Peak II	2.2	36	16.6
Peak III	0.1	60	667.0

a) Samples are as indicated in Figure 5.
b) Values were determined on concentrates of pooled column fractions.

Figure 5: Fractionation of Ammonium Sulfate Precipitated BPH Extract on a Column of Sephadex G-75 with Low and High Salt-containing Buffer

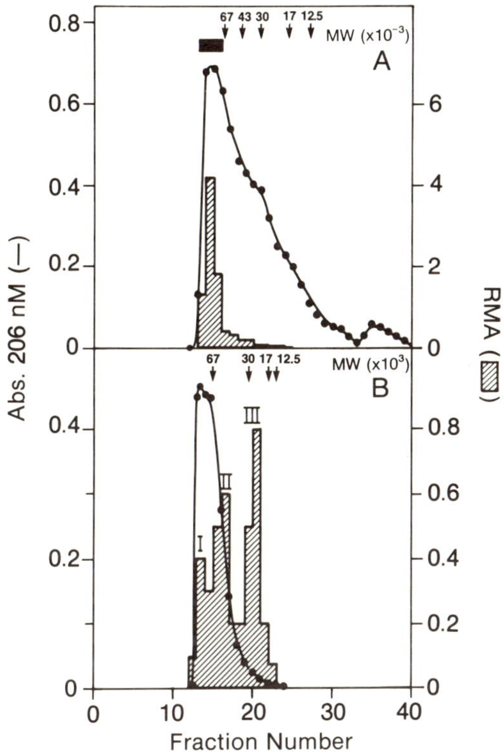

A) Ammonium sulfate precipitated BPH extract (47.4 mg, 2Ø81 units) was fractionated on a 2.6 x 96 cm column of Sephadex G-75 equilibrated with Tris buffer (Ø.Ø5 M Tris with Ø.Ø5 M NaCl, pH 7.6). The sample was eluted with the same buffer at 2Ø ml/hr. Fractions (14.1 ml) were assayed for growth factor activity. The elution position of bovine serum albumin (67,000), ovalbumin (47,000), carbonic anhydrase (30,000), myoglobin (17,000), and cytochrome C (12,500) are indicated. The fractions denoted by the bar were pooled and concentrated by ultra-filtration. Sodium chloride was added to a final concentration of 1.55 M and a portion of the sample (16.5 mg, 754 units) was fractionated on a 2.6 x 95 cm column of G-75 equilibrated with Tris buffer with 1.55 M NaCl, pH 7.6 (B). Fraction size was as indicated in A. Fractions were dialyzed against Tris buffer and assayed for growth factor activity.

DISCUSSION

Extracts prepared from the human prostate are mitogenic for human foreskin fibroblasts (Jacobs and Lawson 1980), human prostate-derived fibroblasts (unpublished observations),and rat calvaria cells in culture (Jacobs et al 1979). The mitogenic activity is not due to epidermal growth factor, EGF, (Story et al 1983); although guinea pig prostate contains EGF and nerve growth factor (Harper et al 1979). In addition, the mitogenic activity of human prostatic extract is not a result of the high content of acid phosphatase or polyamines in these preparations (Jacobs and Lawson 1980) nor is the activity a component of the lipid fraction or associated with the large class of glycoproteins that bind to concanavalin-A (Table 3). The factor is a heat (Jacobs et al 1979) and acid (Figure 1) sensitive component that is susceptible to the action of trypsin (Jacobs and Lawson 1980) and is easily inactivated by the dissociation agents urea and guanidine-HCl (Table 1). These studies were performed with crude tissue extracts or ammonium sulfate precipitated material. In this state the factor appears predominately in a large molecular weight form. The finding that PrGF can be dissociated into a lower molecular weight component (see below) raises the possibility that these properties may not describe the active molecule.

Several preparative fractionation techniques were evaluated for the isolation of PrGF from BPH extract. The growth factor activity after electrofocusing was found in the same pH range as the major contaminating proteins (Figure 4). The technique requires the removal of carrier ampholyte and resulted in a low recovery of growth factor activity. Poor recovery of activity was most likely related to inactivation at acid pH (Figure 1). The growth factor activity did not bind to Con-A and the technique produced only a modest increase in activity (Table 3).

Fractionation of BPH extract by ammonium sulfate precipitation, gel filtration, and ion exchange chromatography strongly suggested that the mitogenic activity was associated with several components in the preparation. The conditions used to prepare extract may have contributed to the heterogenicity. The ionic strength of BPH preparations was kept low (0.05 M Tris with 0.05 M NaCl) to avoid exchanging the buffer before ion exchange chromatography. However, low ionic strength solutions promote protein-protein interaction. Several observations suggest that under the low ionic strength conditions, PrGF may aggregate or bind to specific or non-specific "carrier" proteins. 1) On Sephadex G-200 the growth factor activity was distributed in several MW fractions ranging from 17,000 to over 100,000 (Figure 2). When the ionic strength was increased (0.05 M Tris with 1.55 M NaCl) the predominate growth factor activity was found in the MW range of 17,000 to 30,000 (Figure 5B). 2) About 20% of the growth factor activity did not bind to DEAE and thus differed in charge from the major growth factor activity (Figure 3). However, this fraction behaved in an identical fashion to the fraction that bound to DEAE on gel filtration in high ionic strength buffer, i.e., the activity was recovered in the low molecular weight form (unpublished observation). 3) The distribution of growth factor activity following ammonium sulfate precipitation (Table 2) suggests that PrGF may be associated with proteins that differ widely in their solubility. Alternatively, the distribution of growth factor activity may be related to the pH (7.6) that precipitation was performed. Proteins are more readily salted out at their isoelectric point (PI). The growth factor activity was recovered between pH 4.7 and 5.3 after electrofocusing (Figure 4). However, salt precipitation was not performed at this pH because of the loss of activity at acid pH (Figure 1). The activity that precipitated at 33% saturation and the activity that was not precipitated at 67% saturation eluted in the large MW range in low ionic strength buffer and in the low MW form in high ionic strength buffer (unpublished observations).

A number of other growth factors are know to interact with proteins in a manner resembling PrGF. Endothelium-derived growth factor behaved like a protein with an MW greater than 150,000 in 25 mM Tris or in isotonic phosphate buffer. When exposed to detergent or high concentrates of chaotropic ions the growth factor activity was predominately found in 14,000 to 24,000 MW fractions (DiCorleto et al 1983). Platelet-derived growth factor exhibited similar gel filtration properties. The growth factor activity was distributed in several MW regions ranging from 10,000 to over 100,000 in borate buffer. However, gel filtration in 6 M guanidine-HCl produced a more discrete active fraction corresponding to a MW of 12,000 to 24,000 (Heldin et al 1979). Other growth factors such as EGF (Taylor et al 1970), multiplication-simulating activity (Knauer et al 1981), and nerve growth factor (Varon et al 1967), are known to possess specific carrier proteins of considerably larger MW than the active growth factor. It has not been determined if specific binding proteins are present for PrGF.

Finally, in light of the many enzymes described in prostatic tissue, it would not be surprising if growth factor heterogenicity was, in part, a result of proteolytic activity in these preparations. We have relied on low temperature (0° to 4°) to reduce enzyme activity; as the addition of protease inhibitors would interfere with the bioassay for growth factor activity.

With the information on the properties of PrGF as prerequisite, sequential use of ammonium sulfate precipitation, gel filtration in low ionic strength buffer, ion exchange chromatography, and gel filtration in high ionic strength buffer resulted in greater than a 225-fold increase in growth factor activity (manuscript in preparation).

REFERENCES

Bartsch G, Muller HR, Oberholzer M, Rohr HP (1979). Light microscopic stereological analysis of the normal human prostate and of benign prostatic hyperplasia. J Urol 122:487.

Byyny RL, Orth DN, Cohen S, Doyne ES (1974). Epidermal growth factor: Effects of androgens and adrenergic agents. Endocrinology 95:776.

DiCorleto PE, Gajdusek CM, Schwartz SM, Ross R (1983). Biochemical properties of the endothelium-derived growth factors. J Cell Phy 114:339.

Harper GP, Barde YA, Burnstock G, Carstairs JR, Dennison ME, Suda K, Vernon CA (1979). Guinea pig prostate is a very rich source of nerve growth factor. Nature 279:160.

Hayflick J (1973). Subculturing human diploid fibroblast cultures. In Kruse PF Jr, Paterson MR Jr (Eds) "Tissue Culture: Methods and Applications", New York: Academic Press, p 220.

Heldin CH, Westermark B, Wasteson A (1979). Platelet-derived growth factor: Purification and partial characterization. Proc Natl Acad Sci 76:3722.

Ishii DN, Shooter EM (1975). Regulation of nerve growth factor synthesis in mouse submaxillary gland by testosterone. J Neurochem 25:843.

Jacobs SC, Lawson RK (1980). Mitogenic factors in human prostate extracts. Urology 16:488.

Jacobs SC, Pikna D, Lawson RK (1979). Prostatic osteoblastic factor. Invest Urol 17:195.

Knauer DJ, Wayner FW, Smith GL (1981). Purification and characterization of multiplication-stimulating activity (MSA) carrier protein. J Supramol Struct 15:177.

Lawson RK, Story MT, Jacobs SC (1981). A growth factor in extracts of human prostatic tissue. In Murphy GP, et al (Eds) "The Prostatic Cell: Structure and Function", Part A, New York: Alan R. Liss, p 325.

Lowry OH, Rosebrough NJ, Farr AL, Randall RJ (1951). Protein measurement with the Folin phenol reagent. J Biol Chem 193:265.

Moore RA (1943). Benign hypertrophy of the prostate. A morphological study. J Urol 50:680.

Story MT, Jacobs SC, Lawson RK (1983). Epidermal growth factor is not the major growth-promoting agent in extracts of prostatic tissue. J Urol 130:175.

Taylor JM, Cohen S, Mitchell WM (1970). Epidermal growth factor. High and low molecular weight forms. Proc Natl Acad Sci 67:164.

Varon S, Nomura J, Shooter EM (1967). The isolation of the mouse nerve growth factor protein in a high molecular weight form. Biochemistry 6:2202.

Winter A, Perlmutter H, Davies H (1975). Preparative flat-bed electrofocusing in a granulated gel with the LKB 2117 Multiphor. "Application Note 198", Stockholm: LKB-Produkter AB.

Discussion:

Li: How is this growth factor different from the growth factor from other organs, e.g. mammary glands or uterus? How does this growth factor differ from that in normal prostate?

Story: I'm sorry, we have only limited data on that. We have shown the presence of a mitogen in our fibroblast assay system in extracts of normal prostates. These were postpubertal prostates. We have also shown the presence of a factor which is mitogenic in lymph node metastasis from patients with prostatic cancers. Now, we have not examined the material that might be present in any other tissue. We have used muscle extracts as controls, which in our hands did not stimulate growth. We found that extracts of kidney and liver had varying degrees of activity, but much less, when titered out, than the prostate. We plan on addressing the specificity of this factor after we isolate it.

Schwende: Have you investigated the zinc content or concentration of the high molecular weight growth factor?

Story: No, we haven't. Some of the other growth factors in their high molecular weight form contain zinc. As you know, the prostate contains a lot of zinc. I don't know if it is involved in forming the high molecular weight complex of our growth factor.

Wicha: You stated that this factor is different from epidermal growth factor. Can you demonstrate on any of the target cells you use that there are additive effects of your factor and other known growth factors?

Story: When we test epidermal growth factor in the presence of our factor, we do not get a response that is any greater than with our factor alone. As a matter of fact, the response we see to prostate growth factor, as the labeling of nuclei on autoradiographs, or incorporation of the label into either acid perceptible material or into total uptake of the tritiated label, is much greater with our growth factor than EGF (epithelial growth factor). The response to prostate growth factor is 4.6 times that seen with 20 ng of purified EGF. However, there is one thing that is misleading in this comparison. Our growth factor is not purified. If we fortify EGF with serum, since our preparation contains many serum components, one can see similar degrees of stimulation. When we see maximum stimulation with our growth factor, the addition of EGF does not give an additional response. I don't know if that answers your question.

Wicha: Do you think that means EGF and the prostate growth factor are acting by the same mechanisms?

Story: I would speculate that this prostate growth factor is a mitogen and EGF is a known mitogen, and both are certainly turning on cell replication. If our factor is turning it on maximally, we wouldn't expect to see an added response to EGF. EGF and our growth factor are not competing for the same EGF receptor.

Ofner: You made the very interesting point that EGF and the nerve growth factor are androgen sensitive, and that in actual fact they have been used as assays for androgen inactivity. Can the prostatic factors be stimulated by androgen?

Story: Since we are attempting to isolate prostate growth factor from human tissue, we have not tested the sensitivity to androgens. We really haven't investigated the presence of this factor in a rat model system. Both our group and Dr. Parrish's agree that there is a factor in canine prostate, which is mitogenic. However, we have no information that this is the same factor that we are looking at, and Dr. Parrish has indicated that it may, in fact, be a different factor.

Katzenellenbogen: Since you have done some purification and have some evidence of molecular weight, can you give us some idea of about how much growth factor you think is there per gram of prostate?

Story: If the material has a molecular weight of about 17,000, which we see on gel filtration chromatography, and if we assume that the growth factor is as active as epidermal growth factor, then we estimate that there is about 700 mcg. of this material per kilogram of prostate.

Bhuyan: You mentioned that autoradiographic studies indicate that there is an increase in DNA synthesis. Are you increasing the percent of S cells that are moving from G-1 into the DNA synthesis phase, or are you allowing the cells that are already in S-phase to synthesize more DNA when you add the growth factor?

Story: More cells are going from the G-1 or a G-0 state into the S phase. We have shown an increase in labeled mitoses after addition of the growth factor, so this is not simply an increase in uptake of the label. The growth factor is turning on a round of replication which can quantitated by autoradiography and by monitoring cell number.

Mawhinney: Would you comment on similarities or differences between your growth factor and the prostate secretory protein that seems to be a nonspecific type of binding protein?

Story: I am unfamiliar with the properties of that secretory protein.

New Approaches to the Study
of Benign Prostatic Hyperplasia, pages 217–234

COMMON CHARACTERISTICS OF HUMAN AND CANINE BENIGN PROSTATIC HYPERPLASIA

John T. Isaacs

Depts. of Urology and Oncology, Johns Hopkins University School of Medicine
Baltimore, Maryland 21205

INTRODUCTION

While benign prostatic hyperplasia (BPH) is the most common neoplastic disease in man, the exact etiology of this disorder is presently unknown. Numerous theories have been postulated over the last 40 years to explain the spontaneous development of BPH in man, however, only two facts have been well established for the disease. The first is that the presence of functioning testes is required for the natural development of the disease (Moore 1947; Huggins 1947). Whether the testes play a permissive or active role in the development of BPH is uncertain, however, the fact that pre-pubertal castration prevents the subsequent development of BPH suggests that there are at least some endocrinological determinants in the etiology of BPH. The second fact is that the incidence of BPH increases with advancing age such that nearly all men eventually develop BPH if they live long enough (Moore 1943; Swyer 1944; Franks 1954; Harbitz, Haugen 1972; Pradhan, Chandra 1975)). While these two facts suggest that aging and endocrinological factors are indeed important in the process of BPH development, the exact manner in which these two factors are involved in the etiology of BPH is not clear. In order to delineate how these important factors are involved in the etiology of BPH, it would be very helpful if studies could be performed in which the incidence of BPH development could be determined following the experimental manipulation of the endocrinological state of the host at various ages. Unfortunately, such human studies are too expensive, require too much time and are ethically impossible to perform. Therefore, there is an urgent need for appropriate animal models for BPH in which such experimental manipulation of the host animal at various ages can be performed. In order for any such potential animal models to have any relevance to the human disease, the animal should develop spontaneous prostatic hyperplasia with an incidence which increases with age and the animal should require the presence of testes for such development, thus mimicking the important characteristics of human BPH. While not an absolute requirement for an appropriate animal model for BPH, it would be very helpful, from a practical standpoint, if the spontaneous incidence of prostatic hyperplasia in the animal is rather high so that excessively large numbers of animals would not have to be used.

At present, the only species which meets all of the above requirements for an appropriate model for human BPH is the dog. In the dog, a spontaneous benign hyperplastic overgrowth of the prostate occurs with increasing incidence with advancing host age (Brendler et al. 1983) and development of the disease requires the presence of the testes (Zuckerman, McKeown, 1938; Huggins 1947). Therefore, canine prostatic hyperplasia is believed by many investigators to be an appropriate model for the study of human BPH, although there are important differences between the conditions in the two species (Ofner 1968; DeKlerk et al. 1979). For example, the human disease is often a focal process thought to arise uniquely in the periurethral portion of the gland as a stromal nodule, which is then secondarily invaded by glandular elements (Pradhan, Chandra, 1975). In contrast, canine prostatic hyperplasia is a diffuse process occurring throughout the entire gland involving predominantly the glandular-epithelial cells with less stromal involvement (DeKlerk et al 1979). These differences may explain the different clinical symptoms in the two species. In man, the prostate is anatomically fixed between the symphysis pubis and the rectum and therefore hyperplastic growth of the periurethral nodules compresses inwardly on the urethra producing urinary obstruction. In contrast, in the dog, the prostate is not anatomically fixed and therefore hyperplastic growth expands the prostate in all directions outwardly producing little urinary retention but instead, produces obstruction of the rectum and thus constipation. Recognizing these differences, the dog still remains the best animal model presently available to study BPH experimentally. In this paper, data will be presented to further support the relevance of the dog as an appropriate model system for the study of BPH. In addition, a summary of what has been learned concerning factors involved in BPH development will be presented.

Androgen and the Normal and Abnormal Growth and Maintenance of the Human and Canine Prostate

The human prostate weighs approximately 1 gram at birth. Little net proliferative growth of the human prostate occurs between birth and ten years of age, Figure 1. After the age of ten, however, the prostate begins to proliferatively grow reaching its normal adult size by the age of twenty Figure 1. After the age of twenty, if the individual does not develop BPH, the prostate stops its proliferative growth and is subsequently chronically maintained at this 20 gram size (Leissner, Tisell 1979). By plotting the growth of the human prostate on a semi-logarithmic scale vs. age, it can be demonstrated that, during the active growth phase of the normal prostate between 10-20 years of age, the prostate is growing exponentially with a constant doubling time of 2.78 years, Figure 1. This period of exponential growth corresponds to the time period when the serum testosterone levels are rising from their initially low levels seen before the age of 10, to the high levels seen in an adult male, Figure 2. If an individual is castrated before the age of 10, the serum testosterone levels do not rise to their normal adult level and the proliferative growth of the human prostate between 10 and 20 years of life is completely blocked. These results clearly demonstrate that a physiological level of androgen is required for the normal growth of the human prostate. In addition, if an adult male who already has a fully grown prostate is castrated, the serum testosterone levels rapidly decrease to the low value seen in intact males younger than ten years of age and as a result, the prostate rapidly involutes to less than 20% of its normal size. These results demonstrate that a physiological level of androgen is chronically required to maintain the normal adult size of the human prostate.

Like the human prostate, the prostate of the dog (all data presented in the paper for the "dog" is based upon the

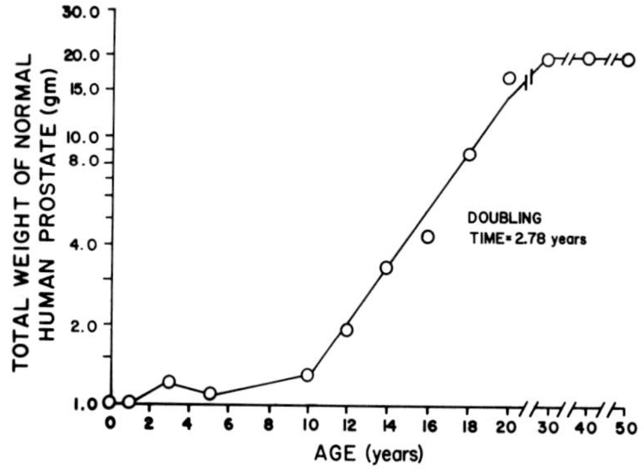

Figure 1. Growth of the normal human prostate from birth to adulthood. Data from Boyd (1962).

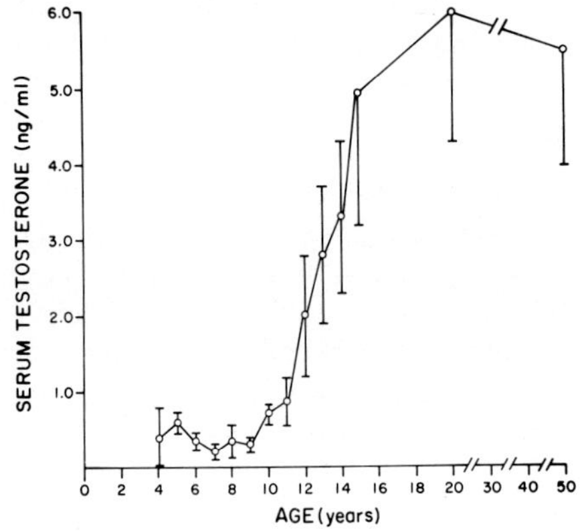

Figure 2. Serum testosterone levels during the aging of the man. Data from Frasier et al. (1969).

purebred beagle) undergoes a period of exponential growth during which the prostate grows to its normal adult size, Figure 3. For the beagle, this occurs between 4 and 16 months of age during which time the prostate grows with a constant doubling time of 0.64 years. Like the human prostate, this period of active prostatic growth in the dog corresponds to the time period when the serum testosterone level is rising to its normal adult level, Figure 3. If this rise is prevented by early castration, then the subsequent normal prostatic growth period in the dog is completely inhibited, demonstrating that, like the human prostate, the canine gland requires a physiological level of androgen for its normal growth (Zuckerman, McKeown, 1938). Also like the human prostate, the beagle prostate stops its exponential growth once it has reached its normal adult size and is subsequently maintained at about 12-14 grams for the remainder of the dog's life if serum testosterone levels are chronically maintained at their normal adult levels and if prostatic hyperplasia does not develop. If serum testosterone levels are not maintained at their normal adult values, the canine prostate, like the human, involutes to about 20% of its normal adult size (Huggins 1947). The data presented demonstrates that the human and canine prostate share the common characteristic that for both glands a critical level of androgenic stimulation is required for normal prostatic growth and maintenance.

While the data supporting the requirement of androgen for the initial development of the abnormal hyperplastic overgrowth of the human prostate is substantial, the question of whether or not human BPH, once established, continuously requires androgenic stimulation for its maintenance is presently unresolved. Theoretically, the most direct way of answering this question would be to demonstrate regression of established human BPH following castration. In the 1890s, there were several large clinical studies which reported that indeed BPH does show rapid regression following castration (White 1895; Cabot 1896). However, there were additional studies performed in the 1890s which failed to confirm these early findings (Kelsey 1896; Robinson 1896). The use of castration as therapy for BPH became obsolete with the improvements in prostatectomy techniques in the 1900s and therefore the purposeful castration of large numbers of men with BPH has never been performed in the modern era. In a small study,

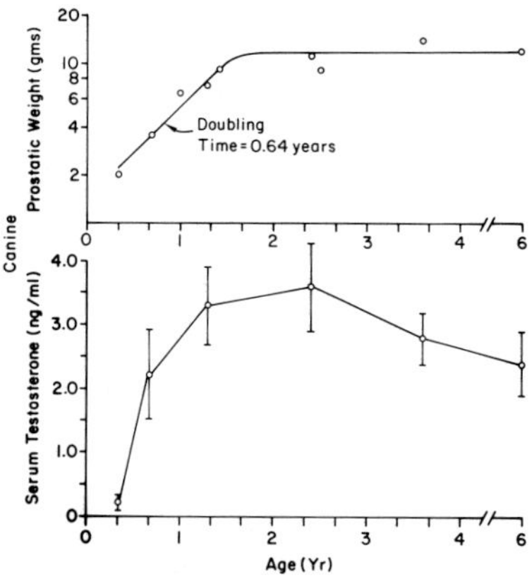

Figure 3. (Upper) Growth of the normal beagle prostate from birth to adulthood. Data from Berry et al. (1984) and James, Heywood (1979). (Lower) Serum testosterone levels during the aging of the beagle. Data from Cochran et al. (1981) and Crook, Heywood (1979).

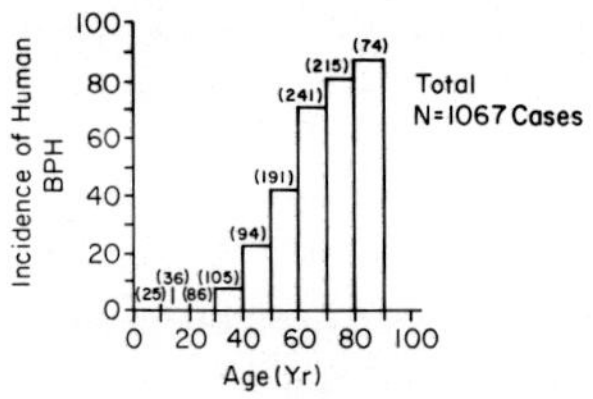

Figure 4. The age-related incidence of human BPH. Data from Berry et al. (1984).

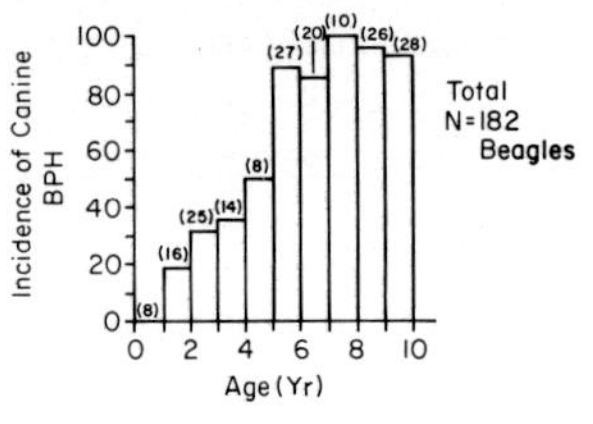

Figure 5. The age-related incidence of BPH in the beagle. Data from Berry et al. (1984).

Huggins and Stevens (1940) obtained pre-castration prostatic biopsies for histological study from 3 patients, 2 of whom had BPH alone and 1 of whom had BPH and prostatic cancer. These 3 men were then castrated and repeat biopsies of their BPH tissue were obtained at various times post-castration. In the one patient who was biopsied at 29 days post-castration, no atrophy of the BPH epithelial cells was observed, however, in the other 2 patients biopsied at 86 and 91 days after castration respectively, substantial involutionary changes were observed in BPH epithelium. In addition, in one patient whose original pre-castration biopsy demonstrated BPH of a primary fibromuscular stromal nature, prostatic size actually decreased and urinary obstructive symptoms were greatly relieved following castration. This study of Huggins and Stevens was followed with a study by Pierson (1946) on the effects of diethylstilbestrol (DES) on established BPH. Using an X-ray technique for the measurement of prostatic size which he developed, Pierson demonstrated that in 10 of 13 cases of BPH studied, androgen deprivation by means of DES treatment resulted in measureable decreases in prostatic size within 1.5 to 6 months of treatment. Wendel et al. (1972) compared the histology of BPH tissue from patients with prostatic cancer who had been treated with castration and/or estrogen therapy with the histology of BPH tissue from patients with prostate cancer who had not been treated with androgen ablation therapy. These studies demonstrated that following androgen ablation therapy, there is a substantial atrophy of the glandular epithelium in BPH tissue as compared to androgen maintained BPH tissue. The specific atrophic changes in BPH tissue which were documented following androgen ablation were: 1) a decrease in the number of epithelial acini per unit amount of BPH tissue, 2) a decrease in the epithelium infolding of BPH acini, and 3) a virtual absence of secretory ability of the epithelial cell lining BPH acini. Taken together, these studies suggest that at least a portion of human BPH tissue requires androgen for its abnormal maintenance.

In the dog, prostatic hyperplasia has been definitively shown to require a continuous supply of androgen for its maintenance. This androgen requirement was illustrated originally by Charles Huggins (1947), who demonstrated in dogs with established prostatic hyperplasia that there was a rapid involution by over 70% in the abnormally enlarged size of the hyperplastic prostate following simple castration. In addition, Huggins further demonstrated that if dogs with abnormally enlarged hyperplastic prostates are castrated and the prostates allowed to regress to 70% of their original size, and then exogenous androgen given continuously to the dog, that the involuted prostates rapidly regrow back, not to the size of normal non-hyperplastic glands, but instead to the original abnormally enlarged size of the pre-castration hyperplastic gland. Once regrown, this abnormally enlarged hyperplastic gland can be maintained in these castrated dogs as long as exogenous androgen treatment is continued. These classic studies demonstrate that the growth and maintenance of canine prostatic hyperplasia requires continuous androgenic stimulation.

In more recent years, it has been learned additionally that prostatic hyperplasia can in fact be experimentally induced in young dogs which have no starting indication of BPH, simply by the exogenous treatment of the animals for 3-4 months with androgen alone or in combination with 17ß-estradiol (E_2). Walsh and Wilson (1976) were the first to demonstrate that enlargement of the prostate comparable to that seen in spontaneously occurring canine prostatic hyperplasia could be produced experimentally by endogenously treating castrated dogs continuously with 5α-androstane-3α,17ß-diol (3α-diol), a potent androgen, in combination with E_2 for 3 to 4 months. These results have subsequently been confirmd and extended by other groups. For example, studies by DeKlerk et al. (1979) and Moore et al. (1979) have demonstrated that besides 3α-diol, DHT alone or in combination with E_2 can experimentally induce the development of prostatic hyperplasia in the dog.

Taken together, these results demonstrate that man and dog share the common characteristic of requiring androgenic stimulation for the development, growth and chronic maintenance of prostatic hyperplasia. Whether this requirement is merely permissive or directly causal in the etiology of BPH in these two species, is not firmly established. Hopefully, advantage will be taken of the ability to experimentally induce the disease in the dog, as well as the ability to manipulate other factors in the dog, so that the question of the essential vs. permissive role of androgen in the etiology of BPH can be answered in the near future.

Significance of the Age-Related Increase in the Incidence of human and canine BPH

Besides the question of the involvement of androgen in the etiology of BPH, another major unanswered question concerning BPH is, why does the incidence of the disease increase with advancing age? The data in Figure 4 has been compiled by Berry *et al*. (1983) from 5 major autopsy series comprising a total of 1067 human specimens in which histological criteria have been utilized to define the presence of BPH at various ages. Histologically, BPH is rarely identified in man under the age of 40 years. However, beginning in the forties, the incidence of BPH increases from an average of 23% to 88% by the 9th decade. Like man, the dog develops prostatic hyperplasia with increasing incidence with age, Figure 5. The data presented in Figure 5 is from the study of Berry *et al*. (1983) which examined the incidence of prostatic hyperplasia in the aged purebred beagle. In the beagle, prostatic hyperplasia is rarely observed before the age of 1 year but thereafter the incidence rises rapidly approaching 100% by the 7th to 8th year of life.

The fact that in both man and dog the incidence of BPH characteristics increase with advancing age raises the question as to what this might mean with regard to the etiology of BPH. In the 1950s, Armitage and Doll (1954) developed the concept that for any disease state which increased with age, a mathematical relationship could be derived from which one could determine whether or not the particular disease process required a single or multiple events for the development of the disease. The basis for the method is that the incidence (I) of a disease at any particular time point (t) can be mathematically expressed as a function of probability of occurrence of an event or events required for the disease to develop per unit time (p) multiplied by the total elapsed time (t). If a disease requires only a single event to occur, then the incidence (I) of the disease at a particular time would equal the probability of occurrence of the event per unit time x the particular time (i.e., I = pt). Alternatively, if a disease requires a series of multiple events to occur, then the incidence (I) at time t of the disease = p(1)t x p(2)t x p(3)t x .... p(N)t, where N is the number of events required and p(1), p(2), p(3) ... p(N) are the individual probabilities of occurence for each of the respective required events occurring per unit time. This mathematical formula can be simplified to $I = (p(1) \times p(2) \times p(3) \times \ldots p(N))t^N$. By means of a logarithmic transformation, this equation becomes $\log I = N \log t + \log (K)$, where K is equal to the product of the multiplication of the various probabilities (i.e., $k = p(1) \times p(2) \times p(3) \ldots p(N)$). If one plots the log of disease incidence at various ages (i.e., time) vs. the log of respective age (i.e., time) and the relationship obeys a straight line relationship (i.e., $y = m x + b$), then the value of N, the number of events required for the disease to occur, can be mathematically determined from the slope (i.e., m) of the line.

If the data on the incidence of human BPH vs. age presented in Figure 4 are replotted as the log of incidence vs. log of age, a straight line relationship is indeed obtained, Figure 6. From the slope of this linear relationship, the number of events requied for human BPH to develop is found to be three. This result strongly suggests that the development of human BPH is a multistep process requiring at least three distinct events. Similarly, if the data on the incidence of canine BPH vs. age presented in Figure 5 is replotted as a double log plot, a straight line relationship is likewise obtained, Figure 7. From the slope of this linear relationship, the number of events required for canine BPH to develop is, however, not three but one. This suggests that the development of canine BPH is not as complex a process as that for the human disease. The observation that the development of canine BPH may be a simpler process requiring fewer events as compared to human BPH, may help to explain the anatomical differences in the disease state in these two species. In the dog, prostatic hyperplasia develops as a diffuse disease involving most, if not all, of the gland while in man, the disease develops as a focal nodule, involving only a small portion of the gland. If the development of human BPH requires that a series of at least three distinct events occur before the disease is evident, then from a statistical probability point of view, while a large portion of cells present in the prostate may undergo one of the three events required for BPH development, only a small subset of these cells would be expected to undergo the second event, and only an even smaller subset of these cells which have undergone the second event would be expected to undergo the third event needed for the development of the disease. This would lead

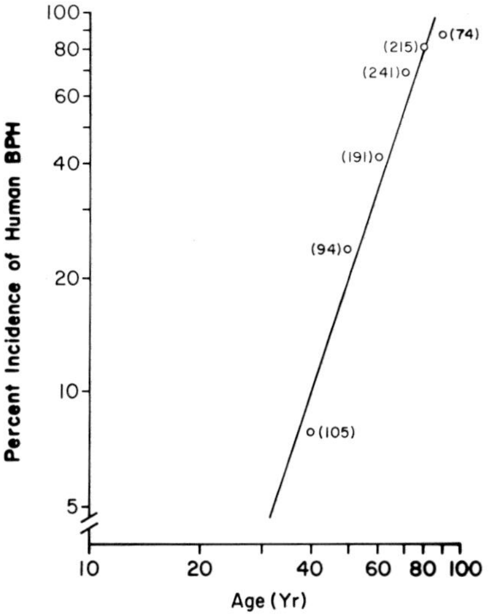

Figure 6. The relationship between the logarithm of BPH incidence *versus* the logarithm of host age in man (based upon the data in Figure 5).

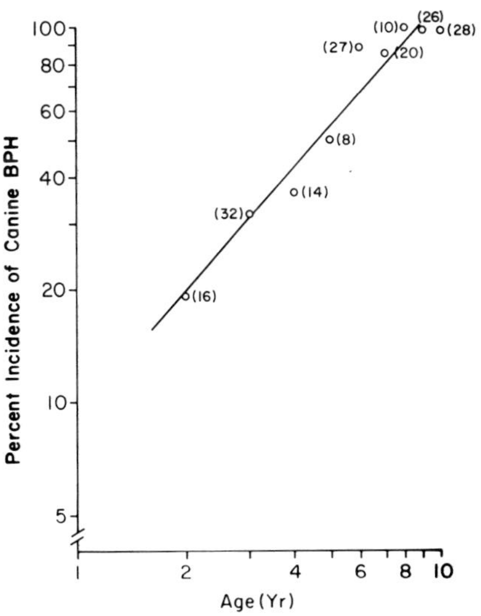

Figure 7. The relationship between the logarithm of BPH incidence *versus* the logarithm of host age in the beagle (based upon the data in Figure 6).

to the initial development of the disease within the prostate in discrete focal sites produced by the abnormal overgrowth of an initially small group of cells which have undergone all three events required for the disease. In contrast, in the dog, if the development of prostatic hyperplasia requires the occurrence of only a single event, then from a statistical probability standpoint, potentially large numbers of cells throughout the canine prostate simultaneously could undergo the event leading to a diffuse rather than a focal origin of the disease.

Biochemical Differences Between Normal and Hyperplastic Prostatic tissue in Man and Dog

A fundamental question concerning BPH is whether BPH is due to: 1) a reaction of normal prostatic cells to a temporally abnormal inductive environment, 2) a reaction of substantially altered (i.e., abnormal) prostatic cells to the normal environment, or 3) a reaction of abnormal prostatic cells to an abnormal inductive environment. At present, the answer to this important question is not entirely known. It is known, however, that both human and canine hyperplastic prostatic cells are not completely normal from a biochemical standpoint. For example, this biochemical abnormality can be illustrated using the ability of hyperplastic vs. the normal prostatic tissue to metabolize dihydrotestosterone (DHT) as a marker. In the prostate, testosterone is irreversibly metabolized by the 5 -reductase enzyme to DHT and numerous studies have demonstrated that it is DHT which is the active intracellular androgen responsible for the hormonal stimulation of the gland. In addition, DHT itself can be further metabolized reversibly by three separate hydroxysteroid oxidoreductase (HSOR) pathways giving rise to a large series of androgen metabolites, Figure 8. Due to the reversibility of the prostatic HSOR activities, each has both a distinct ketosteroid reductase and hydroxysteroid oxidase activity. This means that there are 7 distinct metabolic pathways for androgens in the prostate (i.e., 5α-reductase, 3α-HSOR reductase, 3ß-HSOR reductase, 17ß-HSOR reductase, 3α-HSOR oxidase, 3ß-HSOR oxidase, and 17ß-oxidase activities). The quantitative levels of each of these seven pathways are characteristic for the prostate and thus these levels can be used as phenotypic markers for the normal prostate. In human BPH, there is an abnormal increase in the 5α-reductase activity and an abnormal

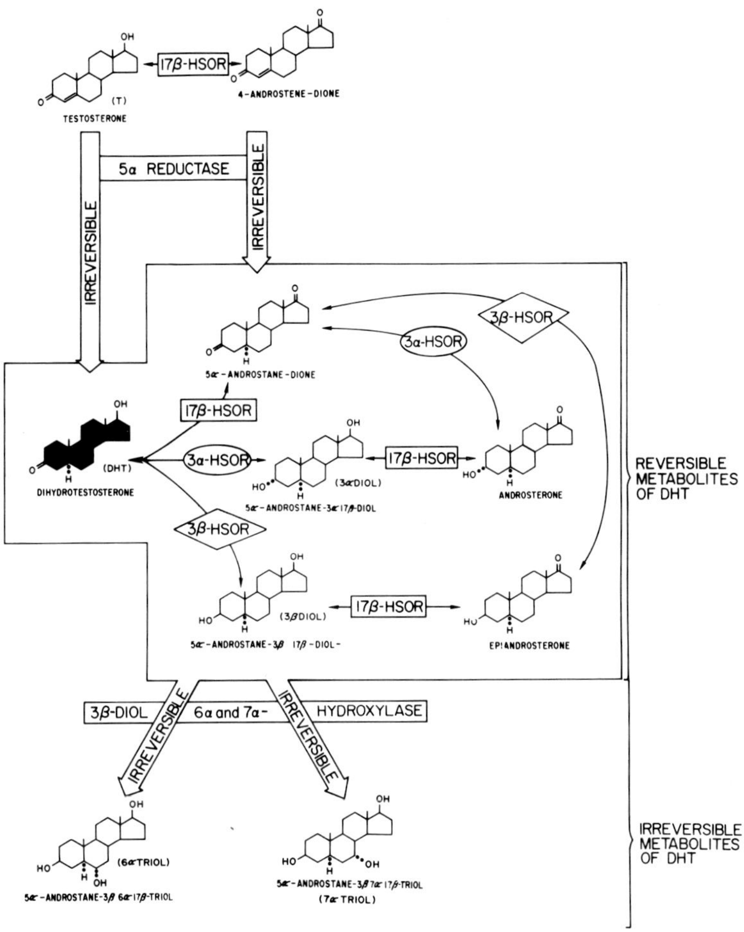

Figure 8. Overview of the complex pathways for androgen metabolism in the prostate. HSOR = hydroxysteroid oxidoreductase.

decrease in the 3α- and 3ß-HSOR reductase and 17ß-HSOR oxidase activities compared to normal non-hyperplastic human prostatic tissue demonstrating that biochemically, human hyperplastic prostatic cells are indeed abnormal (Isaacs et al. 1983). Similarly, comparison of the quantitative levels of these 7 metabolic activities for androgen metabolism in the hyperplastic vs. normal beagle prostate has demonstrated that canine BPH tissue is likewise abnormal (Isaacs, Coffey 1981; Isaacs, 1983; Berry, Isaacs, 1984). The specific abnormalities are an increased 5α-reductase, 3α-HSOR oxidase, and 17ß-HSOR reductase activities in the hyperplastic vs. normal prostatic tissue. These results demonstrate that hyperplastic prostatic tissue of both man and dog is phenotypically abnormal. This suggests that BPH in these two species is not explainable simply as a reaction of normal prostatic cells to an abnormal inductive environment. Whether besides this abnormality in the prostatic cells themselves there is also an abnormal inductive environment in BPH tissue, is presently unknown. Additional studies into this latter possibility are urgently needed to resolve this important issue.

Conclusions

At present, the dog appears to be the best available animal model for the experimental study of BPH. This conclusion is based on the fact that the dog is the only known animal species which spontaneously develops prostatic hyperplasia with increasing incidence with advancing age and in the dog, this spontaneous development requires the presence of functioning testes. The dog thus mimics the two most well established characteristics of human BPH. Analysis of the incidence of BPH vs. host age for man and dog do, however, reveal that the etiology of BPH may be more complicated in man than dog. The development of prostatic hyperplasia in man appears to involve a complex multistep process, while in the dog, the process appears to require fewer steps. This difference may be of experimental value for it suggests that while BPH in man and dog may differ in several steps in the hyperplastic process, the fundamental step involved in the pathogenesis of the disease is likely to be shared in common by the two species. Elucidating the most fundamental step in the process of BPH development may thus be technically easier to do in the dog than in man, not only because the dog is much more amenable to experimental manipulation and control than man, but also because there are fewer steps involved in the development of prostatic hyperplasia in the dog.

Acknowledgments

This work was supported by Grant AM 19300 awarded by NIAMDD. The present study is part of a large ongoing cooperative study on benign prostatic hyperplasia involving a large number of independent investigators at Johns Hopkins. The work presented in this paper could never have been accomplished without the generous support and cooperation of the entire group. In particular, I would like to thank Drs. Donald S. Coffey, Larry L. Ewing, John D. Strandberg, William W. Scott, Patrick C. Walsh and Evelyn R. Barrack for their constant interest and invaluable help without which such a study would have been impossible. In addition, I would like to especially acknowledge the gifted help of Ruth Middleton.

References

Armitage P, Doll R (1954). The age distribution of cancerand a multi-stage theory of carcinogenesis. Brit J Cancer 8:1.

Berry SJ, Isaacs JT (1984). Comparative aspects of prostatic growth and androgen metabolism with aging in the dog versus the rat. Endocrinol (in press).

Berry SJ, Ewing LL, Coffey, DS (1984). A comparison of prostatic growth and the development of benign prostatic hyperplasia in man and dog. Manuscript in preparation.

Boyd E (1962) Growth, including reproduction and morphological development. In Altman, Dittmer (eds) Biological Handbooks, Federation of American Societies for Experimental Biology, Washington, D. C., pp. 346-348.

Brendler CB, Berry SJ, Ewing LL, McCullough AR, Cochran RC, Strandberg JD, Zirkin BR, Coffey DS, Wheaton LG, Hiler ML, Bordy MC, Scott WW, Walsh PC (1983). Spontaneous benign prostatic hyperplasia in the beagle: Age-associated changes in serum hormone levels and morphology and secretory function of the canine prostate. J Clin Invest 71:1114-1123.

Cabot AT (1896). The question of castration for enlarged prostate. Ann Surg 24:265.

Cochran RC, Ewing LL, Niswender GD (1981). Serum levels of follical stimulating hormone, leuteinizing hormone, prolactin, testosterone, 5α-dihydrotestosterone, 5α-androstane-3α,17ß-diol, 5α-androstane-3ß,17ß-diol, and 17ß-estradiol from male beagles with spontaneous and induced benign prostatic hyperplasia. Invest Urol 19:142.

Crook JD, Heywood R (1979). Canine pituitary-testicular function in relation to toxicity testing. Toxicology 13:237.

DeKlerk DP, Coffey DS, Ewing LL, McDermott IR, Reiner WG, Robinson CH, Scott WW, Strandberg JD, Talalay D, Walsh PC, Wheaton LG, Zurkin BR (1979). Comparison of spontaneous and experimentally induced canine prostatic hyperplasia. J Clin Invest 64:842.

Franks LM (1954). Benign nodular hyperplasia of the prostate: A review. Ann R Coll Surg 14:92.

Frasier SD, Gafford F, Horton R (1969). Plasma androgens in childhood and adolescence. J Clin Endocrinol 29:1404.

Harbitz T, Haugen OA (1972). Histology of the prostate in elderly men. A study in an autopsy series. Acta Path Microbiol Scand Section A80:756.

Huggins C, Stevens R (1940). The effect of castration on benign hypertrophy of the prostate in man. J Urol 43:705.

Huggins C (1947). The etiology of benign prostatic hypertrophy. Bull NY Acad Med 23:696.

Isaacs JT, Coffey DS (1981). Changes in dihydrotestosterone metabolism associated with the development of canine benign prostatic hyperplasia. Endocrinol 108:445.

Isaacs JT, Brendler CB, Walsh PC (1983). Changes in the metabolism of dihydrotestosterone in the hyperplastic human prostate. J Clin Endocrinol Metabol 56:139.

Isaacs JT (1983). Changes in dihydrotestosterone metabolism and the development of benign prostatic hyperplasia in the aging beagle. J Steroid Biochem 18:749.

James RW, Heywood R (1979). Age-related variations in the testes and prostate of beagle dogs. Toxicology 12:273-279.

Kelsey CB (1896). Castration for enlarged prostate. Med Rec 49:283.

Leissner KH, Tisell LE (1979). The weight of the human prostate. Scand J Urol Nephrol 13:137.

Moore RA (1947). Benign hypertrophy and carcinoma of the prostate. In Twombly G, Packs G (eds). Endocrinology of

Neoplastic Diseases. Oxford Press, London and New York, pp. 194.
Moore RJ, Gazak JM, Quebbeman JF, Wilson JD (1979). Concentration of dihydrotestosterne and 3α-androstanediol in naturally occurring and androgen induced prostatic hyperplasia in the dog. J Clin Invest 64:1003.
Ofner P (1968). Effects and metabolism of hormones in normal and neoplastic prostatic tissue. Vitamin and Horm 26:237.
Pierson EL (1946). A study of the effect of stilbestrol therapy on the size of the benignly hypertrophied prostate gland. J Urol 55:73.
Pradhan BK, Chandra K (1975). Morphogenesis of nodular hyperplasia-prostate. J Urol 113:210.
Robinson WJ (1896). Failure of castration to cause atrophy of the prostate. Med Rec 49:822.
Swyer GTM (1944). Post-natal growth changes in the human prostate. J Anat 78:130.
Walsh PC, Wilson JD (1976). The induction of prostatic hypertrophy in the dog with androstanediol. J Clin Invest 57:1093.
Wendel EF, Brannen GE, Putong PB, Grayhack JT (1972). The effect of orchiectomy and estrogens on benign prostatic hyperplasia. J Urol 108:116.
White JW (1895). The results of double castration in hypertrophy of the prostate. Ann Surg 22:1.
Zuckerman S, McKeown T (1938). The canine prostate in relation to normal and abnormal testicular change. J Path Bact 46:7.

Discussion

Mawhinney: John, I wonder if your data on androgen metabolism might not be also be consistent with the interpretation that there is no change in individual cell types, but rather a shift in the population of cells?

J. Isaacs: If all we had were my data, that would be a legitimate interpretation. But, Georg Bartsch has assayed the 5-alpha reductase and 3-alpha hydroxyteroid oxidoreductase activity in prostate tissue with different stromal-epithelial ratios and still gets the same amount of activity per gram of tissue.

Mawhinney: I have some problems with how Cowen and colleagues are preparing their epithlium and stroma, but they claim that the 5-alpha reductase is much higher in human prostate stroma than it is normal epithelial cells. In our measurements in dog prostatic tissue and guinea pig seminal vesicle epithelium versus stroma we found greater 5-alpha reductase in the epithelium than in the stroma. I think at this point unless we isolate individual cells and compare normal versus BPH, we also have to consider we may be dealing with ratios in cell types.

Story: Following castration and replacement therapy with testosterone, one sees an increase in DNA synthesis both in vivo and in vitro. Are these normal cells or abnormal cells that are proliferating?

J. Isaacs: Those studies were prefaced on previous ones in the rat. In those animals nothing other than a castration was done. This response of the involuted prostate to androgenic stimulation can be demonstrated at an early age, or late in life. There is no indication that the cells which respond are abnormal, in the sense that when one gives tritiated thymidine and looks at what cells are labelled, they are the normal epithelial cells of the glandular acini. Biochemically, the restored prostate of a castrated rat treated with exogenous androgen has the same enzymatic level as intacts do. So, there's no indication that they're abnormal.

New Approaches to the Study of Benign Prostatic Hyperplasia, pages 235–255

BENIGN PROSTATIC HYPERPLASIA IN THE NONHUMAN PRIMATE

Ronald W. Lewis, M.D.

Associate Professor of Urology and Research Scientist, Tulane University Delta Regional Primate Research Center, Covington, Louisiana

In the development of an animal model for a particular human disease there are certain questions to be considered: Is the organ in which the disease occurs anatomically and functionally homologous to the human counterpart? Does the disease naturally occur in the animal? Can experimental manipulation produce the disease in the animal? Is the experimental disease the same as the natural disease? Are the pathophysiologic effects of the disease the same for the animal and man? Can similar diagnostic modalities be used to detect the presence of the disease? Finally, can the disease process in the animal be modified with preventive or therapeutic manipulations, which can be later applied to man?

For the disease benign prostatic hyperplasia (BPH), some of these criteria have not been dealt with extensively in the nonhuman primate. Each point will be addressed in this presentation. A great deal of information is available to answer the first question for the nonhuman primate prostate. A detailed summary of this work is presented below.

COMPARATIVE ANATOMY

Although a prostate gland is present in all mammals, major anatomical differences from the prostate of man is an obstacle for most comparative biological studies (Price 1963). However, the prostate in the nonhuman primate consists of two histologically distinct areas, the cranial and caudal lobes. Indeed a single-lobed prostate has been reported in two species of nonhuman primates, a marmoset (*Callithrix jacchus*) and an orangutan (*Pongo pygmaeus*) (Miralgia 1970; Roberts 1972). This makes homologous relationships to man much less complex in comparison to rodents which have multiple-lobed prostates.

The prostate and seminal vesicle have been dissected at the Delta Regional Primate Research Center from fifty-eight nonhuman primates (Table 1). In all of these, except for the patas and chimpanzee, there was a definite grossly evident distinction between the cranial and caudal lobes. In these latter animals there was a more intimate association of the two lobes of the prostate (Fig. 1). Although histological sections clearly showed two lobes (Fig. 2). A similar relationship was seen in illustrations of

Table 1. GROSS DISSECTION OF PROSTATE AND SEMINAL VESICLE

Macaque species	
Macaca fascicularis	15
Macaca nemestrina	14
Macaca mulatta	8
Macaca arctoides	3
Baboons	
Papio cynocephalus	8
Papio comatus	1
Papio papio	1
Patas (*Erythrocebus patas*)	5
Squirrel (*Saimiri sciureus*)	2
Chimpanzee (*Pan troglodytes*)	1
Total	58

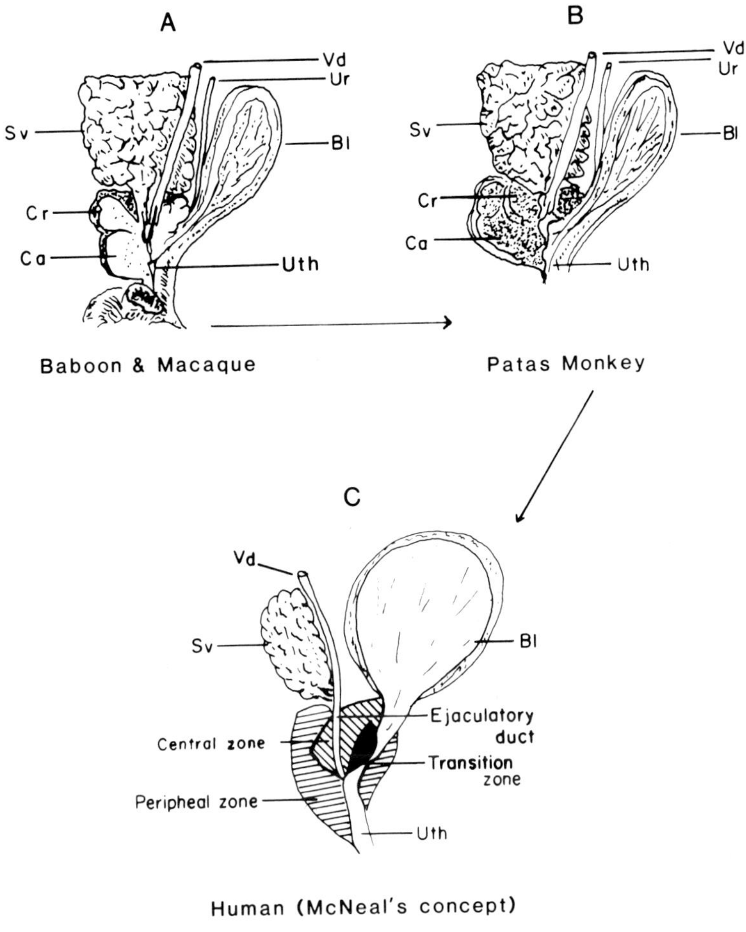

Fig. 1 - Comparative Anatomy of the Prostate in the Primate: Ca, caudal lobe; Cr, cranial lobe; Bl, bladder; Sv, seminal vesicle; Ur, ureter; Vd vas deferens; Uth, urethra.

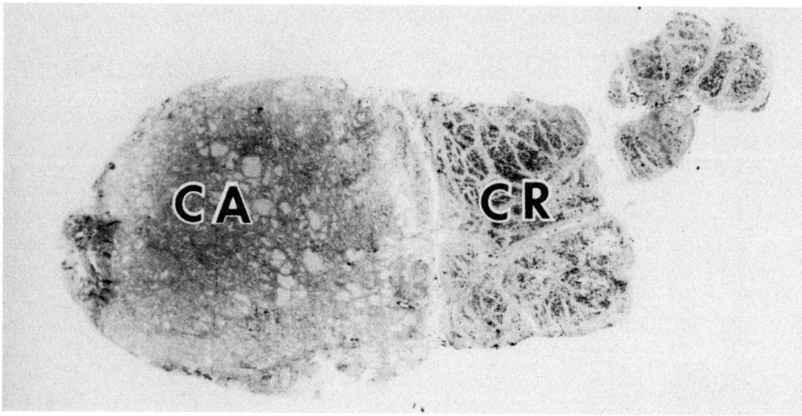

Fig. 2 - Sagittal section of the cranial (CR) and caudal (CA) lobes of the prostate in a chimpanzee showing the intimate association of the two lobes. X 2.

the prostate in the Cape chacma baboon (*Papio ursinus*) (Schoonees, DeKlerk 1968).

The surface of the cranial lobe is lobulated or furrowed resembling the seminal vesicle in appearance. This lobe lies inferior to the seminal vesicles, surrounds the terminal vas deferens and ducts of the seminal vesicles, and lies superior to the caudal lobe from which it can be separated easily except at the antero-medial junction of these lobes. The caudal lobe surface is smooth and more closely applied to the urethra, surrounding it on its posterior and lateral surfaces. The ejaculatory ducts pass through the upper portion of this lobe to exit at the verumontanum of the urethra.

The cranial lobe acini are larger and more irregular and enfolded than those in the caudal lobe. There is a prominent fibromuscular stroma dividing the lobe into a lobular configuration with blood vessels in the deep intralobular clefts. The epithelial cells lining these cranial acini are single-layered, tightly packed, tall columnar cells with oval or elongate, darkly staining nuclei. The nuclei are oriented with their long axis perpendicular to the prominent basement membrane. The cytoplasm of the epithelial cells is granular and strongly eosinophilic. Nerve bundles are prominent in the capsular area. Other investigators have shown a difference in the ultrastructure of the epithelial cells of the lobes of the prostate (Muntzing et al. 1976; Chai et al. 1981). In the epithelial cells in the cranial lobe cytoplasm was more electron dense, secretory granules were homogenous and of a uniform density, and surface microvilli were rarely seen.

The caudal lobe acini are for the most part regular simple tubules lined by low columnar to cuboidal epithelial cells with paler staining nuclei whose long axes are parallel to the basement membrane. The cytoplasm is not granular and demonstrates pale eosinophilic staining. The fibromuscular stroma is diffuse and does not divide the acini into a lobular configuration. Blood vessels and nerve bundles are found scattered throughout the lobe. At the ultrastructure level microvilli on the surface of the caudal epithelial cells are prominent and secretory granules have diversified characteristics (Muntzing et al.1976; Chai et al. 1981).

There is a striking similarity of the acini and stroma in the cranial lobe of the nonhuman primate to the central zone of the human prostate (McNeal 1968; Blacklock, Bouskill 1977; Lewis et al. 1981). Similarly the caudal lobes have been anatomically compared to the peripheral zone of the human prostate (McNeal 1968; Blacklock, Bouskill 1977; Lewis et al. 1981).

McNeal feels that the anatomic region homologous to the region of origin of human BPH is absent in primates. He feels that BPH in man arises exclusively in the pre-prostatic tissue, the transition zone and periurethral subregion (McNeal 1983). However, the duct structure of the cranial and caudal lobes in the nonhuman primate prostate has not been described in as great a detail as in man. McNeal has also shown the striking anatomic dissimilarities between canine and human prostate, and points out that BPH in the dog is of a different morphological type than that seen in man (McNeal 1983).

McNeal has presented the idea that the central zone of the human prostate may derive from the Wolffian duct system because of the: 1) anatomic proximity to the Wolffian-duct-derived ejaculatory ducts; 2) histologic similarity of the central zone epithelium to that of the ejaculatory ducts and seminal vesicles; and 3) relative immunity of both the central zone and the seminal vesicle to carcinoma and BPH (McNeal 1983). Many of the same arguments could be made for the cranial lobe of the nonhuman primate prostate.

COMPARATIVE BIOLOGY

Semen coagulation appears to be a main function of the cranial lobe of the prostate in the monkey. Van Wagenen (1936), in an experimental study of the interaction of secretions from the various accessory sex organs in the rhesus monkey (*Macaca mulatta*), showed that secretions from the cranial lobe when mixed with the secretion of the seminal vesicle caused the formation of a firm white coagulum. It is of interest that secretions from the coagulating gland of the rat also produced a coagulum when mixed with the seminal vesicle fluid of the rhesus (van Wagenen 1936). Greer et al. (1968) prevented coagulation of electroejaculated semen from two rhesus monkeys by prior surgical removal of the cranial lobe.

Zinc is heavily concentrated in the prostate in both normal and abnormal tissue (BPH) (Kirchheim 1983). Uptake of zinc (^{65}zinc chloride) in the caudal lobe exceeds that of the cranial lobe in the baboon (*P. ursinus*) (Schoonees et al. 1969). A similar concentration gradient is found in the human prostate when the lateral and posterior regions are compared to the anterior and central regions. Castration significantly diminished zinc uptake in the caudal prostate but not in the cranial. Testosterone treatment significantly increased zinc uptake in both lobes (Schoonees et al. 1969). The administration of growth hormone to intact baboons (*P. ursinus*) resulted in a statistically significant reduction of cranial and caudal Zn uptake, but not in testosterone treated animals (Schoonees et al. 1970). Rhesus monkeys have been shown to concentrate $^{67}ZnCl_2$ in the prostate at levels 15 times greater than that found in dogs (Johnston et al. 1966).

Other biochemical studies in primates have shown that the cranial lobe of the prostate resembles the caudal lobe of the prostate in some instances and the seminal vesicles in others (Kaack et al 1983; Lewis et al. 1983). Protein content and maltase activity are similar for all of these tissues. The same was true for citric acid in baboons. Tissue content of prostatic acid phosphatase was higher in the caudal lobe of the prostate compared to both cranial lobe and seminal vesicle. This had been previously reported in the baboon (Muntzing et al. 1976). Citric acid and total lactic dehydrogenase were seen in lower concentrations in the seminal vesicles of the nonhuman primate.

LDH isoenzymes in the nonhuman primate migrated in the same pattern as those in man (Kaack et al. 1983). The seminal vesicles showed a higher concentration of fraction 3 and less fraction 1 than in both prostate lobes. The cranial lobe had less concentration of fraction 5, similar to the seminal vesicle when compared to the caudal lobe. (Fig.3)

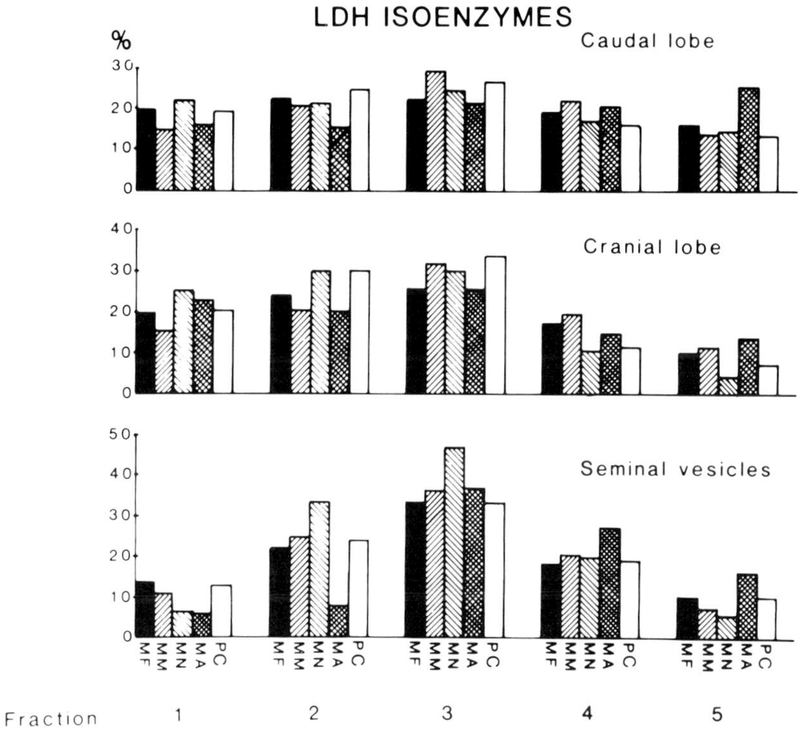

Fig. 3 - Concentrations of lactic dehydrogenase (LDH) isoenzymes in the prostate and seminal vesicle in 37 macaques and baboons. The ordinate represents the percentage of the total area under the curves for each fraction; the abscissa represents the 5 LDH functions. (7 cynomolgus, MF; 5 rhesus, MM; 14 pigtail, MN; 3 stumptail, MA; and 8 baboon, PC).

Steroid hormone uptake and androgen receptor studies have been prominent in the recent evaluation of the prostate. However, technical problems in localizing receptors by biochemical assay systems have made histochemical techniques more promising. However, technical problems exist here also (Karr, Murphy 1983; Kirchheim 1983). Some studies in this area have been performed in the monkey. However, a rhythmic variation of plasma androgen levels in the noncastrate primate may affect androgen study data (Ghanadian 1981).

The major metabolites found in both lobes of the prostate of the rhesus monkey are dihydrotestosterone and androstanediol. Both of these are reductive pathway products (5α reductase) showing that the conversion of testosterone in the prostate differs from such tissue as the liver where oxidative pathways are dominant, producing such products as androstenedione (Ghanadian, Smith 1981).

Ghanadian et al. showed there was a significantly higher uptake of ^{3}H-testosterone in the caudal lobe of prostate compared to the seminal vesicle in rhesus monkeys (*Macaca mulatta*). The cranial lobe was similar to the seminal vesicle (Ghanadian et al. 1977b). When excess unlabeled testosterone (100 fold) was added to the incubation media the uptake of radioactivity in both lobes of the prostate was significantly reduced whereas uptake was unaffected in liver or muscle. With 1000-fold excess of unlabeled testosterone, the uptake of radioactivity was further suppressed in the caudal lobe, not in the cranial.

In another study Ghanadian et al. (1977a) found the concentration for the total, free, and bound cytosol androgen receptor content of the caudal lobe to be higher than in the cranial lobe in rhesus monkeys - most significantly in the two mature animals compared to the two younger animals. Similarly cytosol androgenic receptor content was found to be higher in the caudal lobe than in the cranial lobe in an adult male baboon (*Papio anubis*) which had been castrated 24 hours before the prostate studies (Karr 1979). Karr et al. have reported the uptake of ^{3}H oestradiol-17β to be 2-3 times higher in the cranial compared to the caudal lobe in the baboon, in contrast to that seen with the androgens mentioned above (Karr et al. 1978).

In summary, the caudal prostate in the nonhuman primate

very closely resembles the peripheral zone prostate of man, both from an anatomical and biochemical standpoint. What remains to be established is the human homology of the cranial lobe. It is very possible that this area is a derivative of the Wolffian duct system. There is ample evidence that the cranial lobe resembles the seminal vesicle using many criteria; however, similarities to the caudal prostate certainly exist, as well. What happens to this region in man is the major question. Does a similar region exist? Is it the area that McNeal has called the central or transition zones? Further characterization is needed.

BPH IN THE NONHUMAN PRIMATE

BPH as a natural disease has been infrequently reported in the literature (Fox 1923; Roberts 1972; Adams, Bond 1979; Lewis et al. 1981). The rarity of reported disease may be due to the small number of primates studied, incompleteness of autopsies, and the infrequent study of aged primates.

This author has reviewed the histology of the cranial and caudal prostates in 100 mature adult nonhuman primates in 12 different species (Table 2) (Lewis 1981). Findings

TABLE 2. HISTOLOGIC STUDIES OF THE PROSTATE IN NONHUMAN PRIMATES

Animal species	Number of prostates examined
Macaca mulatta	25
Pan troglodytes	13
Macaca fascicularis	10
Callicebus moloch	10
Erythrocebus patas	9
Saimiri sciureus	8
Macaca arctoides	8
Cercocebus (species unknown)	2
Papio (comatus and papio)	2
Ateles geoffroyi	1
Hylobates lar	1
Macaca radiata	1
Unknown species (genus or species not indicated on stained slides)	10
Total	100

of glandular (or cystic) hyperplasia were found in 13 of the animals, often associated with areas of fibromuscular hyperplasia. Isolated fibromuscular hyperplasia was seen in five animals. The fibromuscular hyperplasia was characterized by a marked proliferation of smooth muscle fibers replacing glandular epithelium. This was found in both lobes of the prostate equally (Fig. 4).

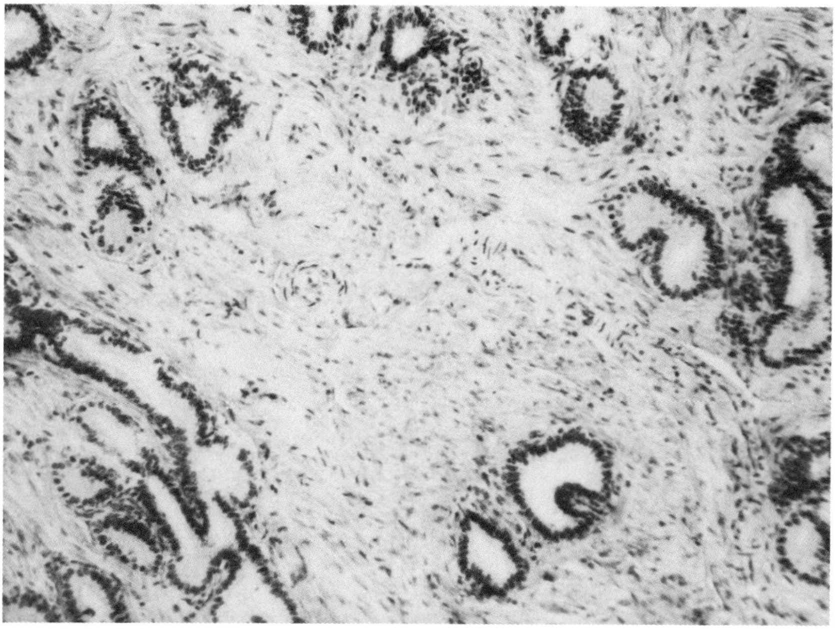

Fig. 4 - Fibromuscular hyperplasia in the caudal lobe of an older mature patas monkey (*Erythrocebus patas*). PTAH staining. X 40.

Cystic or glandular hyperplasia was more commonly seen in the cranial lobe but in three species (5% of the total animals) an isolated area of cystic hyperplasia in the caudal lobe was also seen. In these species (*Pan troglodytes*, *Erythrocebus patas* and *Callicebus moloch*) the cystic enlargement resembled the cystic enlargement reported in the dog, being nodular and localized to one hemisphere of the caudal lobe, rarely impinging upon the urethral lumen (Fig. 5). Dilated acini appear to be located for the most part in the peripheral area of the lobe. There was no compression of normal prostatic tissue against the true prostatic capsule. The association of eosinophilic secretions in some ducts with cystic areas of enlargement suggests obstruction of the distal duct area, but these eosinophilic inclusions were not present in all specimens. More importantly, the areas were not associated with dilated ducts. This suggests that this cystic hyperplasia is akin to that seen in the dog.

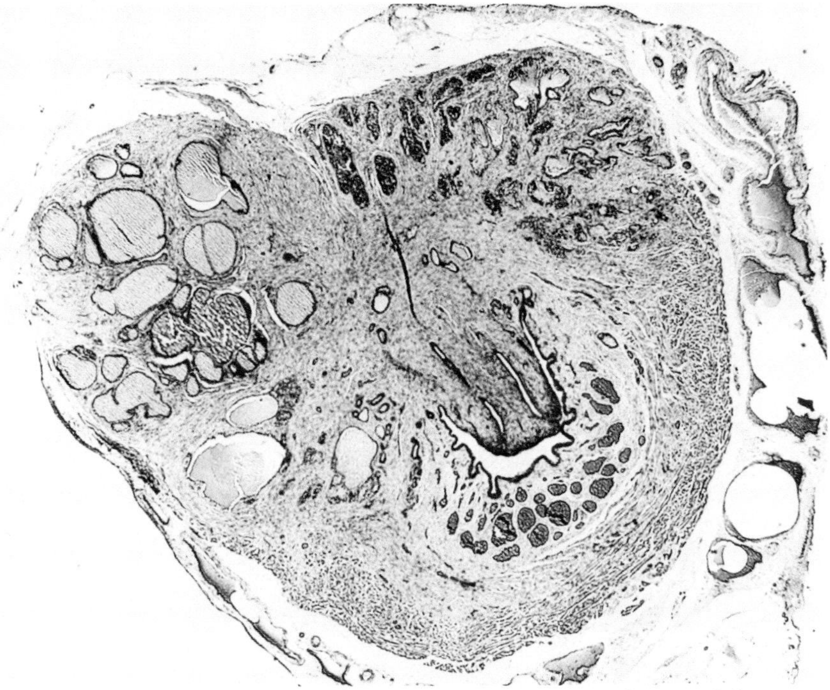

Fig. 5 - Transverse section of caudal lobe of an adult callicebus (*Callicebus moloch*) showing a cystic hyperplastic nodule. X 5.

Adams and Bond (1979) reported nodular enlargement in three of four regions of the prostate in a squirrel monkey (*Saimiri sciureus*) estimated to be 11 years of age. This nodular enlargement of right and left portions of the cranial lobe and right portion of the caudal lobe (the left caudal lobe appeared normal) was characterized histologically by hypertrophic and hyperplastic glands surrounded by hyperplastic smooth muscle.

A nonhuman primate model of prostatic hyperplasia does not exist. Elegant hormonal manipulation studies to produce hyperplasia such as in the dog have not been done (Wilson 1980). However, several studies of the effects of various hormones on the nonhuman primate are reported and the results of these markers have shed some light on ways to develop a model of BPH in the monkey. Many of these studies are similar to the early hormonal manipulation model of prostate hyperplasia in the dog.

Van Wagenen as early as 1935 reported an increase in fibromuscular tissue in the seminal vesicles and prostate (more pronounced in the cranial lobe than the caudal) in two macaque monkeys (testicles intact) which received injections of an estrogen daily for 34 to 42 days compared to two controls. (Table 3)

Parkes and Zuckerman in 1935 (Parkes, Zuckerman 1935) gave estrogen to 10 immature male rhesus monkeys for periods from 6 to 28 days. This produced a diminution in the number of true prostatic glands with corresponding increase in fibromuscular stroma and epithelial growth in the uterus masculinus. Zuckerman (1938) gave estrogen to two castrated rhesus monkeys for a year and found "prostate" enlargement mainly due to fibromuscular growth in the utricular bed, thus substantiating the above report by van Wagenen that estrogen caused little change in the glandular epithelium. In a later paper, Zuckerman and Sandys (1939) discussed the effect of steroid hormones on the prostates of juvenile rhesus monkeys. Short term treatment (14-15 days) was with either estrogen, testosterone, both, or estrogen and progesterone. Although estrogen in the short term study increased the size of the whole organ significantly, there was no change in the relative percentage of utricular, urethra or glandular tissue compared to controls.

In a small series of adult intact baboons (n = 4, controls, n = 4) given 5 mgm of oral diethylstilbesterol (DES) daily for three weeks, Chai et al. (1981) found variable caudal epithelial cell changes. Atrophy of the apical region of epithelial columnar cells of some acini or parts of acini, with these cells taking on a cuboidal appearance, occurred. In addition, there was a marked reduction in the formation of secretory granules in the caudal lobe epithelial cells. In contrast, in the cranial lobe there was only a moderate decrease in epithelial cell height. Secretory

Table 3. STUDIES OF EFFECTS OF ESTROGEN ON THE NONHUMAN PRIMATE PROSTATE

Study	Animal/Intact or Castrate	Hormone/Duration	Result
Van Wagenen (1935)	2 mature rhesus/intact	estrogen/34 & 42 days (injection)	Increased fibromuscular tissue in prostate and seminal vesicle (greatest in cranial lobe)
Parkes & Zuckerman (1935)	10 mature rhesus/intact	estrogen/6-28 days (injection)	Dimunition in number of true prostatic glands increase in fibromuscular stroma & epithelia in uterus masculinus
Zuckerman (1938)	2 mature rhesus/castrate	estrogen/1 yr (injection)	Fibromuscular growth in utricular bed
Zuckerman & Sandys (1939)	6 juvenile rhesus/intact	estrogen/14-15 days (injection)	Increased size of total prostate with no change from normal in percentage of utricular, uretha, or glandular tissue
Chai et al. (1981)	4 mature baboons/intact	Diethylstilbesterol (oral, 5 mgm)/21 days	Reduction in total prostate weight, marked atrophy of caudal epithelial cell, fibromuscular stroma increased in cranial lobe

vacuoles were reduced but numerous inclusion bodies in lysosomes (2° lysosomes) appeared increased in number and were concentrated in the vicinity of Golgi complexes. Most significantly the fibromuscular stroma appeared to increase in mass in the cranial lobe only with resultant widening of spaces between adjacent acini.

Zuckerman and Parkes in 1936 (Zuckerman, Parkes 1936) gave androgens to six immature rhesus monkeys from 10 to 20 days. They reported rapid growth in the size of the prostate with increase in fibromuscular and glandular tissue in these immature animals with transformation to a mature type of prostate. In the same report Zuckerman and Parkes were able to block the effect of estrone injection by simultaneous androstanediol injection in three immature rhesus monkeys. In a later report Zuckerman and Sandys (1939) showed that testosterone increased the size of the whole prostate by increasing the size of the glandular zone and reducing the relative contribution of the urethra and utricular regions. This increase was only slightly more than in those treated with estrogen alone. (Table 4)

Karr and Murphy reported an increase in prostate weight (mainly caudal lobe) in six non-castrated mature baboons given 200 mg of testosterone enanthate for three to six months (Karr, Murphy 1983). They reported definite glandular and marked stromal hyperplasia with fibrosis of the caudal lobe. In contrast only glandular hyperplasia occurred in the cranial lobe with minimal or no effect on stromal tissue. Serum testosterone, dihydrotestosterone, androstanediol and estradiol-17ß were increased in these animals. Androgen receptor content was increased in the cytosol and decreased in the nuclei of both lobes of the animals. Scanning and transmission electromicroscopy revealed heavy deposition of collagen fibers (fibrosis) in the central and periureteral regions of the caudal lobe. (See discussion by Dr. Karr in this book).

In summary, in response to estrogen, fibromuscular hyperplasia appears to occur in the utricular region of immature non-castrated rhesus monkeys, and in the cranial lobe of mature non-castrated baboons. In contrast, testosterone and other androgens produce an increase in size of both caudal and cranial prostate in immature rhesus and mature baboons. Glandular hyperplasia occurs in both lobes of the prostate but stromal hyperplasia is seen in only the

Table 4. STUDIES OF EFFECTS OF ANDROGEN ON THE NONHUMAN PRIMATE PROSTATE

Study	Animal/Intact or Castrate	Hormone/Duration	Result
Zuckerman & Parkes (1936)	6 immature rhesus/intact	androsterone androstanediol (injection)/10-20 days	Rapid growth of prostate - transformation to "mature" prostate (fibromuscular & epithelial)
Zuckerman & Sandys (1939)	6 immature rhesus/intact	testosterone propionate (injection)/14 days	Increased size of prostate - primarily in glandular zone
Karr et al. (1983)	6 mature baboons/intact	testosterone enanthate (200 mgm weekly)/3-6 months (injection)	Total increase in prostate weight (most in caudal lobe), glandular & marked stromal hyperplasia (later fibrosis) of cranial lobe, glandular hyperplasia only in cranial lobe

caudal lobe of baboons treated with testosterone. A nonhuman primate model for benign prostatic hyperplasia is not yet available, but hormonal manipulation holds promise as a method to produce the disease

UROLOGICAL EVALUATION OF THE NONHUMAN PRIMATE

The size of the nonhuman primate and its physiologic similarity to man makes this animal an excellent choice of studies involving the genitourinary system. Evaluation of prostatic size can be accomplished by rectal examination of the gland while the animals are sedated. In addition, a rectal probe can easily be introduced for ultrasound evaluation of the prostate. We have used probes of similar size for electroejaculation for many years. In our current studies we have demonstrated that the space occupied by the prostate can be demonstrated by comparing retrograde urethrograms and voiding urethrograms (Fig. 6).

The effects of obstruction on the urinary system can be evaluated by several studies. We have used a quantitated radioscintillation camera study for determining effective renal plasma flow and excretion time of the nuclide by each kidney in many urological studies in the nonhuman primate. In particular, bladder neck obstruction has been created in some of our studies of vesicoureteral reflux and an obstructive picture of renal function has been shown by decreased effective renal plasma flow and increased time of excretion of the radionuclide by each kidney. In current studies we are able to measure intravesical pressure as the bladder is perfused suprapubically. We also are able to get a voiding flow rate as the sedated animal voids spontaneously after the bladder is adequately filled suprapubically. Each of these parameters are able to evaluate adequately the functional effects of urinary obstruction in the nonhuman primate if they are produced by experimentally induced BPH.

The cranial and caudal lobes of the prostate in the nonhuman primate is readily accessible for repeat open surgical biopsy without having to terminally sacrifice the animal.

In conclusion, the nonhuman primate is an excellent potential model for studies of BPH. There is a major need for studies to determine the natural occurrence of this disease in the older nonhuman primate. Clearly anatomical and biochemical studies have shown the great physiologic similarity of the nonhuman primate prostate to the prostate of man. Some preliminary studies have shown that hormonal manipulation in the nonhuman primate produces anatomic changes similar to BPH in man. The nonhuman primate can be studied by every diagnostic test used in man for the evaluation of BPH.

ACKNOWLEDGMENT

Supported by USPHS grant 5 P06 RR 00164-19 and NIH grants 5 T32 AM 07212-03 and 5 S07 RR0544417.

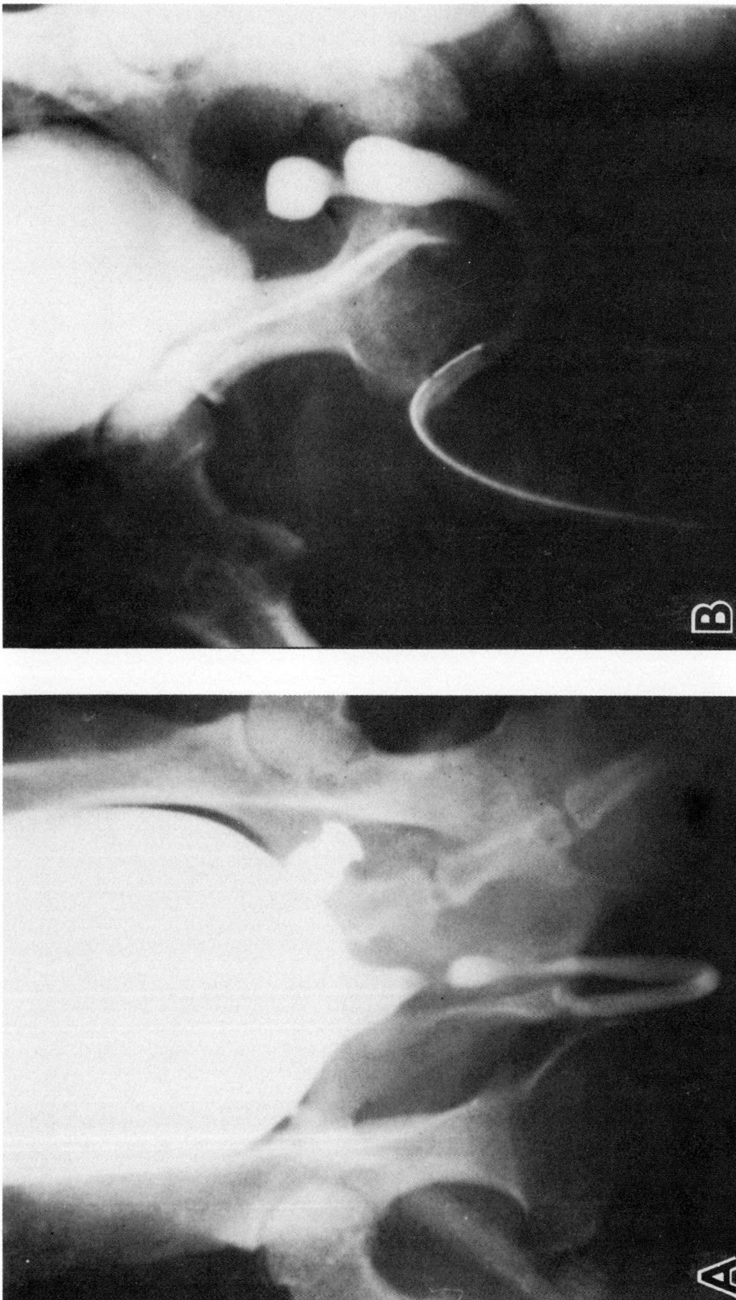

Fig. 6.- Voiding urethrogram (A) and retrograde urethrogram (B) in a cynomolgus monkey (*Macaca fascicularis*).

Adams MR, Bond MG (1979). Benign prostatic hyperplasia in a squirrel monkey (*Saimiri sciureus*). Lab Anim Sci 29: 674.

Blacklock NJ, Bouskill V (1977). The zonal anatomy of the prostate in man and in the rhesus monkey (*Macaca mulatta*). Urol Res 5:163.

Chai LS, Karr JP, Murphy GP, Sandberg AA (1981). Effect of DES on the morphology of the lobes of the baboon prostate. Invest Urol 19:202.

Fox H (1923). "Diseases in Captive Wild Mammals and Birds." Philadelphia: Lippincott, p 314.

Ghanadian R (1981). Androgen regulation in the prostate of rhesus monkey (*Macaca mulatta*). In Hafez ESE, Sprug-Nile E (eds): "Próstate Carcinoma - Biology and Diagnosis," Boston: Martinus Nishoff Publishers, p 160.

Ghanadian R, Smith CB (1981). Androgen metabolism within the lobes of rhesus monkey prostate. Eur Urol 7:89.

Ghanadian R, Auf G, Smith CB, Chisholm GD, Blacklock NJ (1977a). Androgen receptors in the prostate of the rhesus monkey. Urol Res 5:169.

Ghanadian R, Smith CB, Chisholm GS, Blacklock NJ (1977b). Differential androgen uptake by the lobes of the rhesus monkey prostate. Brit J Urol 49:701.

Greer WE, Roussel JD, Austin CR (1968). Prevention of coagulation in monkey semen by surgery. J Reprod Fertil 15:153.

Johnston GS, Gibbons RP, Schmidt JD, Murphy GP, Scott WW (1966). Fluid and tissue kinetics of ^{65}zinc in the dog and monkey. Invest Urol 3:419.

Kaack B, Lewis RW, Resnick MI, Roberts JA (in press). Biochemistry of the nonhuman primate prostate and seminal vesicles. I. Some chemical parameters. Arch Androl.

Karr JP, Sufrin G, Kirdoni RY, Murphy GP, Sandberg AA (1978). Prostatic binding of oestradiol 17β in the baboon. J Steroid Biochem 9:87.

Karr JP, Kirdani RY, Murphy GP, Sandberg AA (1979). The baboon prostate as a model for steroid hormone receptors in the human gland. In Murphy GP, Sandberg AA (eds): "Prostate Cancer and Hormone Receptors," New York: Alan R Liss, p 165.

Karr JP, Murphy GP (1983). Cellular growth and hormone receptor. In Hinman F Jr (ed): "Benign Prostatic Hypertrophy," New York: Springer Verlag, p 193.

Kirchheim D (1983). Histochemistry. In Hinman F Jr (ed): "Benign Prostatic Hypertrophy," New York: Springer-Verlag, p 90.

Lewis RW, Kim JCS, Irani D, Roberts JA (1981). The prostate of the nonhuman primate: normal anatomy and pathology. The Prostate 2:51.

Lewis RW, Resnick MI, Kaack B, Roberts JA (in press). Biochemistry of the nonhuman primate prostate and seminal vesicles. II. Molecular weights of soluble proteins. Arch Androl.

McNeal JE (1968). Regional morphology and pathology of the prostate. Am J Clin Pathol 49:347.

McNeal JE (1983). Relationship of the origin of benign prostatic hypertrophy to prostate structure of man and other mammals. In Hinman F Jr (ed): "Benign Prostatic Hypertrophy," New York: Springer-Verlag, p 152.

Miralgia T, Telles FM, Branco AL (1970). The male reproductive system of the common marmoset (*Callithrix jacchus*). Acta Anat 76:594.

Muntzing J, Myhrberg H, Saroff T, Sandberg AA, Murphy GP (1976). Histochemical and ultrastructural study of prostatic tissue from baboons treated with antiprostatic drug. Invest Urol 14:162.

Parkes AS, Zuckerman S (1935). Experimental hyperplasia of the prostate. Lancet 1:925.

Price D (1963). Comparative aspects of development and structure in the prostate. Natl Cancer Inst Monogr 12:1.

Roberts JA (1972). The male genital system. In Fiennes RNT-W (ed): " Pathology of Simian Primates," Basel: S Karger, p 878.

Schoones R, DeKlerk JN (1968). Anatomy, radioisotopic blood flow and glandular secretory activity of the baboon prostate. S Afr Med J (Suppl) 42:87.

Schoones R, DeKlerk JN, Murphy GP (1969). Correlation of prostatic blood flow with ^{65}zinc activity in intact, castrated and testosterone-treated baboons. Invest Urol 6: 476.

Schoonees R, DeKlerk JN, Mirand EA, Murphy GP (1970). The effect of bovine growth hormone on zinc-65 metabolism and prostatic blood flow of intact, testosterone treated, and castrated adult male chacma baboons. Invest Urol 8:103.

Van Wagenen G (1936). The coagulating function of the cranial lobe of the prostate gland in the monkey. Anat Rec 66:411.

Van Wagenen G (1935). The effects of oestrin on the genital tract of the male monkey. Anat Rec 63:387.

Wilson JD (1980). The pathogenesis of benign prostatic hyperplasia. Am J Med 68:745.

Zuckerman S, Parkes AS (1936). Effects of sex hormones on

the prostate of monkeys. Lancet 230:242.
Zuckerman S (1938). The effects of prolonged oestrogenic stimulation of the prostate of the rhesus monkey. J Anat 72:264.
Zuckerman S, Sandys OC (1939). Further observations on the effects of sex hormones on the prostate and seminal vesicles of monkeys. J Anat 73:597.

Discussion

McNeal: I would like to comment on your statement that man and the dog are the only species with spontaneously occurring benign prostatic hyperplasia. Although other species haven't shown it so far, there are an awful lot of species that haven't been looked at.

New Approaches to the Study of Benign Prostatic Hyperplasia, pages 257–289

BENIGN PROSTATIC HYPERPLASIA IN THE BABOON

James P. Karr, Ph.D., Untae Kim, M.D., Gerald P. Murphy, M.D.,D.Sc. and Avery A. Sandberg, M.D.
Departments of Experimental Surgery, Pathology and Genetics and Endocrinology
Roswell Park Memorial Institute
Buffalo, New York 14263 (USA)

INTRODUCTION

Because of the phylogenetic proximity of primates to man (Washburn 1982), the baboon has certain anatomical and physiological features which allow investigators to more readily extend their research findings to the human. For this reason, a colony of baboons (Papio cynocephalus) has been maintained for biomedical research at Roswell Park Memorial Institute (RPMI) for nearly 15 years. Baboons had been used extensively for drug and steroid metabolism studies at RPMI, and, in recent years, studies of prostatic biochemistry have suggested the relevance of this species as a model for studying human BPH (Karr et al 1983). The baboon, belongs to those species of primates classified as New World Monkeys, and thus has certain behavioral and postural characteristics which are indeed remarkably human-like in nature. For example, in order to accommodate the natural preference of baboons to sit and stand upright, and to even practice bipedalism on occasions, Federal regulations stipulate that baboon cages be constructed in such a manner as to allow the animal ample room to stand in an erect position. Whether such postural characteristics of the baboon are relevant to the usefulness of this species as a model for studies of BPH is not known. Nevertheless, we present in this chapter our findings that the hormonal induction of BPH in the baboon also causes urethral obstruction, as determined through urodynamic analyses performed on the baboons supported in a sitting position.

Gross and Microscopy Anatomy

Figure 1 is a dorsal or posterior view of the prostate and adjacent structures which were removed en bloc from an adult baboon. The prostate consists of two discrete structures, the cranial and caudal lobes, which are closely bound together and partly fused and enclosed by a thin condensation of endopelvic fascia (Schoonees 1968). The seminal vesicles in the baboon are large and the cranial lobe, which lies above and behind the caudal lobe, is superficially lobulated. The caudal prostate is comprised of two well defined and prominent lateral lobes which lie mainly dorsolateral to the posterior urethra. These prominent lobes are joined together on the dorsal side of the prostate by a narrow dorsal isthmus of caudal prostatic tissue which is also fused at this point to the cranial lobe of the prostate. Note the shallow dorsal median groove and that one can readily visualize the line of demarcation through which the caudal and cranial lobes are easily separated with blunt dissection. Figure 1 also illustrates the well developed bulbourethral glands of the baboon reproductive tract.

In cross section (Figure 2), the compact caudal prostate lobes are seen to have a granular appearance and yellow pigmentation, which is in contrast to the white and vesiculated appearance of the cranial prostate. The cranial prostate, which is principally related to the posterior wall of the urethra above the level of the verumontanum, is cone-shaped extending from the verumontanum in a dorso-cranial direction towards the base of the bladder. The ejaculatory ducts (not shown) are completely surrounded by cranial prostate throughout their course and open on the verumontanum along with caudal and cranial prostatic ducts. Note that the verumontanum appears as a conical elevation on the posterior urethra wall and that a small utricle can be seen at the apex of the verumontanum (Schoonees 1971).

The fibromuscular stroma is well developed in both the cranial and caudal lobes of the baboon prostate (Figures 3 and 4), but note that the acini are generally larger and more irregular in shape in the cranial lobe than are those of the caudal prostate. The glands of both lobes are lined with a simple columnar epithelium with a well defined basement membrane. Moreover, in the normal adult baboon, the ratio of fibromuscular stroma to the glandular tissue is greater in the caudal than the cranial prostate (Schoonees et al 1968; Muntzing 1976; Chai et al 1981). Ongoing

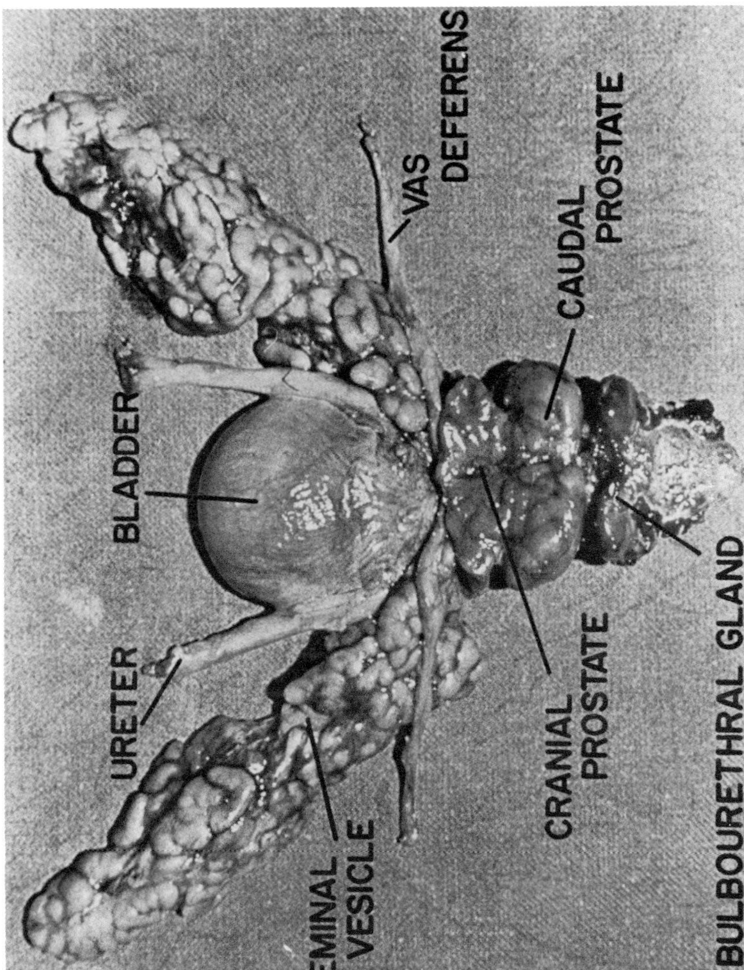

Figure 1. Dorsal view of the adult baboon prostate.

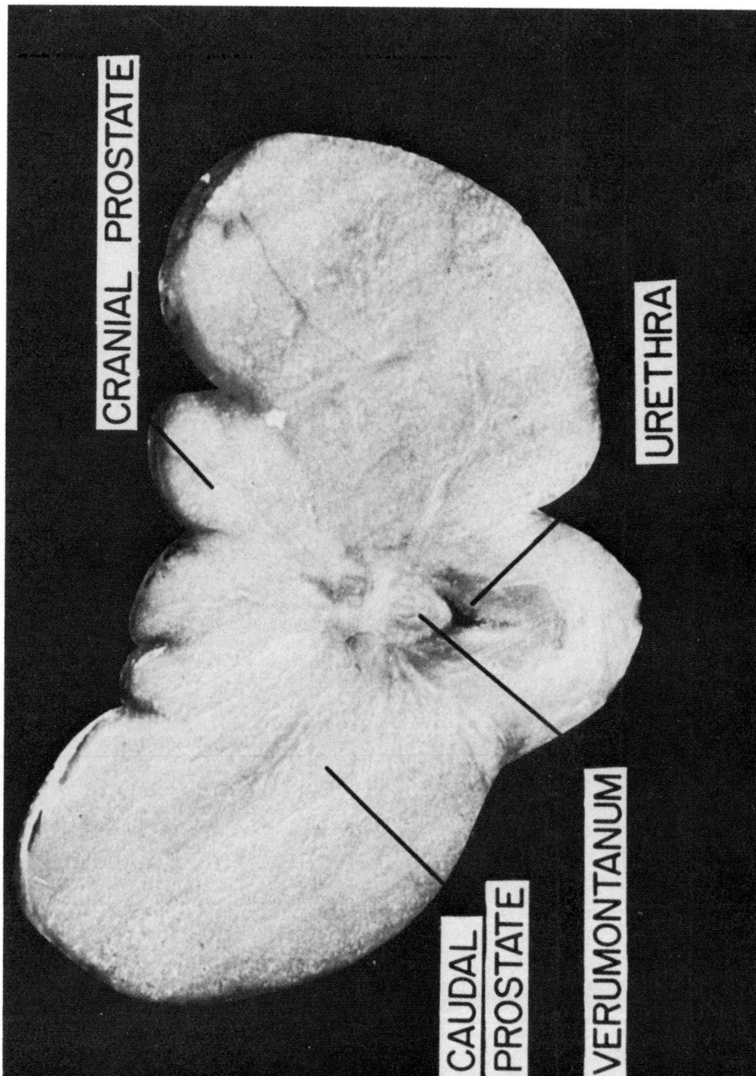

Figure 2. Cross section of the baboon prostate.

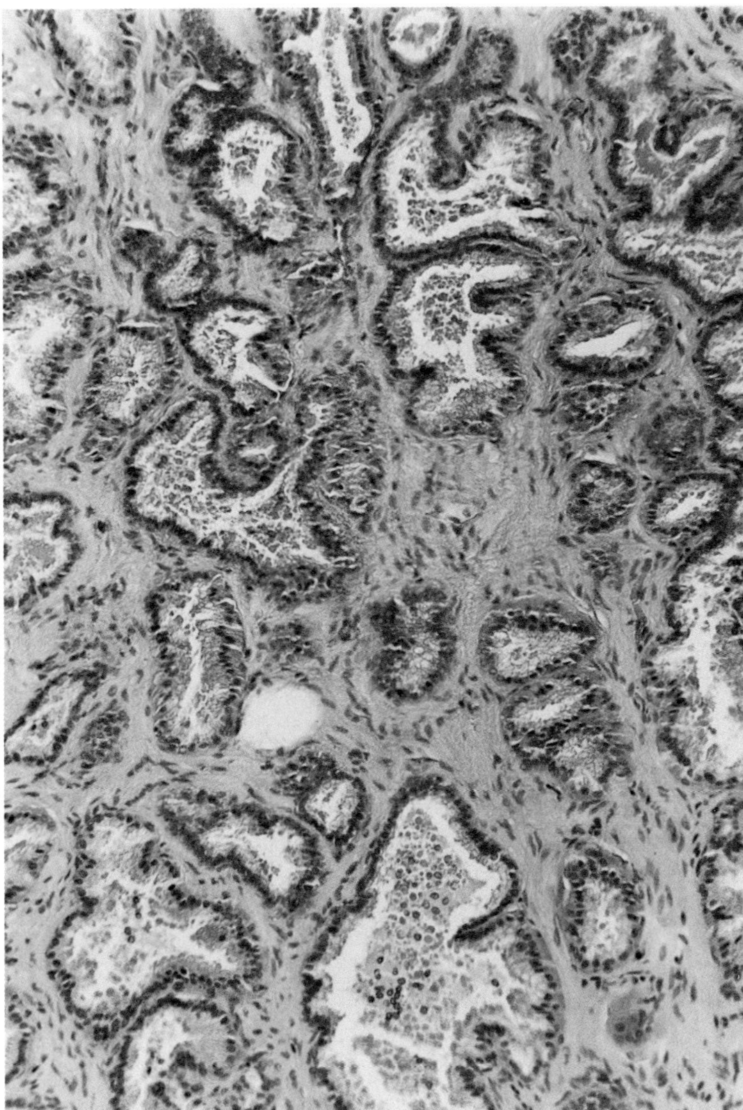

Figure 3. Cranial prostate of the noncastrated baboon, 160x.

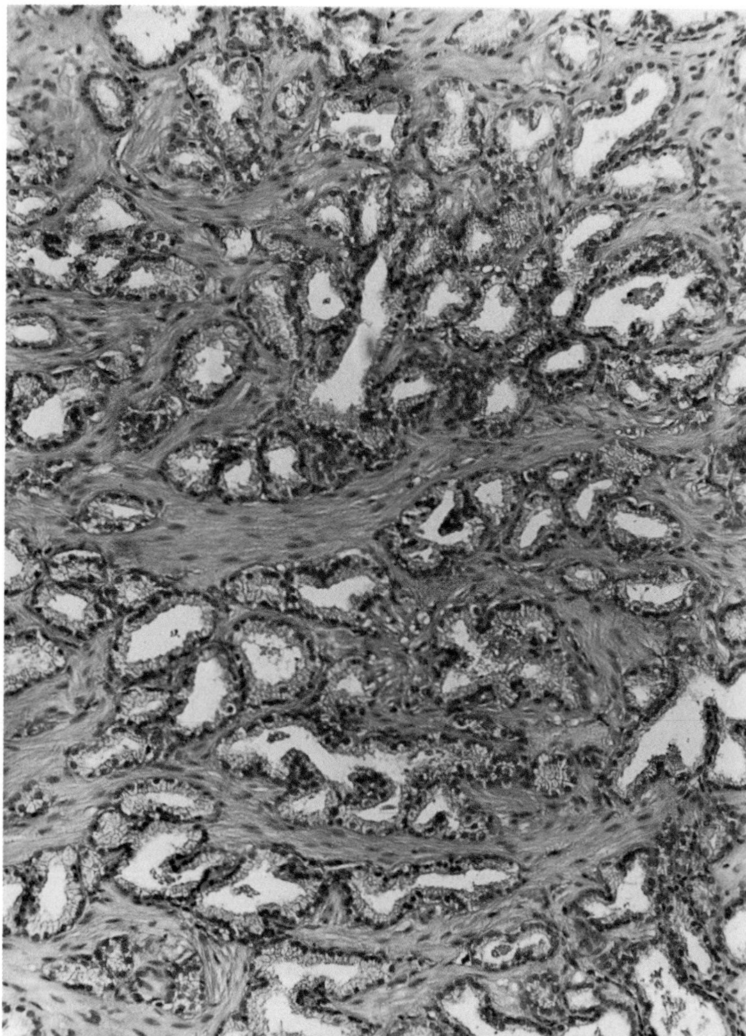

Figure 4. Caudal prostate of the noncastrated baboon, 160x.

quantitative morphometric and stereological studies of baboon prostates (Rohr 1980), have been undertaken to determine whether such detailed analyses of step sections will reveal zonal or regional differences in the relative amounts of stromal and epithelial tissue within the caudal and cranial lobes. Identification of distinct histologic differences in specimens obtained from different portions of the baboon prostate lobes would indeed bring to mind the distinct histologic differences associated with the zonal anatomy of the human prostate, as reported by McNeal (1981).

Hormonal Induction of BPH

We have recently reported (Karr et al 1983) the results of our induction of prostatic hyperplasia in noncastrated adult male baboons with the long-acting androgen, testosterone enanthate (TE, 200mg i.m./week). Eight adult males (six treated, two controls) were treated for up to 28 weeks with TE or vehicle only. At the beginning of the study and every two weeks thereafter serum samples were collected for determination of steroid hormone levels. Baboons are safe to handle when tranquilized with ketamine hydrochloride (5-7.5mg/kg i.m.) and valium (diazepam, 5-10mg, i.v.). Plasma testosterone (T) and dihydrotestosterone (DHT) were maintained at high levels in the TE injected baboons during the duration of the study. The control levels were in the range of 10 ng/ml for T and 2-3 ng/ml for DHT, whereas the levels of these steroids in the baboons treated with TE were 30-40 ng/ml and 5-6 ng/ml, respectively. Moreover, there was a 3-4 fold increase in androstenedione levels in the treated baboons, with the control values ranging between 0.5 and 1 mg/ml versus plasma concentrations of 3-4 ng/ml in the treated animals. Probably the most important change in plasma steroid levels with regard to the induction of BPH was the remarkable increase in plasma 17β-estradiol (E_2), the levels of which increased from 20 pg/ml in the control animals to 80-90 pg/ml in the TE treated baboons. It is known from other studies that aromatization of androstenediol and T to estrone in peripheral tissue in man accounts for up to 90% of the estrogen available to the prostate (Bullough 1965; Hemsell et al 1974; Kley et al 1974; Zumoff et al 1976). The high concentrations of plasma E_2 in the androgen stimulated baboons undoubtedly plays an important role in the induction of the histologically defined BPH after relatively short treatment periods, i.e. no longer than six months.

Stromal and Glandular Hyperplasia in the Baboon Prostate

A convincing and useful animal model for studies of human BPH should share several fundamental features in common with the human condition, not the least of which is histologic evidence of a hyperplastic condition in terms of both stromal and glandular proliferation. For the purpose of comparative illustration, the predominant histologic characteristics which are typical of human BPH are shown in Figures 5-8. Figure 5 illustrates the crowding and tortuous appearance of the glandular acini that is characteristic of the glandular hyperplasia seen in human BPH. The hyperplastic glands of human BPH are frequently outlined by stromal fibrosis giving the proliferating glands a nodular appearance (Figure 6). In 1980, Rohr and Bartsch reported that human BPH, when assessed with quantitative morphologic techniques, appears to be a stromal disease, with the stromal component accounting for 60% of the volume density of the gland as compared to 45% in the normal gland. Thus, as shown in Figures 7 and 8, human BPH is a condition that is typified by marked proliferation of the fibromuscular stroma. By way of comparison, Figures 9-12 are photomicrographs of specimens removed from the prostates of noncastrated male baboons which were chronically treated with testosterone enanthate. Figure 9 is from a section of the caudal lobe following 15 weeks of treatment. Note that the marked glandular hyperplasia with crowding of the glandular acini bears a remarkable resemblance to the glandular features of human BPH illustrated in Figure 5. Figure 10 is a photomicrograph of caudal prostate after 20 weeks of TE treatment and this Figure, when compared to Figure 9, indicates that stromal fibrosis has become a more noticeable feature of the caudal lobe. At the same time, as illustrated in Figure 11, there is a manifestation of a marked epithelial hyperplasia as evidenced by crowding of the columnar epithelial cells linings the acini, giving the appearance of pseudostratification and some nuclear hyperchromatism and/or atypia. Note that similar areas are seen in human BPH (Figure 6). After 28 weeks of testosterone enanthate treatment (Figure 12) there is considerably more stromal fibrosis, such that there is an uncanny similarity of human BPH and the caudal lobe of the TE treated baboon with regard to the histological manifestation of the disease.

Ultrastructural changes were also prominent after six months of TE treatment. Figure 13 is an example of caudal prostate from a control animal and illustrates that secretory

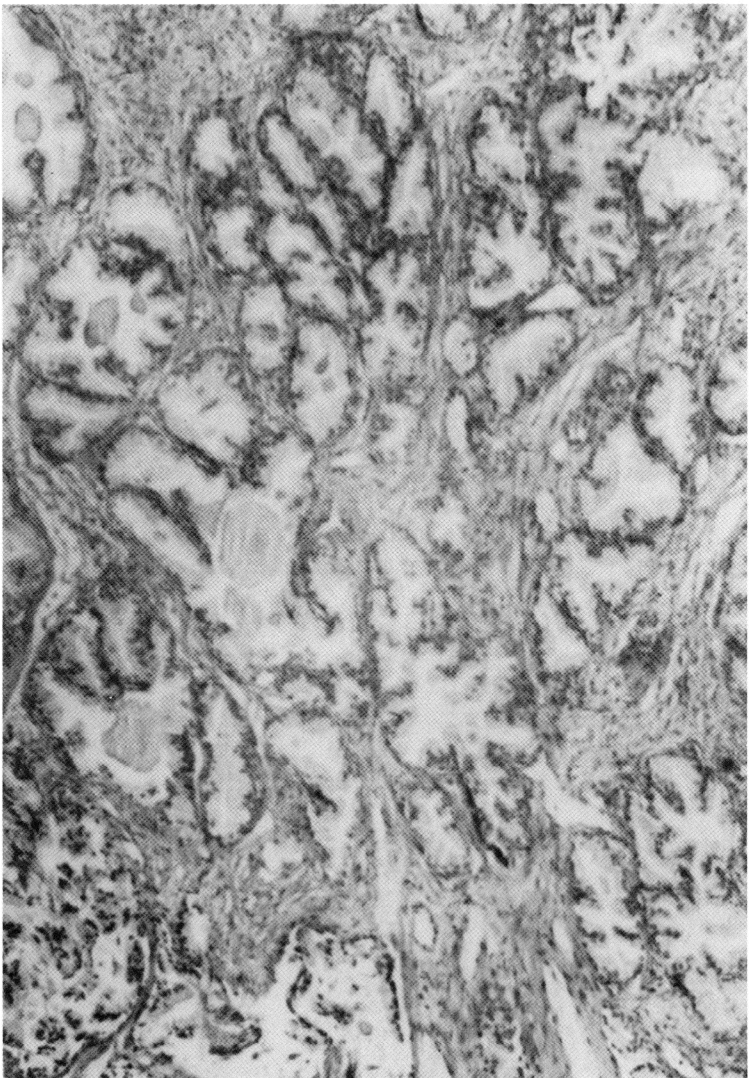

Figure 5. Glandular hyperplasia of human BPH.

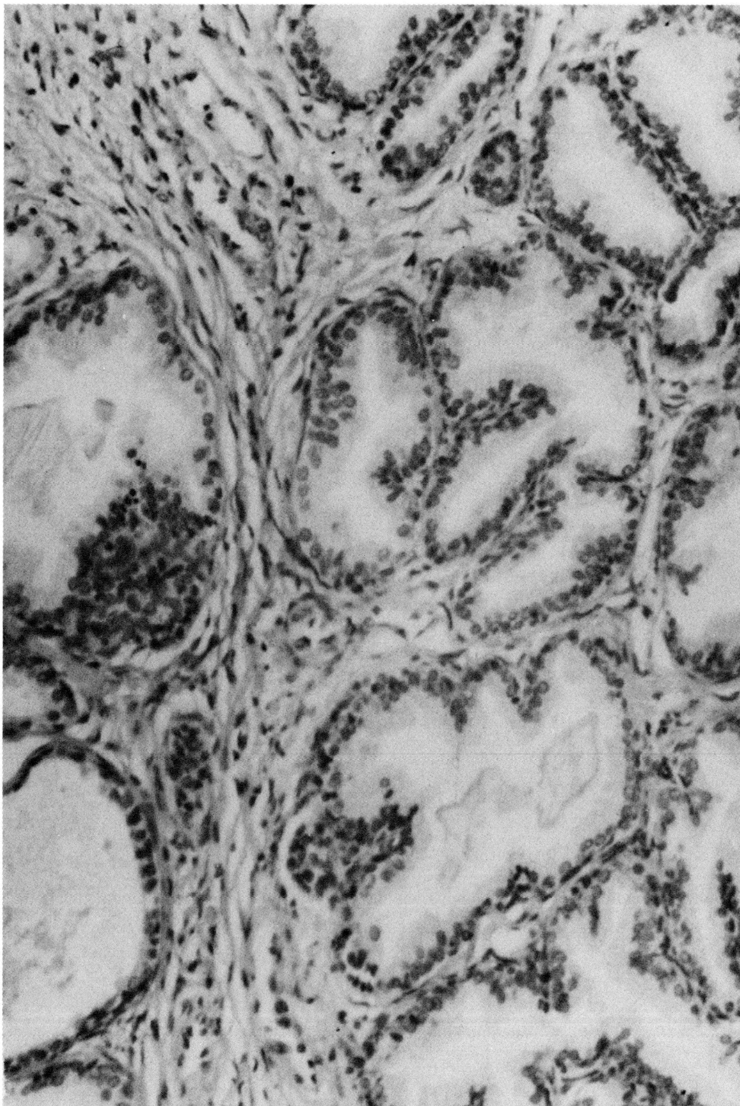

Figure 6. Stromal fibrosis and glandular nodularility of human BPH.

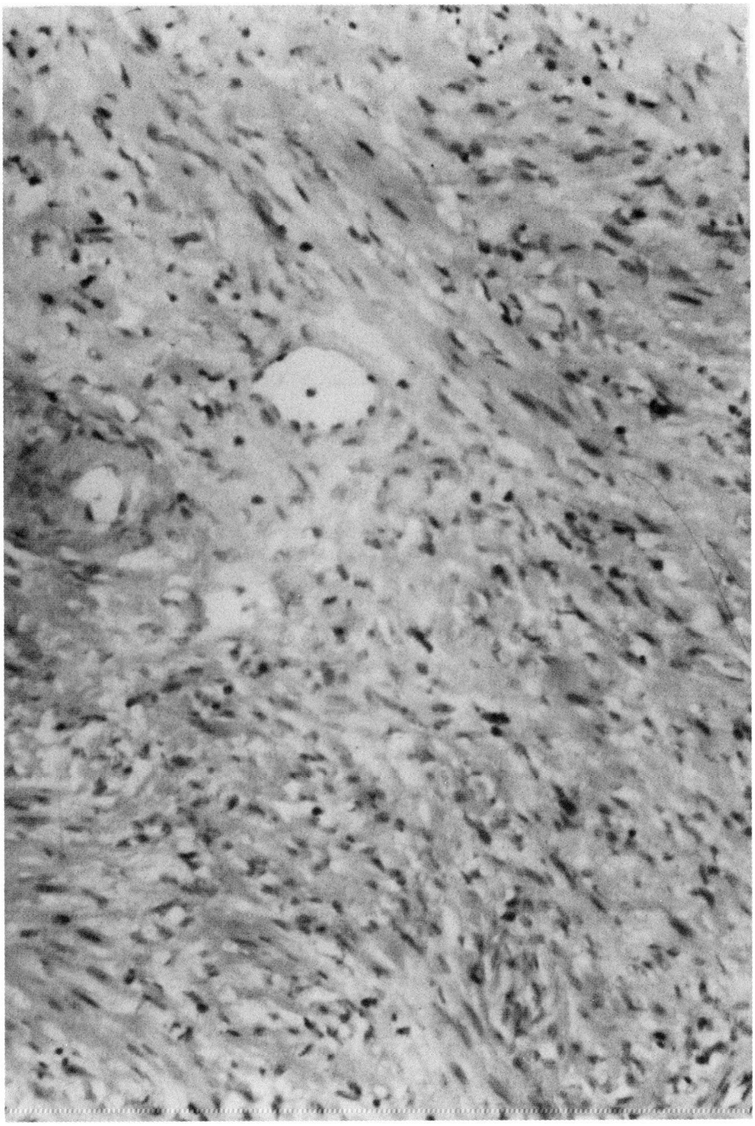

Figure 7. Stromal proliferation in human BPH, low power.

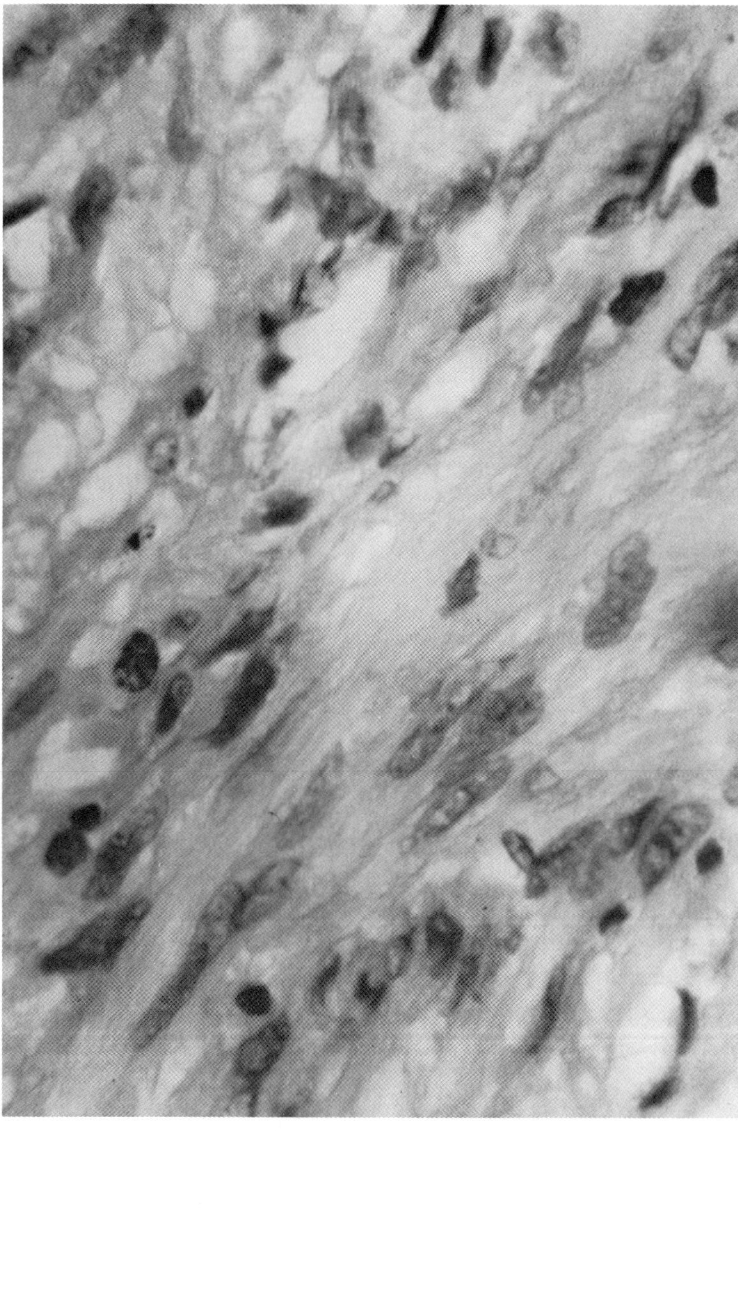

Figure 8. Fibromuscular stroma of human BPH, high power.

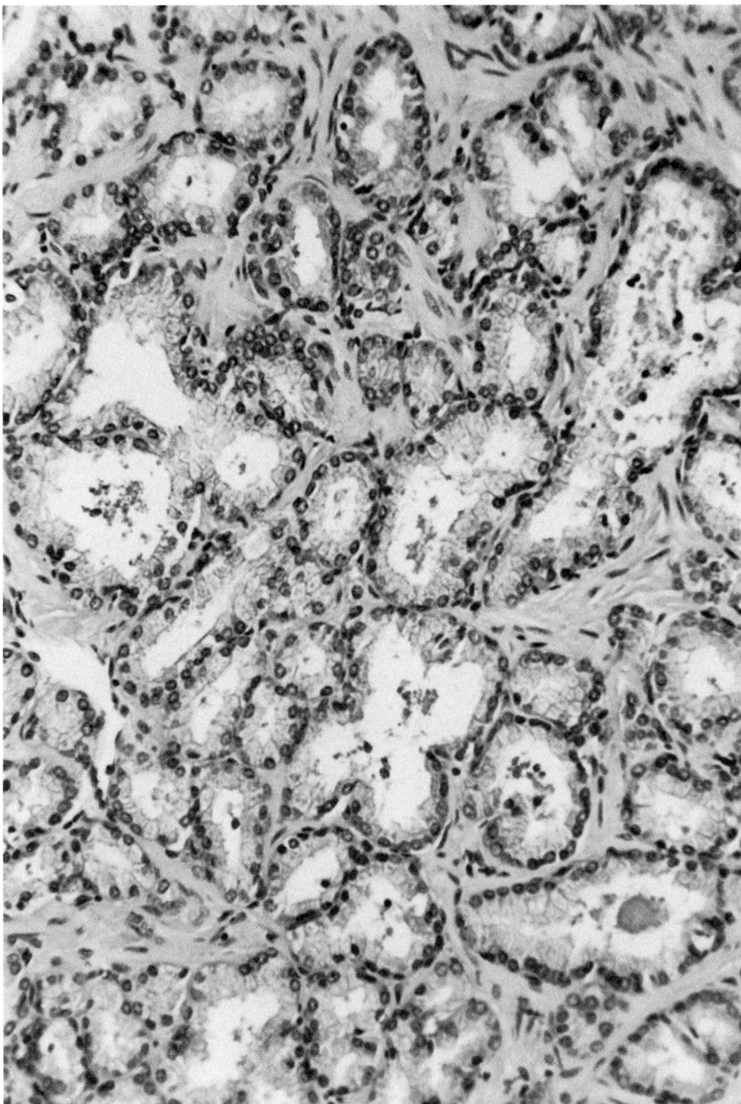

Figure 9. Glandular hyperplasia in baboon BPH.

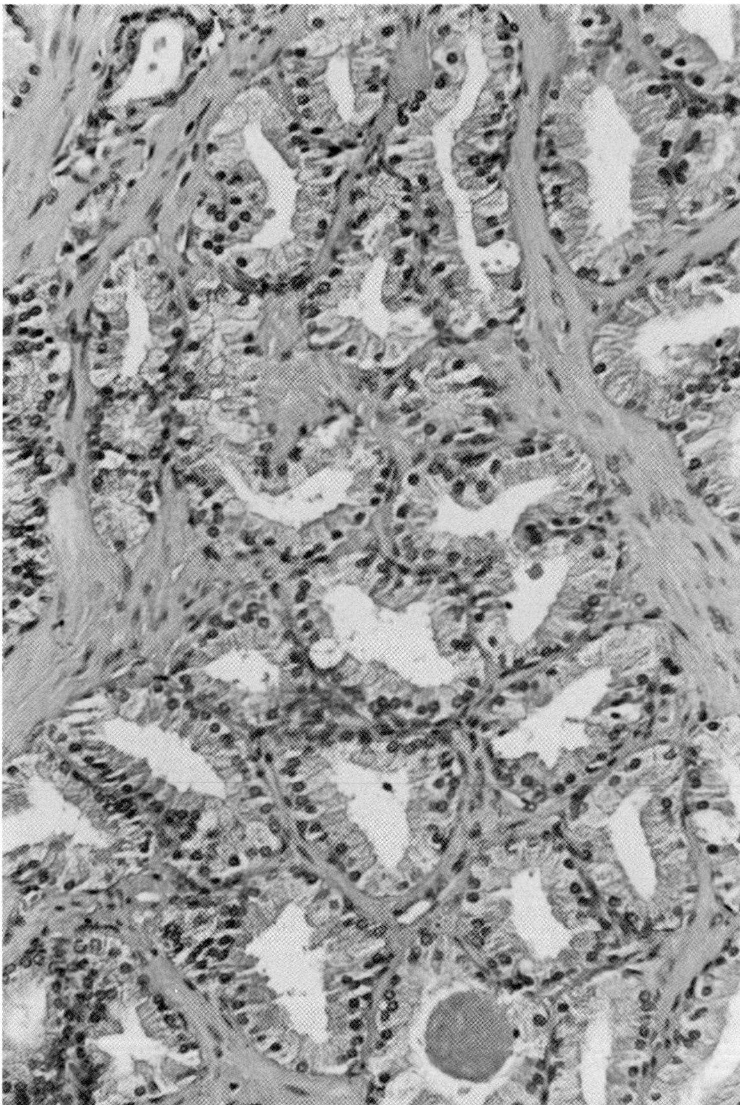

Figure 10. Stromal fibrosis in baboon BPH.

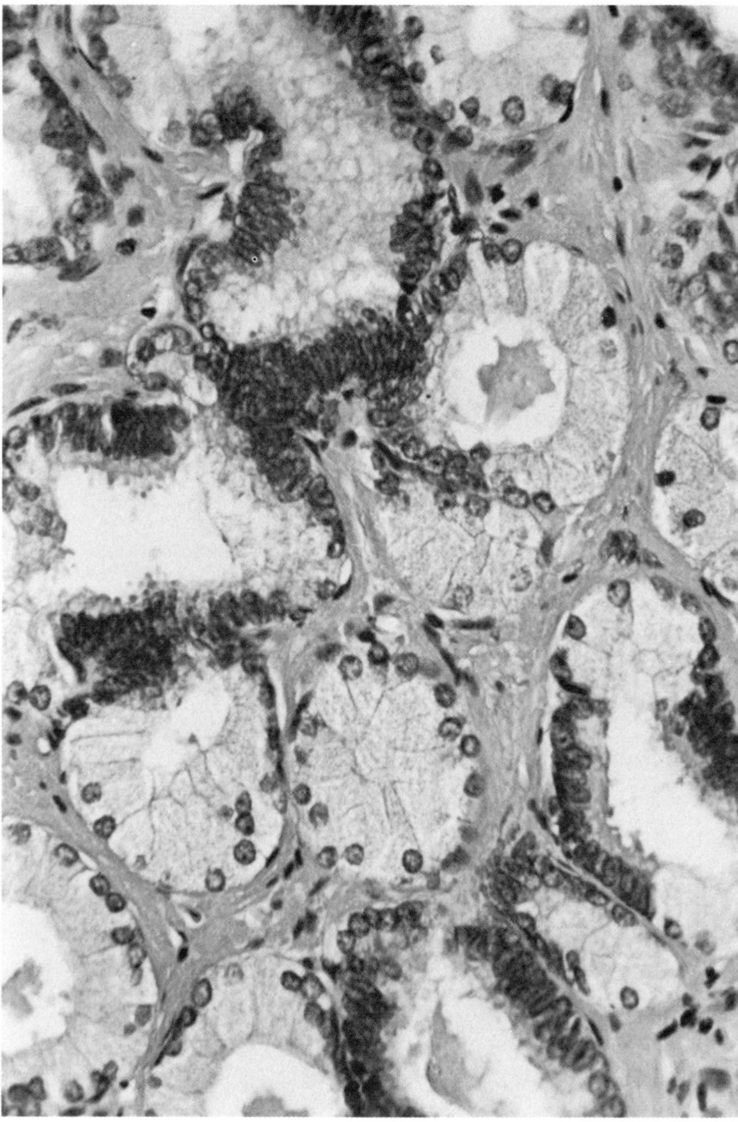

Figure 11. Epithelial hyperplasia in baboon BPH.

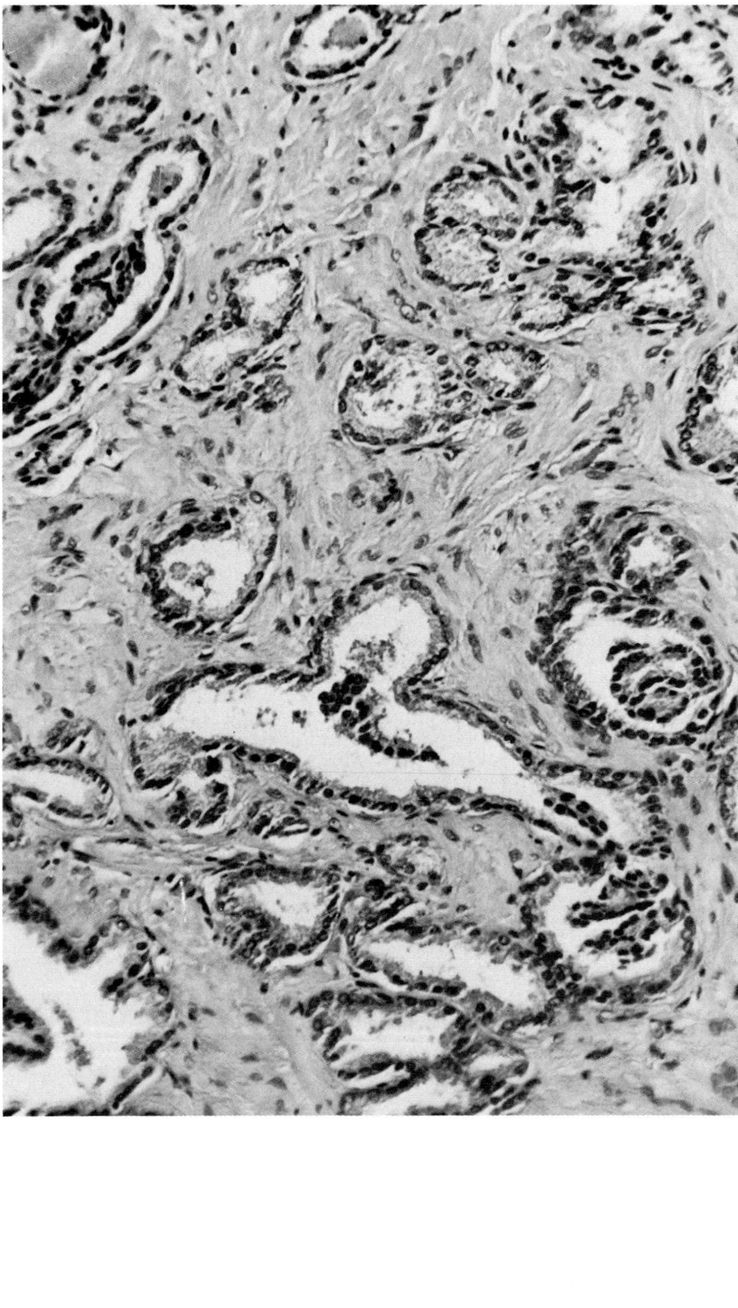

Figure 12. Stromal hyperplasia and glandular nodularity in baboon BPH.

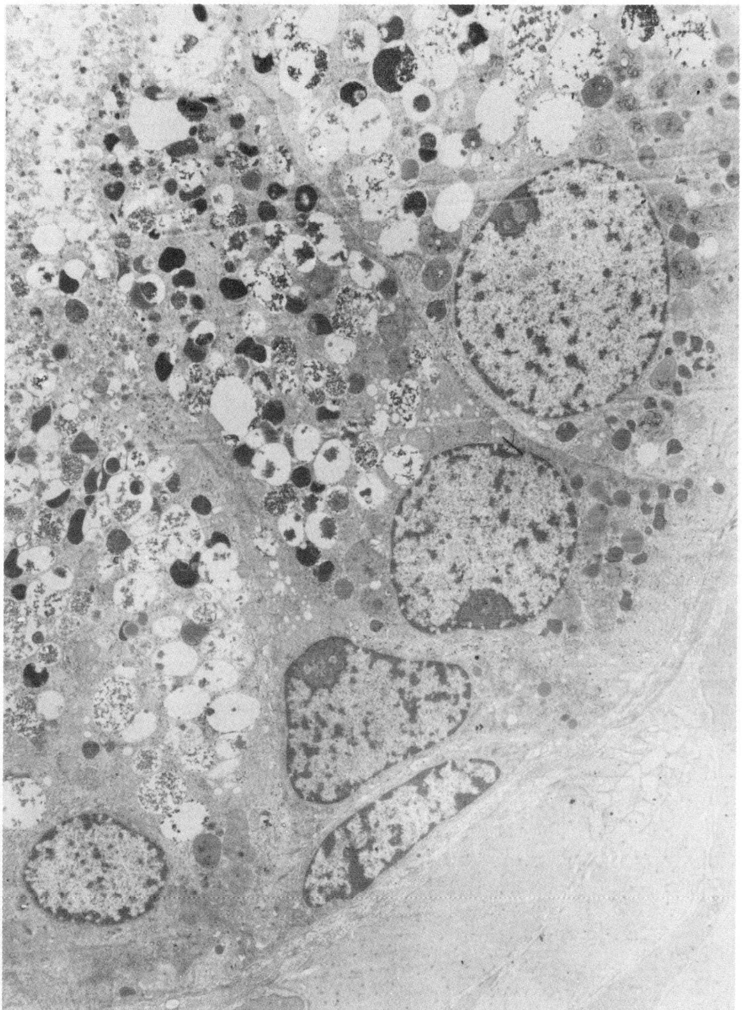

Figure 13. Ultrastructure of normal cadual prostate, 6000x.

granules and vacuoles are abundant, and that the nucleus is generally round and that the basal cells, connective tissues, and muscle cells appear to be intact. After six months of treatment, the glandular epithelial cells of the caudal lobe appear to be disrupted, having electron dense irregularly shaped nuclei as well as electron dense granular-like structures in the cytoplasm (Figure 14). Moreover, as illustrated in Figure 15, there is a particularly prominent increase in the amount of stromal elements and decreased secretory activity of the caudal lobe, and while there was an increase in connective tissue in some areas, the connective tissue in order areas appeared to be disorganized. This distortion and expansion of the connective tissue undoubtedly effects the organization of the glandular elements (Figure 16). Scanning electron microscopy also revealed some interesting changes. For example, when compared with a representative section of the caudal lobe of a control baboon (Figure 17), after four months of TE treatment one can see areas of glandular and epithelial hyperplasia, as seen in Figure 18, which illustrates the epithelial lining of a section taken from the peripheral zone of the caudal lobes as being arranged in a tightly packed cobblestone pattern. In contrast, a heavy deposition of collagen fibers or fibrosis was noted in specimens taken from the central and periurethral regions of the caudal lobes (Figure 19).

Prostatic Weight and Volume

The gross effects of TE on the baboon prostate were evidenced quantitatively in terms of both volumetric and gravimetric increases measured in the caudal and cranial lobes at the end of the 6-month period of study. The caudal lobe contributed more to the increases recorded than did the cranial lobe. The mean weight of the caudal lobes from the two control animals were 3.4 grams, whereas the mean weight of the caudal lobes from two animals each treated with TE for 3, 4.5, and 6 months were 6.7, 5.8 and 5.2 grams, respectively. In contrast, the mean cranial lobe weight of the two control animals was 2.5 grams as compared to mean cranial weights of 3.1, 2.4, and 3.6 grams, respectively, following 3, 4.5 and 6 months of TE treatment. Similar increases in volume, as determined by fluid displacement, were measured in both prostatic lobes. Obviously, the apparent differences in the volume and weights measured in

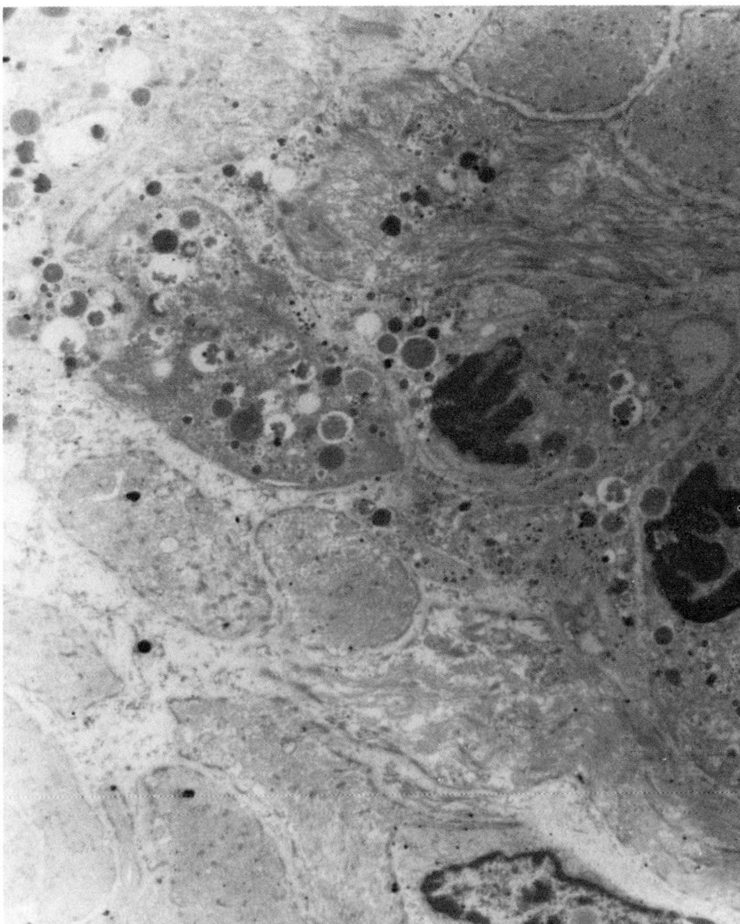

Figure 14. Electron micrograph of disrupted glandular epithelial cells in baboon BPH.

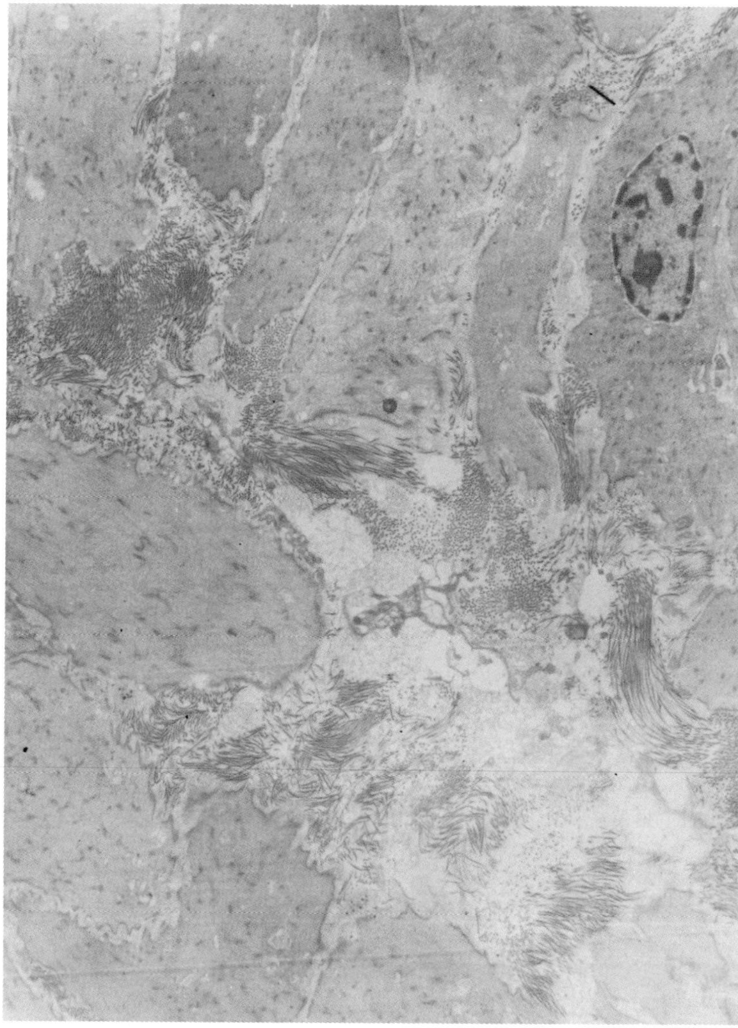

Figure 15. Electron micrograph showing proliferation of fibromuscular elements in baboon BPH.

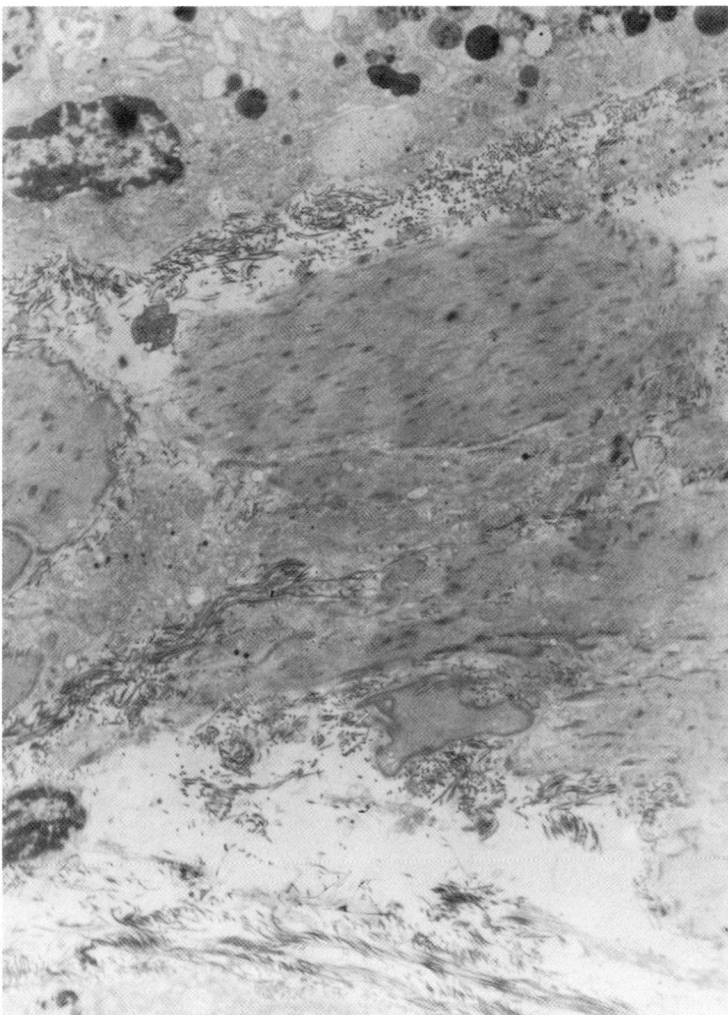

Figure 16. Electron micrograph illustrating the expansion of connective tissue elements in baboon BPH.

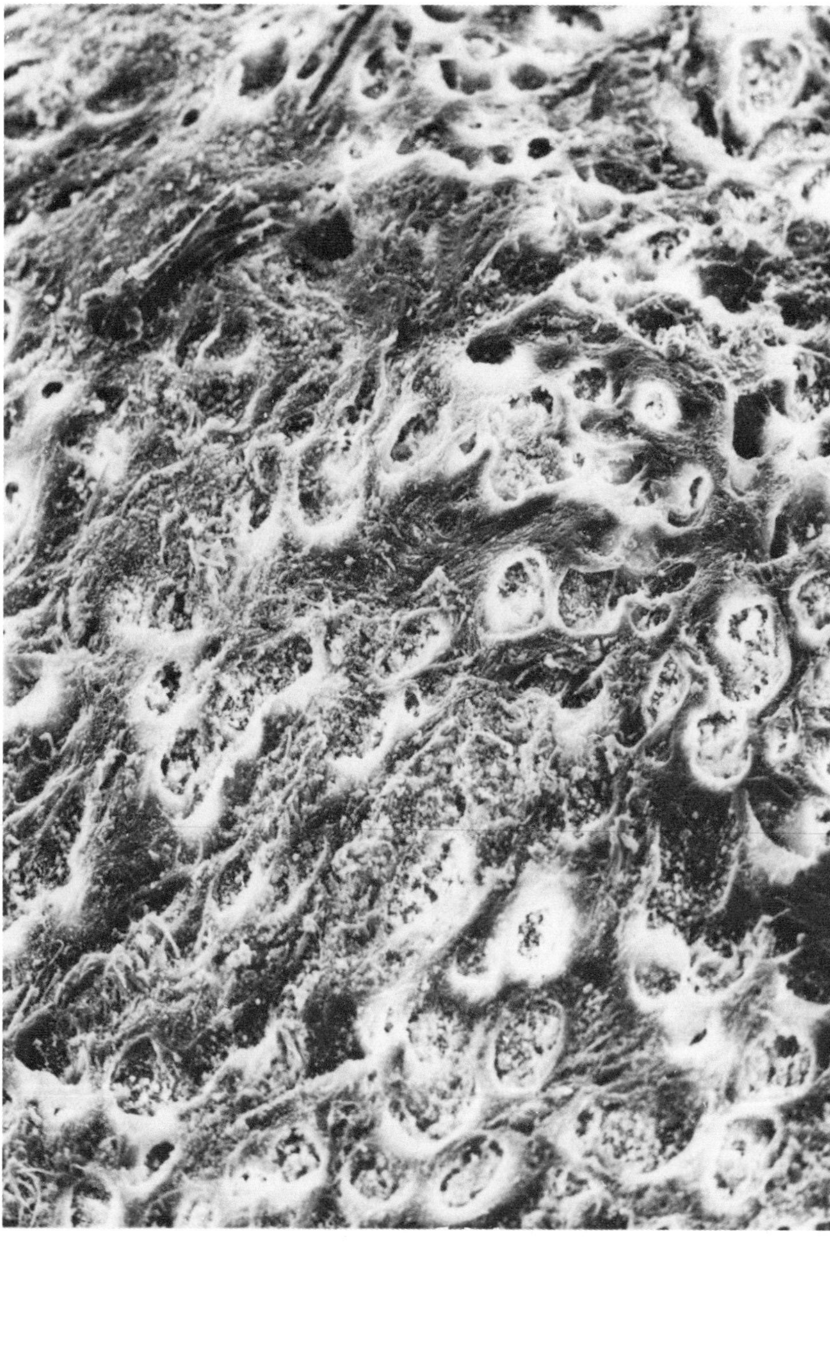

Figure 17. Scanning electron micrograph of the caudal prostate of a noncastrated baboon.

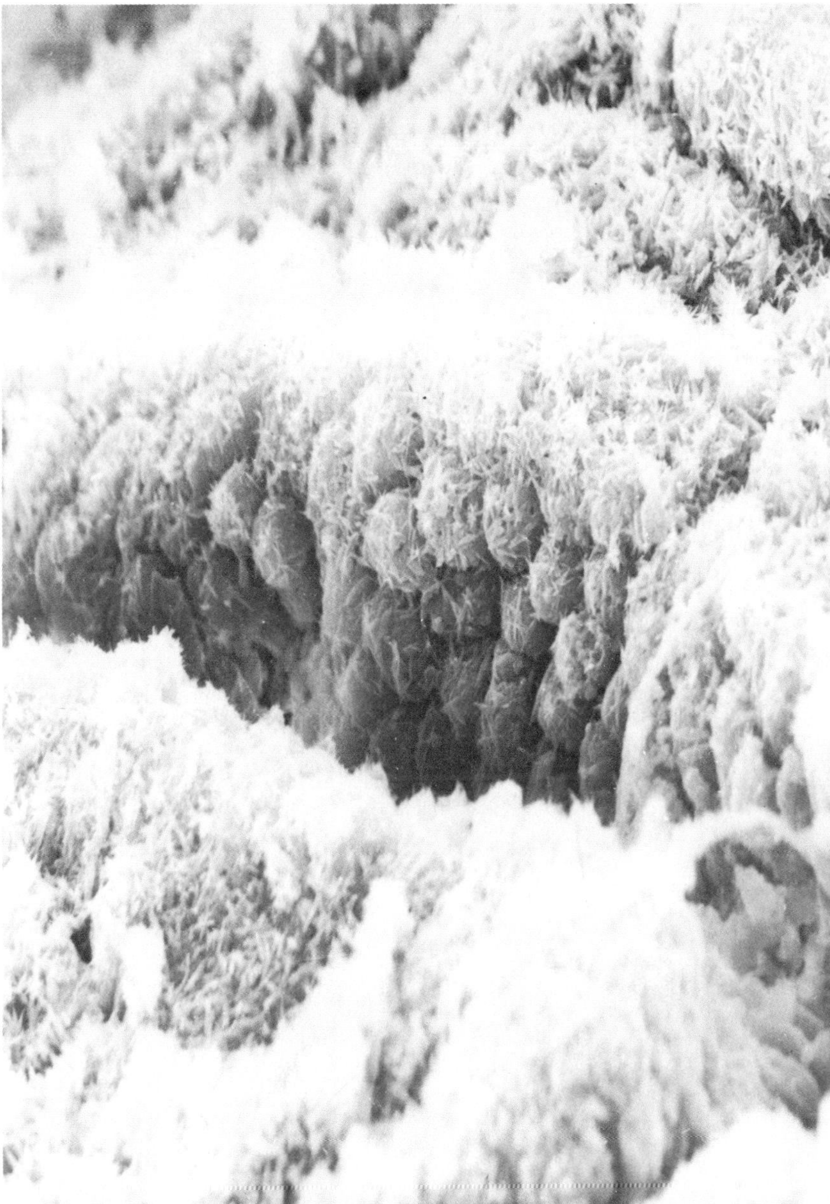

Figure 18. Scanning electron micrograph of glandular and epithelial hyperplasia in baboon BPH.

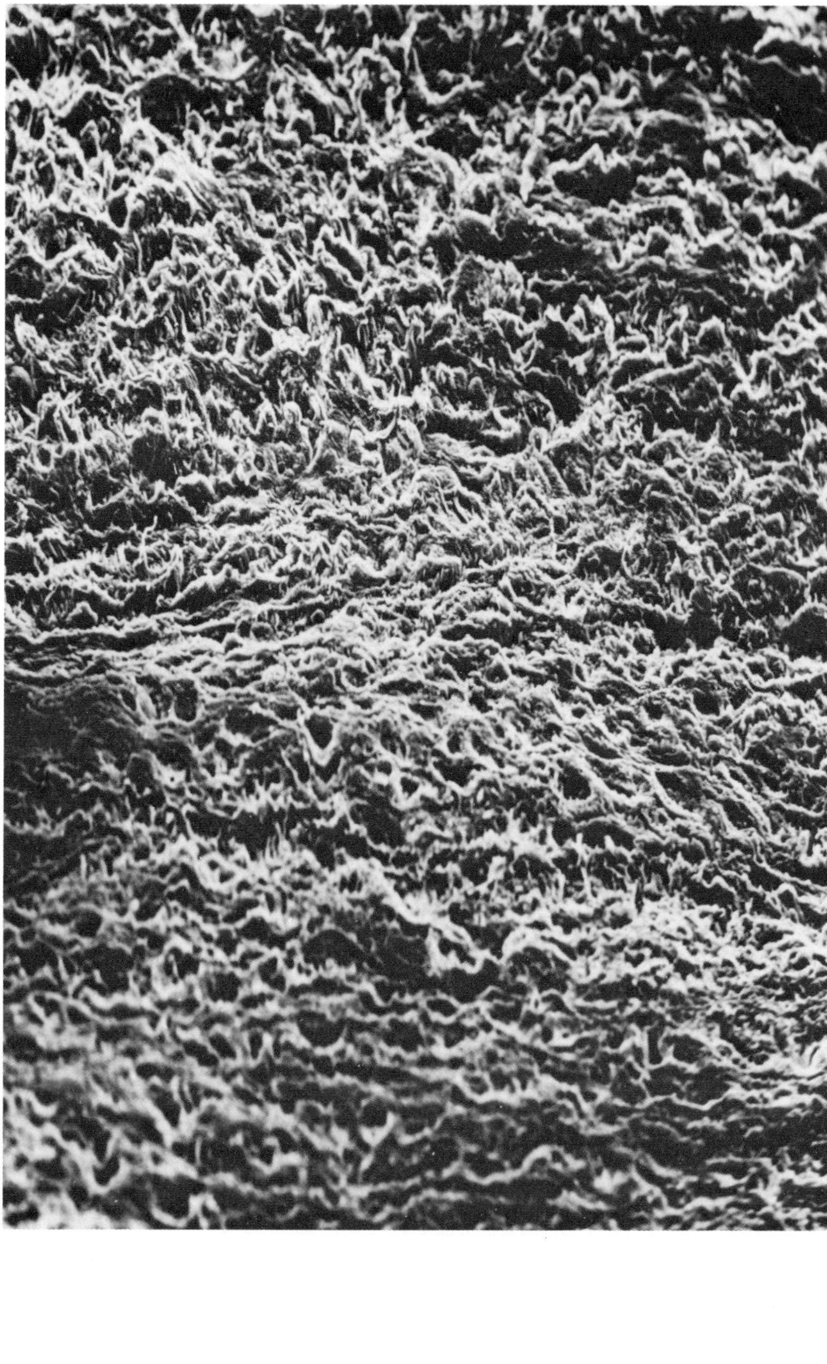

Figure 19. Scanning electron micrograph of stromal fibrosis in baboon BPH.

the treated and control animals would be more convincing if the data were based on a larger series of animals, thus pointing to one of the limitations of using animals such as baboons, which are so costly to procure and maintain, in biomedical research.

Transrectal Ultrasonography

Recognizing the desirability of having each animal serve as its own control for certain aspects of this research, we have recently begun to use transrectal ultrasonography as a means of monitoring the enlargement of the total prostate in baboons receiving TE. Recently, a group of noncastrated adult male baboons, consisting of three experimental and two control animals, has been placed on a protocol similar to that just described, and at the time of this writing, the experimental animals have been receiving TE for eight months. Figure 20 is a composite of two sonograms taken of the prostate of a control baboon, the upper panel having been recorded 3.5 months before the lower panel. This Figure illustrates the ease with which differences both in size and in the integrity of the prostatic capsule become readily apparent through the use of ultrasound. In contrast to the control animal, Figure 21 illustrates that a noticeable enlargement of the prostate has occurred over a 3.5 month period of testosterone enanthate stimulation. Methods are currently available and are being tested for determining the actual mass and volume of the baboon prostate with ultrasonography. Other changes have been noted in the baboons during the first half year of TE treatment of the current study, including a noticeable increase in body weight of the experimental animals (Table 1). Thus far, however, no differences have been detected in any of the animals with regard to serum BUN and creatinine values (Table 1), indicating that the TE treatments, as judged by these clinical laboratory parameters, have not caused detectable uropathy. Thus, even though the TE treatment has caused volumetric and gravimetric increases in the prostatic lobes, as determined both at autopsy and by ultrasound, and even though the histologic features of these TE stimulated baboon prostates are consistent with those of human BPH, we have not thus far created a condition in the baboon prostate that has resulted in elevated BUN and creatinine values similar to those measured in men with acute BPH.

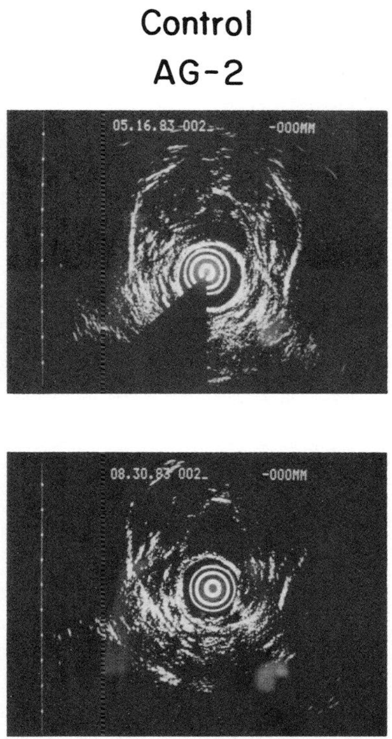

·Figure 20. Transrectal ultrasonogram of the baboon prostate.

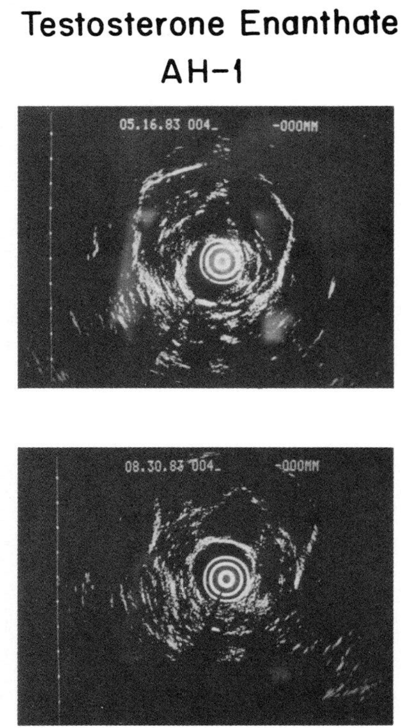

Figure 21. Transrectal ultrasonogram of the prostate of a baboon treated with testosterone enanthate.

Table 1. Effects of Testosterone Enanthate (200 mg Weekly) on Body Weight and Serum BUN and Creatinine Values

	-Body Wt. (kg)-		-BUN (mg %)-		-Creatinine (mg %)-	
Control	2/7/83	9/6/83	2/7/83	9/6/83	2/7/83	9/6/83
AF-10	29.4	30.1	18	17	1.4	1.3
AG-2	34.0	34.0	15	16	1.5	1.4
Rx						
AG-7	27.0	31.0	19	18	1.5	1.3
AG-10	20.6	22.0	11	15	1.1	1.1
AH-1	22.9	26.0	11	16	1.5	1.5

Urodynamics

Since urinary obstruction is a matter of degree and does not necessarily have to be accompanied by elevated serum BUN and creatinine values, we have recently begun to perform urodynamic analyses on the baboon as a means of detecting measurable differences that are associated with the baboon BPH. Perhaps the initial significance of these preliminary studies can be noted in the fact that such urodynamic measurements can be performed on tranquilized baboons (Figure 22). A No. 8 French catheter, used for filling the bladder, can be passed simultaneously through the penile and prostatic urethra with a smaller tube through which the pressure is transmitted to the transducer and recording device. Given in Table 2 are the results of urodynamic analyses performed on a control and TE treated baboon. The bladder of the control baboon received 200cc of warm physiologic saline, at which point, at 60cm H_2O, spontaneous voiding commenced and a peak flow of 2cc per second was reached at a pressure of 50cm H_2O. In marked contrast, the bladder of the TE treated baboon received 300cc and at 60cm H_2O only a few cc's of fluid leaked into the collection vial. At this point voiding was induced through application of manual pressure to the lower abdomen above the pubis. The peak flow thus induced in this treated baboon was also 2cc per second, but note that in order to achieve that flow rate, 98cm H_2O of pressure, transmitted at least in part through the application of external manual force, was registered. The larger capacity of the bladder in the treated baboon is suggestive of some degree of decompensation. Moreover, in this pilot study, the residual volume of the treated baboon was at least 80cc as opposed to 20cc in the control animal.

The pressure/flow relationships of micturition are determined by the combined characteristics of the independent fundamental properties of the bladder and urethra. The relationship of pressure and flow has been described with various urethral resistance factors, the most common of which is an expression of minimal resistance, and relates intravesical pressure to the square of the flow at maximum flow, i.e. $Rmin=Pves/Fmax^2$. In men, the highest acceptable value for urethral resistance is 0.6 (Abrams et al 1983). Values in man above 0.6 are considered to be indicative of abnormal resistance or obstruction. Applying this formula to the values measured in the control and treated baboons,

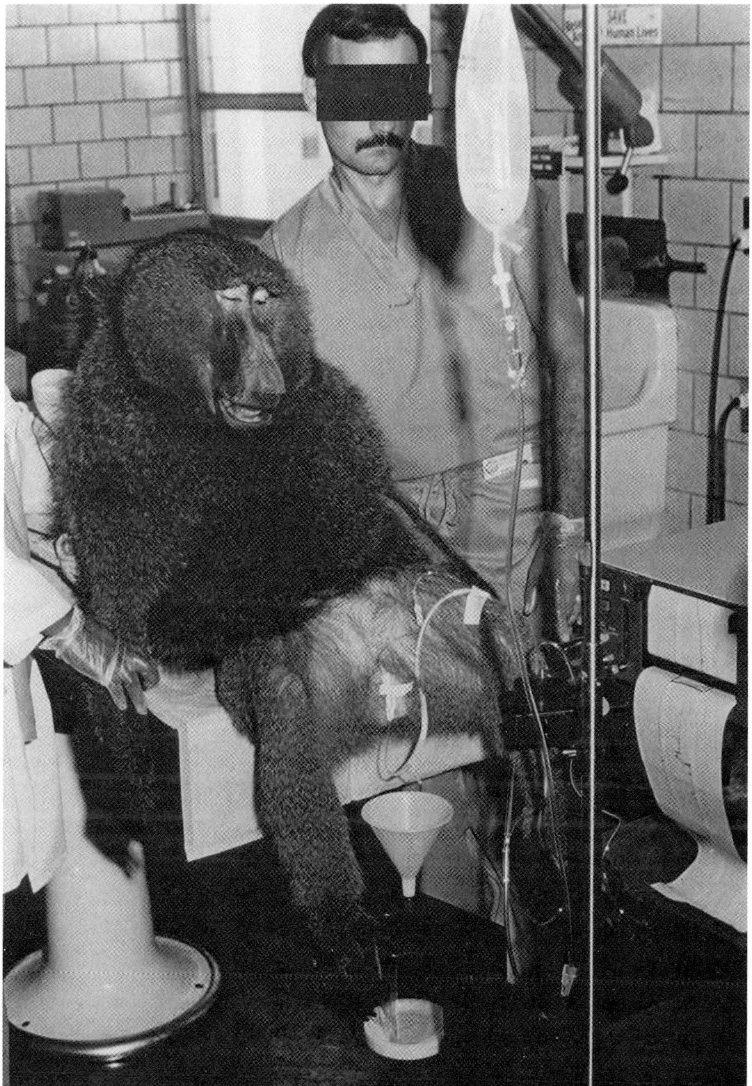

Figure 22. Analysis of urodynamics in a tranquilized baboon.

Table 2. Baboon Urodynamics

	Control AG-2	Treated* AH-1
Filling	200 cc, 60 cm H_2O	300 cc, 60 cm H_2O
	Spontaneous Voiding, 180 cc	Induced voiding, 220 cc
Peak Flow	2 cc/sec, 50 cm H_2O	2 cc/sec, 98 cm H_2O
$R=P/F^2$	12	24
UPP	120 cm H_2O	>160 cm H_2O

*Testosterone enanthate, seven months

the minimal resistance in the treated baboon was calculated to be twice that of the control baboon. While the mean intravesical pressure at maximum flow in the baboon is similar to that of men, the mean maximal flow rate of the baboons, both control and treated, are one order of magnitude less than reported values for man (Abrams 1983) and therefore, this lower factor, as measured in the tranquilized baboon, would account for the very high Rmin value. Obviously, the meaningful interpretation of such future studies of the baboon will have to be based on the development of a table of intravesical pressure and maximum flow rate values in control tranquilized baboons.

The urethral pressure profile (UPP), a measurement that reflects most elements contributing to urethral closure (Abrams 1983), was determined on the control and treated baboons using the internal CO_2 source of the Life Tech, Inc. instrumentation used. As given in Table 2, the UPP value was 120 cm H_2O in the control versus a value greated than 160 cm H_2O in the treated animal. With regard to the latter, it must be noted that this instrumentation is engineered to ensure the safe measurement of UPP in humans, and, as such, the instrument automatically stops the CO_2 infusion at 160 cm H_2O. Thus, with the equipment designed to stop the CO_2 infusion at that pressure, the maximum UPP value in the treated baboon was not determined. Nevertheless, the difference measured between the control and treated baboons was striking and we are most encouraged that these findings may be the first quantitative evidence that the BPH produced by TE injections in the intact baboon is accompanied by measurable obstruction akin to and clinically relevant to that seen in human BPH.

In conclusion, we plan to continue our studies of the hormonal induction of BPH in the baboon. We know of no other species which, based upon histology and apparent urinary obstruction such as that which we have identified in the baboon, so closely resembles the condition of BPH in man.

REFERENCES

Abrams P, Feneley, R, Torrens, M (1983). "Urodynamics". Great Britain: Springer-Verlag, p 225.

Bullough WS (1965). Mitotic and functional homeostasis: a speculative review. Cancer Res 25:1683.

Chai LS, Karr JP, Murphy GP, Sandberg AA (1981). Effects of DES on the morphology of the lobes of the baboon prostate. Invest Urol 19:202.

Hemsell DL, Grodin JM, Brenner PG, Siiteri PK, MacDonald PC (1974). Plasma precursors of estrogen. II. Correlation of extent of conversion of plasma androstenedione to estrone with age. J Clin Endocrinol Metab 38:476.

Karr JP, Kim U, Resko JA, Schneider S, Chai LS, Murphy GP, Sandberg AA (in press, 1983). Induction of benign prostatic hypertrophy in baboons. Urology.

Kley HK, Nieschlag E, Bidlingmaier F, Kruskemper HL (1974). Possible age dependent influence of estrogens on the binding of testosterone in plasma of adult men. Horm Metab Res 6:213.

McNeal JE (1981). Normal and pathologic anatomy of prostate. Urology, Suppl 17:11.

Muntzing J, Myhrberg H, Saroff J, Sandberg AA, Murphy GP (1976). Histochemical and ultrastructural study of prostatic tissue from baboons treated with antiprostatic drugs. Invest Urol 14:162.

Schoonees R (1971). A study of the endocrine control of the prostate gland in relation to the etiology and the treatment of prostatic carcinoma and benign prostatic hyperplasia. Thesis presented for the Degree of Doctor of Medicine (M.D) at the University of Stellenbosch.

Schoonees R, deKlerk JN (1968). Anatomy, radio-isotopic blood flow and glandular secretory activity of the baboon prostate. S Afr Med J, Suppl 42:87.

Rohr HP, Bartsch G (1980). Human benign prostatic hyperplasia: a stromal disease. Urology 16:625.

Washburn SL (1982). Human evolution. Perspect Biol Med 25:583.

Zumoff B, Bradlow HL, Finkelstein J, Boynar RM, Hellman L (1976). The influence of age and sex on the metabolism of testosterone. J Clin Endocrinol Metab 42:703.

Discussion

Buhl: In a previous paper done at your institution, you were using diethylstilbesterol (DES) and claimed, as I remember, that you were getting some nodular disease using that kind of treatment. How do you compare that with your most recent study and why have you abandoned the DES treatment?

Karr: To begin with, the DES study was based on a very short period of treatment (3 weeks). The primary effect with the DES was, as Dr. Lewis mentioned, a decrease in the epithelial height in the caudal lobes and at least the maintenance, or in some areas, an enrichment, of the epithelial elements and particularly the stromal elements of the cranial lobe. I don't recall our noting that it was a nodular condition. As to why we shifted gears, we were studying DES for other reasons. In our current work, the objective was to see if we could induce BPH in the baboon. We felt that the most expeditious way of getting some answers was to first try testosterone injections on a long term basis in intact baboons.

New Approaches to the Study
of Benign Prostatic Hyperplasia, pages 291–306

A NEW MOUSE MODEL FOR PROSTATIC HYPERPLASIA: INDUCTION OF ADULT PROSTATIC OVERGROWTH BY FETAL UROGENITAL SINUS IMPLANTS

Leland W.K. Chung[1 2], Ph.D., James Matsuura[1], Audrey K. Rocco[1], B.S., Timothy C. Thompson[1], B.S., Gary J. Miller[2], M.D., Ph.D., and Meredith N. Runner[1], Ph.D.

[1]University of Colorado
Boulder, CO 80309

[2]University of Colorado Health Sciences Center
Denver, CO 80262

The etiological factors for human benign prostatic hyperplasia (BPH) development have been explained by two hypotheses. First, human BPH develops under conditions of sex steroids imbalance. This hypothesis is supported by the observation that human BPH tissues contain higher (3- to 4-fold) concentrations of the potent androgen, dihydrotestosterone (DHT), than the normal tissues (Siiteri and Wilson, 1970; Geller et al, 1976; Krieg et al, 1977). In the canine BPH model, chronic administration of pharmacological doses of androgen or androgen plus estrogen to non-castrated dogs induces prostatic hyperplasia (Walsh and Wilson, 1976; DeKlerk et al, 1979). In the castrated dog, however, androgen administered with estrogen but not alone promote prostatic hyperplasia (Walsh and Wilson, 1976). The synergism between androgen and estrogen in the castrated host has been explained on the basis that estrogen has direct stimulatory action on the growth of fibromuscular stroma (Mawhinney and Neubauer, 1979). Estrogen also increase the androgen receptor contents in prostatic tissues (Bouton et al, 1981). Estrogen receptors have been detected in human BPH tissues (Hawkins et al, 1975) and reside primarily in the fibromuscular stroma (Krieg et al, 1981; Puah and Ghanadian, 1981). The hypothesis of an imbalance in the levels of sex steroids, however, fails to reconcile the clinical observation that human BPH is initiated during the third and fourth decades of life, whereas altered ratios of plasma sex steroids concentrations occur in the male population after the sixth decade (Wilson, 1980).

Second, human BPH may develop as a result of re-expression of embryonic growth potential of the fibroblasts in the periurethral region of prostate gland (McNeal, 1978). This hypothesis is supported by our recent experimental observation that embryonic mesenchyme derived from fetal urogenital sinuses (UGM) have a growth inductive potential that governs the growth and differentiation of its adjacent adult and fetal epithelium (Cunha and Chung, 1981; Chung and Cunha, 1983). In this report, we extended the previous observations and described a new mouse model for prostatic hyperplasia (Chung et al, 1982). This model was developed with the assumption that tissue interactions occur between fetal and adult prostatic cells <u>in situ</u>. Results showed that indeed adult prostatic cells can be induced by fetal prostatic cells to proliferate as a result of close cellular interactions. Both the intact fetal urogenital sinus (UGS) and its mesenchyme were shown to have growth-promoting functions on the adult prostate. Fetal urogenital sinus epithelium (UGE) appears to play a modulatory role in the expression of the growth inductive capability by the UGM. The growth was recorded in the complete absence of exogenous sex steroids. These findings argue against the hypothesis of sex steroid imbalance as the causative factor(s) for the development of prostatic hyperplasia, and support the second hypothesis that human BPH may be developed as the result of re-expression of embryonic growth potential in the adult prostate gland (McNeal, 1978).

New Mouse Model for Prostatic Hyperplasia

Figure 1 depicts the typical gross morphology of an adult mouse prostate four weeks following implantation of UGS from 3 fetal mice (3 X UGS). The wet weight and DNA content of the uninduced prostate (N=38, VP_C) increased from 5.8 ± 0.3 mg and 14 ± 0.7 μg to 57.1 ± 9.3 mg and 113.6 ± 18.2 μg (N=6, VP_{UGS}, mean ± SE), respectively. This accounts for a 10- and 8-fold increase over the basal

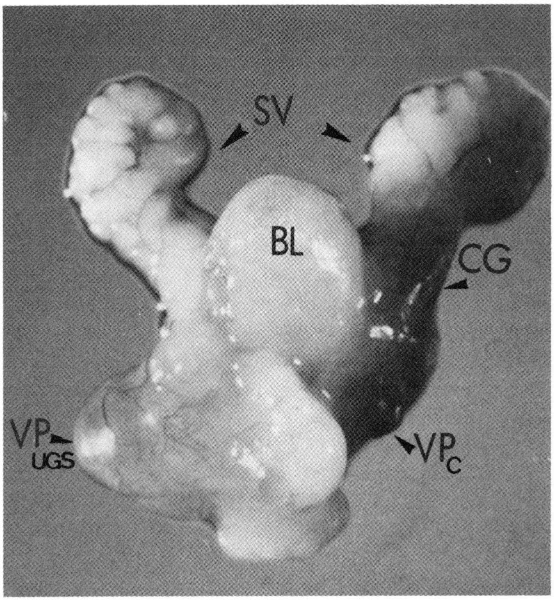

Fig. 1 Gross morphology of the enlarged mouse ventral prostate following direct inplantation of fetal urogenital sinuses (VP_{UGS}). The contralateral lobe (VP_c) served as control. Other organs are seminal vesicles (SV), coagulating gland (CG) and urinary bladder (BL).

levels of wet weight and DNA content of the adult prostate gland. The size of two other prostate glands with 3 X UGS implants increased to a mean wet weight of 240 mg (mean DNA content was 600 μg) at 25 weeks. This represents an enlargement of the adult prostate gland by 40-fold.

The fetal UGS-induced adult prostatic hyperplasia can be accounted for by the ability of fetal UGS to induce adult prostatic cells into proliferation. Figure 2 shows that the resultant UGS-induced overgrowth of the adult mouse prostate and coagulating gland contains both donor (fetal) and host (adult) glucose phosphate isomerase (GPI) isozymes in about equal proportion. Because GPI isozyme profiles customarily are used to quantify the contribution of donor and host cells in chimeric tissues (Illmensee and Mintz, 1976; Gootwine et al, 1982), the equal proportion

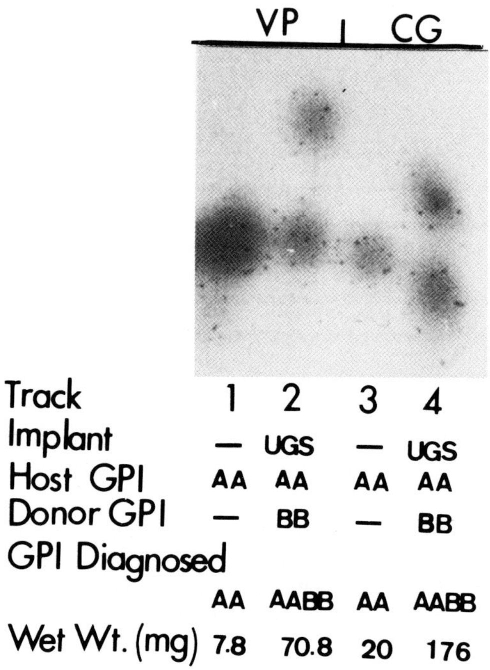

Fig. 2 Glucose phosphate isomerase (GPI) isozymic profiles in the control and UGS-induced growth of adult mouse ventral prostate (VP) and coagulating gland (CG).

of GPI isozymes in the resultant UGS-induced overgrowth of the adult prostate indicates that one-half of the 113.6 μg DNA (or 56.8 μg DNA) was derived from the cells of the adult prostate gland proliferating as a result of their interaction with fetal UGS. This amounts to a 4-fold increase in DNA content (mean DNA content in adult prostate = 14 μg) after 3 X UGS implantation.

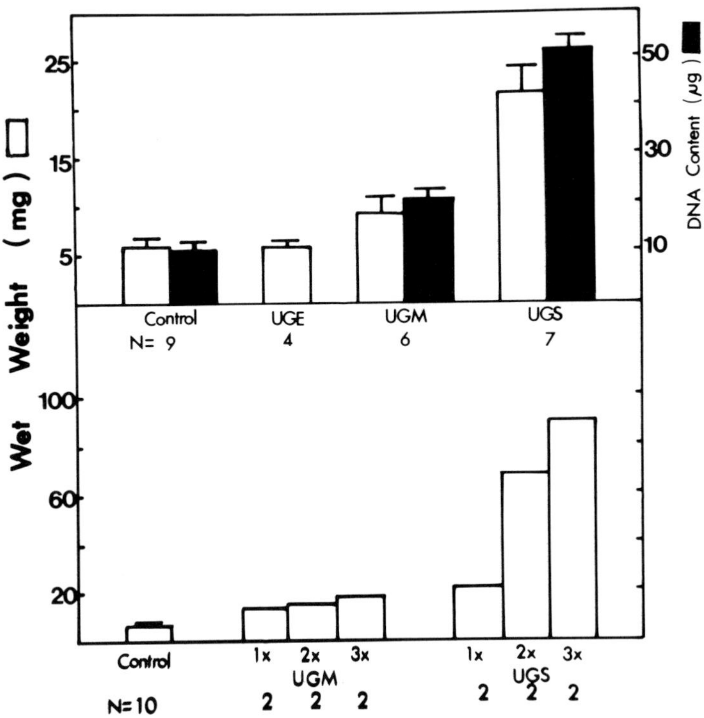

Fig. 3 Comparison of the growth promoting effects of intact urogenital sinus (UGS), urogenital sinus mesenchyme (UGM) and urogenital sinus epithelium (UGE). Top panel indicates the net growth (wet weight and DNA) content of the adult mouse VP observed during a 4-week growth period following implantation of 1 X UGE, UGM or UGS. Panel B shows a dose response relationship between the net growth (wet weight) of the adult mouse VP and the dose (1 X to 3 X) of UGM and UGS during the same growth period. Average or average ± S.E. of 2 to 10 determinations.

Comparison of the Induction of Overgrowth of Adult Prostate Gland by Fetal UGS and Fetal UGM Implants

The fact that UGS implants induce marked adult prostatic overgrowth prompted an investigation into the role of the individual components of UGS, i.e, UGM and UGE, on growth of the adult prostate gland. Figure 3 showed that 1 X UGS induced 2.5-fold more growth than 1 X UGM, and 1 X UGE was completely inactive (top panel). The magni-

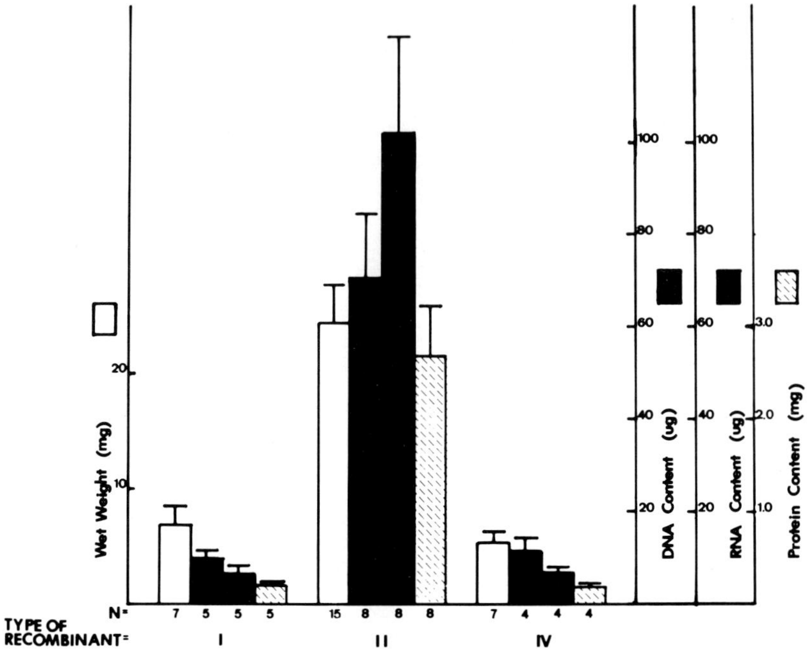

Fig. 4 Comparison of the net growth (wet weight, DNA, RNA and protein content) of homotypic (Group I: UGM_{rat} + UGE_{rat}) and heterospecific (Group II: UGM_{rat} + UGE_{mouse}, and Group IV: UGM_{mouse} + UGE_{rat}) tissue recombinants grown under the renal capsules of adult male athymic mice (Balb/c-nu) for an 8-week period. Average ± S.E. of 4 to 15 determinations.

tude of UGS- and UGM-induced prostatic overgrowth was dose-dependent (bottom panel). It is unlikely that differences in efficacy between UGS and UGM may be due to the irreversible loss of growth inductive substance(s) during UGM isolation, because tissue recombinants consisting of UGM and UGE grew to the same extent as the intact UGS under renal capsules (Chung and Cunha, 1983). Alternatively, UGE may modulate the gene expression of UGM which is responsible for inducing the proliferation of adult prostatic cells. This modulatory role of UGE on the growth inductive capability of UGM has been demonstrated recently by Rocco et al, (1983) in tissue recombination experiments. Figure 4 shows that rat UGM, when recombined heterospecifically with mouse UGE (Group II), induces a 2- to 4-fold more growth than when recombined homotypically with rat UGE (Group I). These results suggest that UGM and UGE may exist in a relationship analogous to the paracrine system (Hakanson and Sundler, 1983) where UGE modulates the gene expression of its adjacent UGM, and hence the ultimate growth inductive potential of UGM on the adult prostate.

Table 1 Inhibition of the initiation of UGS-induced adult prostatic overgrowth by castration, or the administration of estrogen or antiandrogen to intact adult male hosts.

Condition[a]	N	DNA Content (μg) (% Inhibition)
Intact Control	3	---
Castration	3	70 ± 3.1
Estradiol dipropionate-treated	2	61.5
Cyproterone acetate-treated	3	59.3 ± 2.4

[a] 3 X UGS isolated for donor hosts (HS strain) were implanted directly into one lobe of the ventral prostate of the adult Balb/c-nu hosts. Some hosts carrying UGS implants were either castrated or treated every three days with estradiol dipropionate (15 μg) or cyproterone acetate (4 mg) for a period of 10 to 30 days. DNA contents in 3 X UGS-induced prostate under various treatment protocols were determined. Data were expressed as DNA content, % of inhibition ± S.E.

Requirement of Testicular Androgen for Both the Initiation and the Maintenance of UGS-Induced Adult Prostatic Overgrowth

To test the androgen dependency of the UGS-induced adult prostatic overgrowth, hosts receiving 3 X UGS either were castrated or treated with estradiol dipropionate (15 μg/mouse every 3 days) or cyproterone acetate (4 mg/mouse every 3 days) immediately following 3 X UGS implantation. Table 1 shows that the initiation of UGS-induced adult prostatic overgrowth was inhibited as much as 60-70% by these hormonal depletion regimens. These results suggest that androgenic steroids are required for the initation of UGS-induced prostatic overgrowth.

To determine the requirement of testicular androgen for the maintenance of UGS-induced adult prostatic overgrowth, some male hosts receiving 3 X UGS implants for 4 weeks were castrated and allowed to grow for 2 additional weeks. The size of the prostate gland was estimated at the time of castration and was found to be reduced by about 20-30%. Histological examination revealed typical castration-induced changes, such as atrophic epithelial acini and reduced lumenal accumulation of secretory materials as described (Chung and McFadden, 1980). These results suggest that UGS-induced adult prostatic overgrowth depends upon endogenous testicular androgens for its maintenance.

The suggestion that UGS-induced prostatic overgrowth is androgen-dependent is further supported by the assessment of cytosolic androgen receptors in the UGS-induced adult mouse prostate. Scatchard analysis of cytosolic androgen receptors in the UGS-induced overgrowth of adult mouse prostate gland showed the presence of high affinity (Kd=0.73 nM) and low capacity (Bmax=4.7 fmole/mg) androgen binding (R1881 binding) resembling that detected in the host prostate glands (Thompson et al, 1983). These results again are consistent with the suggestion that UGS implants induce an enlargement of host prostate gland.

Specificity of UGS-Induced Overgrowth of Adult Mouse Prostate

Donor tissue specificity. Table 2 shows that the implantation of live fetal bladder, fetal skin, fetal salivary gland or adult prostate gland of comparable size as 3 X UGS results in no overgrowth of the adult host prostate gland. Induction of adult prostatic overgrowths depends upon the implantation of live urogential sinus tissues. Fetal UGS either subjected to heat (100°C for 5 min), freeze and thaw or radiation (5,000 rad for 4.1 min) was completely inactive (Table 2).

Table 2 Donor tissue specificity for the induction of adult prostatic overgrowth.

Donor Tissue[a]	N	Wet Weight (mg)	DNA Content (μg)
None (Sham-operated)	6	5.7 ± 0.4	11.1 ± 0.3
3 X UGS	6	40.4 ± 5.3	80.0 ± 5.5
Adult Prostate	3	5.2 ± 0.6	15.0 ± 1.1
Fetal Bladder	3	4.5 ± 0.4	11.0 ± 1.4
Fetal Skin	3	5.4 ± 1.1	13.4 ± 2.3
Fetal Salivary Gland	3	4.9 ± 1.0	13.2 ± 3.1
3 X UGS (heat-treated)	4	7.5 ± 0.5	---
3 X UGS (freeze thaw-treated)	2	3.8	---
3 X UGS (radiation-treated)	2	3.8	10.1

[a]Donor tissues were obtained from HS mice. Hosts (Balb/c-nu) carrying donor tissues were allowed to grow for 4 weeks. Wet weight and DNA content in the host prostate implanted previously with donor tissues were determined.

Implantation site specificity. Implanting fetal UGS into all of the mouse male accessory sex organs, such as the prostate, coagulating gland and seminal vesicles (Chung et al, 1982) induces prostatic overgrowth. Implantation of fetal UGS or tissue recombinants composed of UGM and UGE under the renal capsules, however, does not induce the overgrowth of the mouse kidneys (Chung and Cunha, 1983).

Table 3 Strain and species specificity for UGS-induced overgrowth of the adult prostate gland.

Donor[a]	Host	N	Ventral Prostatic Wet Weight (mg)	DNA Content (μg)
		MOUSE		
None	C3H	4	12.6 ± 2.4	19.7 ± 2.5
C3H	C3H	4	24.9 ± 2.7	45.7 ± 1.9
None	Balb/c-nu	2	5.4	---
C3H	Balb/c-nu	2	72.4	---
None	Balb/c	2	3.5	3.2
Balb/c	Balb/c	2	49.5	79.8
None	Balb/c-nu	2	7.8	11.9
Balb/c	Balb/c-nu	2	51.0	80.3
		RAT		
None	Nb	4	157.8 ± 21.2	---
Nb	Nb	4	439.7 ± 45	---
None	Hooded-nu	1	70	---
Nb	Hooded-nu	1	350	

[a]Donor UGS isolated from 16 or 18-day old embryos of mice and rats, respectively were used in these studies. One lobe of the ventral prostate of the adult male host was implanted with 3 X UGS and other the lobe was sham-operated. Ventral prostates were harvested from the hosts at the end of 30-day growth period. Wet weight and DNA content were expressed either as average or average ± S.E. of 1 to 4 determinations.

Strain and species specificity. Table 3 shows that the phenomenon of UGS-induced adult prostatic overgrowth is not limited to Balb/c-nu mice. UGS isolated from C3H or Balb/c mice was found to induce adult prostatic overgrowth in their respective inbred strains of mice. In addition, fetal UGS isolated from Nb rats also were found to be capable of inducing adult prostatic overgrowths in both adult male syngeneic and nude (Hooded-nu) rats (Table 3).

Progression of UGS-Induced Adult Prostatic Hyperplasia

Adult mouse ventral prostate glands after UGS-induction were isolated at 3 different intervals (15, 30 and 180 days) and were analyzed by histological methods. At 15 days following the implantation of 3 X UGS, the UGS implants appeared to be markedly swollen and were clearly identified. Thirty days after the initiation of the growth period, areas containing mixed adult and fetal cell populations were identified. Abundant new prostatic acini were formed in these areas. Nests of cell aggregates that have the appearance of urethral were observed. However, when the UGS-induced growth was allowed to proceed for 180 days, there are three distinct elements that can be identified in the histological specimens: 1) the pre-existing adult prostate gland, 2) the hyperplastic adult prostate gland with areas of nodular hyperplasia resembling that observed in human, and 3) the persistence and proliferation of small nests of cell aggregates that resemble the urethral. As described earlier, typical castration-induced changes were observed in UGS-induced prostatic growth following castration.

Summary

A new mouse model for human BPH has been established. This model was developed on the basis that fetal and adult prostatic cells interact to induce the proliferation of adult prostatic cells. A 10- to 20-fold overgrowth of the adult mouse prostate gland can be induced by implantation of fetal UGS into the adult prostate gland. Components of UGS, fetal UGM, and fetal UGE may be involved in the regulation of adult prostatic overgrowth. The androgen dependency and the specificity (donor tissue, site of implantation, and strain and species) of UGS-induced adult prostatic overgrowth have also been established.

The question remains whether the prostatic hyperplasia seen in this mouse model may be representative of human BPH. The observation that fetal UGS implants induce adult prostatic overgrowth in the complete absence of exogenous sex steroids support the hypothesis of McNeal that human BPH may develop as a result of the reactivation of fetal growth potential in the periurethral area of the adult prostate gland. The present mouse model may be used as a test system for the future development of anti-BPH drugs.

Acknowledgement

This work was supported in part by PHS grant AM-25266 awarded to L.W.K.C.

References

Bouton MM, Pornin C, Grandadam JA, (1981). Estrogen regulation of rat prostate androgen receptor. J Steroid Biochem 15:403.

Chung LWK, McFadden DK, (1980). Sex steroids imprinting and prostatic growth. Invest Urol 17:337.

Chung LWK, Matsuura J, Thompson TC, Chao, RCFY, (1982). A new approach to regulation of prostatic growth: Interactions between embryonic urogenital sinuses and adult prostate _in situ_. Proc West Pharmacol Soc 25:141.

Chung LWK, Cunha GR, (1983). Stromal-epithelial interactions. II. Regulation of prostatic growth by embryonic urogential sinus mesenchyme. The Prostate (In Press)

Cunha GR, Chung LWK, (1981). Stromal-epithelial interactions. I. Induction of prostatic phenotype in urothelium of testicular feminized (Tfm/y) mice. J Steroid Biochem 14:1317.

DeKlerk DP, Coffey DS, Ewing LL, McDermott IR, Reiner WG, Robinson CH, Scott WW, Strandberg JD, Talalay P, Walsh PC, Wheaton LD, Zirkin BR (1979). Comparison of spontaneous and experimentally induced canine prostatic hyperplasia. J Clin Invest 64:842.

Geller J, Albert J, Lopez D, Geller S, Niwayama G, (1976). Comparison of androgen metabolites in benign prostatic hypertrophy (BPH) and normal prostate. J Clin Endocrinol Metab 43:686.

Gootwine E, Webb CG, Sachs L, (1982). Participation of myeloid leukaemic cells injected into embryos in haematopoietic differentiation in adult mice. Nature 299:63.

Hakanson R, Sundler F. (1983). The design of the neuroendocrine system: A unifying concept and its consequence. Trend in Pharmacol Sci 4:41.

Hawkins EF, Nijs M, Brassine C, (1975). Steroid receptors in the human prostate. I. Estradiol 17-β binding in benign prostatic hypertrophy. Steroids 26:458.

Illmensee K, Mintz B, (1976). Totipotency and normal differentiaton of single terato-carcinoma cells cloned by injection into blastocysts. Proc Nat Acad Sci USA 73:549.

Krieg M, Bartsch W, Herzer S, Becker H, Voight KD, (1977). Quantification of androgen binding, androgen tissue levels and sex hormone-binding globulin in prostate, muscle, and plasma of patients with benign prostatic hypertrophy. Acta Endocrinol (Copenh) 86:200.

Krieg M, Klotzl G, Kaufmann J, Voigt KD, (1981). Stroma of human benign prostatic hyperplasia: preferential tissue for androgen metabolism and oestrogen binding. Acta Endocrinol 96:422.

McNeal JE, (1978). Origin and evolution of benign prostatic enlargement. Invest Urol 15:340.

Mawhinney MG, Neubauer BL, (1979). Actions of estrogen in the male. Invest Urol 16:409.

Puah CM, Ghanadian R, (1981). Correlative studies between endogenous steroids and stromal-epithelial composition in human benign hypertrophied prostate. Brit J Cancer 244:308.

Rocco A, Matsuura J, Runner M, Chung LWK, (1983). Biochemical characterization of growth induction by fetal urogenital sinus: A new mouse model for studying prostatic hyperplasia. Fed Proc 42:1768.

Siiteri P, Wildon JD, (1970). Dihydrotestosterone in prostatic hypertrophy. I. The formation and content of dihydrotestosterone in the hypertrophic prostate of man. J Clin Invest 49:1746.

Thompson TC, Chung LWK, Cunha GR, Neubauer BL, Shannon JM, (1983). Biochemical characterization of tissue recombinants composed of wild-type fetal urogenital sinus mesenchyme (UGM) and Tfm/y adult bladder epithelium (ABLE) Fed Proc 42:1769.

Walsh PC, Wilson JD, (1976). The induction of prostatic hypertrophy in the dog with androstanediol. J Clin Invest 57:1093.
Wilson JD, (1980). The pathogenesis of benign prostatic hyperplasia. The Am J of Med 68:745.

Discussion

Cuhna: If mice are going to be a valid model for humans, it would be nice to be able to show that the basic developmental mechanisms are similar between the mouse and the human. We recently did a very extensive series of heterospecific prostatic inductions using epithelium and mesenchyme from rat, rabbit, mouse and human tissues. In those we paired mesenchyme from one species with epithelium from another. Some of the tissue recombinants are all what we would call permissive inductions. That is, we used a target urogenital epithelium, which would normally form prostate, and paired it with urogenital mesenchyme from another species. Prostatic or glandular inductions occured very nicely across species lines. The other type of inductions were of the instructive type, those in which a bladder epithelium was reprogrammed to form structures that are distinctly prostatic or that can be identified as glands. We combined mouse urogenital sinus mesenchyme and human fetal bladder epithelium, and grew these recumbinants in athymic nude mice for various periods of time, and found they elicited a glandular differentiation in the human fetal bladder epithelium.

Also, using the starting material of the human fetal bladder epithelium and mesenchyme, we made homotypic recombinations. We took the human bladder epithelium and combined it with its own mesenchyme. We got the kind of histology which is the histology of the human fetal bladder epithelium.

When a heterospecific recombination, mouse mesenchyme, and the human bladder epithelium, was grown for only two weeks we found solid epithelial growths that were beginning to penetrate out into the surrounding stroma. If these recombinants were grown for longer periods of time those outgrowths will continue to expand and then begin to develop lumina. If you looked at slides of human fetal prostate at about 12 weeks of gestation, you would recognize that these structures from the mouse-human recombinant are very similar to, if not identical, to the solid epithelial cords that you find in the human fetal prostate at the stage of cannalization. We let those recombinants go for a slightly longer period of time, and found glandular differentiation. We saw lumina forming and tall columnar epithelial cells. That configuration of epithelium is never found in the human fetal bladder. I think, based upon our series of heterospecific recombinations in rodents, as well as the mouse-human recombinants, we can postulate that the basic mechanism for the development of the prostate has been very highly conserved during the evolution of mammals. The message is that basic mechanisms of interaction between these two cell types are very similar between species. Similar enough that human epithelium can be altered in a rather dramatic way as a result of developmental information coming from a species such as the mouse. I think this speaks strongly for the validity and the applicability of rodent and other animal models, to study human disease and birth defects.

Neil: Does the urogenital sinus have to be present continuously for growth of the adult prostate to occur? Can you implant the urogenital sinus, allow growth to proceed, and then remove it and follow the continued growth of the adult prostate?

Chung: Obviously, I don't know the answer to that question because once you put the implant into the prostate it would be very difficult to remove it. The way that we have approached this problems is to develop an <u>in vitro</u> system to grow the epithelium and stroma, then look for possibly another factor of some kind. It would certainly be interesting to observe if transfection is the mode of action of induction.

McNeal: You showed that combining rat urogenital mesenchyme (UGM) with mouse bladder epithelium showed about twice the growth of combining the rat mesenchyme with the mouse prostatic epithelium. How do you explain that.

Chung: This can be explained by the difference of the intrinsic inductive potential of the rat UGM which is greater than that of the mouse UGM.

McNeal: You mentioned that the overgrowth was confined to the adult prostatic lobe in which the fetal tissue was implanted, but you showed a slide in which the coagulating gland increased from 20 to some over 100 mg.

Chung: In the first experiment isoenzymatic analysis showed that the adult prostatic cells were recruited into cellular proliferation.

In the second experiment, cellular proliferation was induced in the coagulating gland by the same mechanism.

Cunha: Leland, just a comment about the reduction in prostate weight that you saw when you castrated the urogenital sinus (UGS) implanted animals or treated them with estradiol or cyproterone acetate. You noted a reduction of 50-70%, but that there was clearly 30% that was still unaccounted for. That may be explained by the fact that you implanted the whole intact UGS. The types of structures that are going to form from such an implant include, of course, the active acini components of the prostate, but also prostatic urethra and urethral glands. You pointed out those structures in your slides of the UGS implanted adult prostates. The urethra and urethral glands may not atrophy quite as much as the result of androgen deprivation as the active acini components of the prostate will. The prostatic urethra and the urethral glands that you would obtain can be eliminated in large part by grafting only the upper expanded part of the urogenital sinus. It is just recently we have cut the UGS into upper, middle and lower segments. We found that the upper segment is the really strong prostatic inducer and as we move to more caudal regions that the amount of prostate induced by those regions falls off. The lower end is pretty much an urethral gland inductor. By trimming the UGS you may be able to increase the incidence of prostate acini induction.

Chung: That is a good point. I might add that I didn't present the histology of the prostates from castration and cyproterone acetate or estradiol treated groups. There seemed to be substantially more stroma over epithelium in the castrated or drug treated groups as compared to the nontreated group. Possibly the stromal growth is less androgen dependent under these particular experimental conditions.

New Approaches to the Study of Benign Prostatic Hyperplasia, pages 307–331

STRUCTURAL AND FUNCTIONAL COMPONENTS IN NORMAL AND HYPERPLASTIC CANINE PROSTATES

William B. Isaacs

Department of Urology and Pharmacology

Johns Hopkins Univ. Sch. of Med., Balto., Md.

It is becoming increasingly apparent that the structural organization both within a cell and in its surrounding environments plays a crucial role in modulating basic cell processes such as replication, differentiation and expression of differentiated functions. [(For a recent review, see Bissell et al. (1982)]. The structural organization within a given glandular organ such as the prostate resides within three distinct domains or matrices, which collectively can be viewed as forming an overall "tissue matrix" (Figure 1) (Isaacs et al. 1981). The three matrices are the extracellular matrix, the cytoplasmic matrix (or cytoskeleton) and the nuclear matrix. Despite the relatively recent identification and characterization of these various matrix systems and their components, distinct, important biological processes have been demonstrated to be associated with each one. Examples are the nuclear matrix as the site of DNA replication and transcribing genes (Pardoll et al 1980; Robinson et al 1983), the cytoplasmic matrix as the mediator of cell shape and motility, and as the anchorage site for subcellular organelles (Osborn, Weber 1977; Lenk et al 1977), and the extracellular matrix as an important modulator (or even inducer in some cases) of morphogenesis, cell proliferation, and cellular differentiation (Hay 1981; Kleinman et al 1981). Although it is by no means clear how these different matrix systems are integrated within a whole tissue, several models have been proposed which imply a dynamic interaction between nuclear, (Bissell et al. 1982) cytoplasmic and extracellular matrices (Hay, 1982), in which there is bidirectional information transfer (i.e., from nucleus to cytoplasm to extracellular environment and vice versa). Obviously, elucidation of the mechanism by which signals (e.g., a growth factor triggering a mitogenic response) are transmitted by these matrices and the components involved in interfacing one matrix system with another is an exciting area of future research.

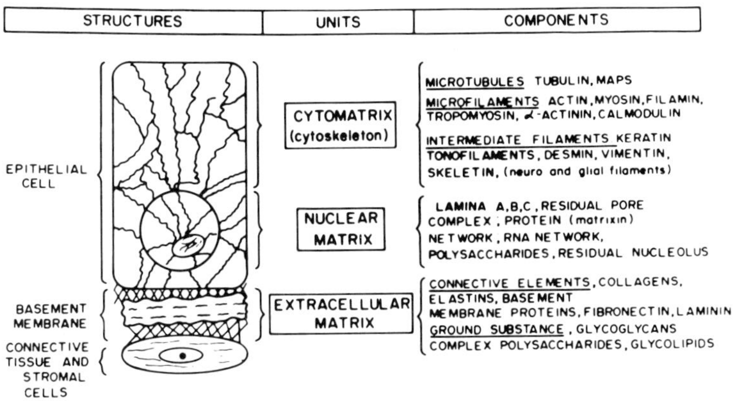

Figure 1. Schematic diagram of the structural organization of various components present in the tissue matrix of a typical glandular organ. From Isaacs et al. (1981).

Recently, the hypothesis that the supranormal accumulation of dihydrotestosterone (DHT) within hyperplastic prostates is an important etiological factor in the development of benign prostatic hyperplasia (BPH) has come into question (Walsh 1983). The demonstration that DHT levels are not elevated in BPH suggests that alternative factors or mechanisms may be involved. McNeal (1978) has proposed that a non-hormonally mediated embryonic reawakening of the inductive potential of prostatic stroma is responsible for the development and maintenance of BPH. This idea has been supported by the work of Cunha and Chung (1981, 1983) demonstrating the potent inductive effect of urogenital sinus mesenchyme to promote differentiation and growth of overlying epithelium. Whether this is due to a diffusible factor released by the mesenchyme or due to a physical and/or geometric influence on cell shape or cell contact of the epithelium remains to be determined. However, it is quite possible that alterations in cell structure (e.g., cell shape changes due to a reorientation of the cytoskeleton) may be important aspects of this inductive influence and the resultant condition of altered growth control that exists in BPH.

It is also interesting to note that some of the most well documented changes that occur with aging are alterations in the extracellular matrix components (e.g., collagen and elastin) of connective tissue (Grahame 1970). The strong correlation between advancing age and the development of BPH may be reflective of such changes occurring in the prostatic stroma of BPH glands. In relation to this, changes in the solubility of various extracellular matrix components ("ground substance") were postulated to be important in regulating prostatic growth almost thirty years ago (Arcadi 1954).

Canine BPH has been recently shown to be associated with a decreased prostatic secretory capability (Brendler et al. 1983), in spite of maintenance of serum androgen levels. This decreased prostatic function may be the result of an altered structural environment at the cellular level. It has been shown that the functional ability of mammary epithelium in vitro is extremely sensitive to the substrate on which these cells are cultured (Emerman et al 1977; Bissell et al 1982). Cells cultured on floating collagen gels allows the cells to assume a cuboidal morphology and express differentiated functions, whereas cells plated on plastic assume a flattened morphology and are non-functional. It would be of interest to examine such phenomenon with prostatic epithelium.

In order to apply some of the ideas outlined above to the study of the prostate and the development of BPH, appropriate methodology and probes need to be acquired. We present in this paper some preliminary work on the identification and localization of some of the major structural proteins present in the canine prostate. In addition, work on the identificaion and characterization of a specific marker of canine prostatic function is reviewed. The dog was chosen for this work because of its propensity to spontaneously develop BPH with a high, age-related frequency.

Materials and Methods

Animals

Animals used in this study were all purebred beagles of known age. Surgical procedures, histological grading of prostates and other details are fully explained elsewhere (Brendler et al 1983; DeKlerk et al 1979).

Immunofluorescence

The antisera used and their sources are as follows: antilaminin and antifibronectin antisera were obtained from Bethesda Research Labs.; antikeratin was a gift of Dr. T. T. Sun, NYU School of Medicine; anti-canine secretory protein antiserum was prepared as described (Isaacs, Shaper 1983a). NBD-phallacidin was obtained from Molecular Probes; fluorescein conjugated goat anti-rabbit IgG was obtained from Cappel Laboratories.

For immunofluorescent staining of laminin, fibronectin, keratin, and actin, frozen sections were cut (6-10 μm), rapidly thawed and dried, and subsequently fixed in absolute methanol at -20°C, followed by equilibration in phosphate buffered saline (PBS). Staining with anti-canine secretory protein was performed on sections of formalin-fixed, paraffin embedded tissues. To save space, control sections stained with preimmune serum are not shown. However, these were uniformly negative.

Other methods are given in the text or found in more detail where noted.

Results

Cell Types of the Canine Prostate

A representative light micrograph of a normal canine prostate in presented in Figure 2. The cells present within the prostate can be divided into two categories - stromal and epithelial. Within the normal epithelium there are at least two morphologically distinct types of cells: 1) secretory epithelial with tall column morphology and profuse secretory granules filling the apical half of the cell and 2) the basal epithelium located sporadically along the basement membrane. The precise role of the basal epithelium is unknown, although several investigators have

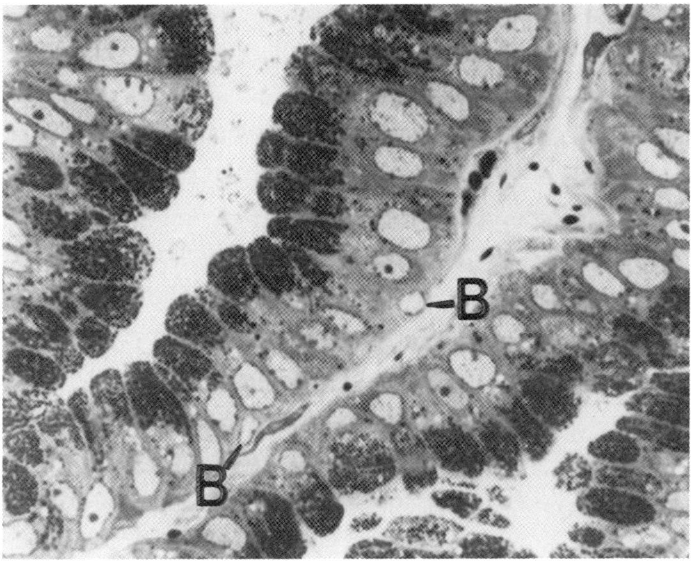

Figure 2. Light micrograph of a normal canine prostate from a two year old beagle. Notice the tall, columnar secretory epithelium with a dense accumulation of secretory granules in the apical portion of these cells. Two basal epithelial cells are denoted by "B". 800X

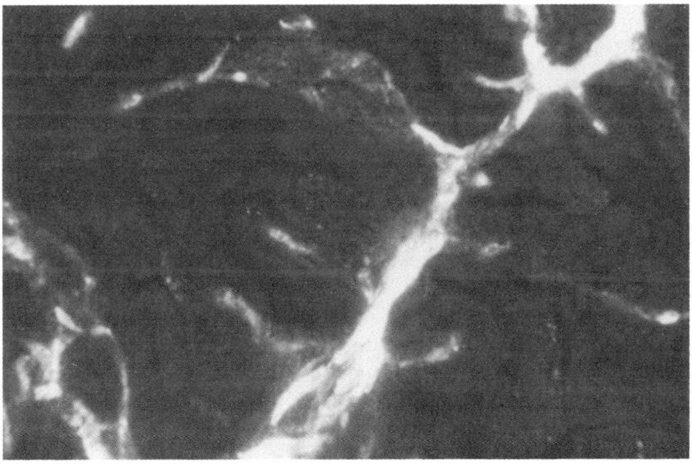

Figure 3. Immunofluorescent (IF) staining of fibronectin in a section of canine prostate. Intense fluorescence is seen in the stroma with fainter fluorescence associated with basement membranes. 130X.

proposed that they are precursors of the secretory epithelium (Mao, Angrist 1966; Timms et al 1976; Merk et al 1982). It is possible that a subpopulation of the basal cells is in fact the prostatic epithelial stem cell. The prostatic stroma consists mainly of fibroblastic and smooth muscle cells enmeshed in extracellular matrix material, primarily collagen. Vascular endothelium and mononuclear inflammatory cells comprise the majority of the remaining stromal cell types.

Immunofluorescent Identification and Localization of Various Structural Proteins in the Canine Prostate

Fibrobronectin: Fibronectin is a large glycoprotein which is thought to mediate attachment of cells, primarily mesenchymal, to their surrounding extracellular matrices (Yamada, Olden 1978). Figure 3 is an example of a section of normal canine prostate stained with anti-fibronectin antiserum. The presence of fibronectin can be seen to be localized exclusively to the stromal component, where it is presumably associated with collagen fibers. Fibronectin can also be seen in lesser amounts associated with basement membranes of the prostatic epithelium, smooth muscle and vascular endothelium.

Laminin: Laminin is another large glycoprotein component of the extracellular matrix which is also thought to be involved in attachment of cells to their respective matrices, specifically in basement membranes (Terranova et al 1980). It is not produced by fibroblasts, but is found in basement membranes of epithelial, smooth muscle and vascular endothelial cells. Figure 4 is an example of a prostatic section stained for laminin. The basement membranes are easily recognizable as ribbons of fluorescence surrounding the acini. The epithelial cells themselves are essentially devoid of laminin, attesting to the strict deposition of laminin synthesized by these cells into their basement membranes. It is interesting to note that in estrogen induced squamous metaplasia, laminin can be localized only to the basement membrane under the basal layer of epithelium, apparently indicating that the superficial epithelial cells do not synthesize laminin. Laminin associated with the basement membranes of both smooth muscle and vascular endothelium can be seen in the stromal component in Figure 4.

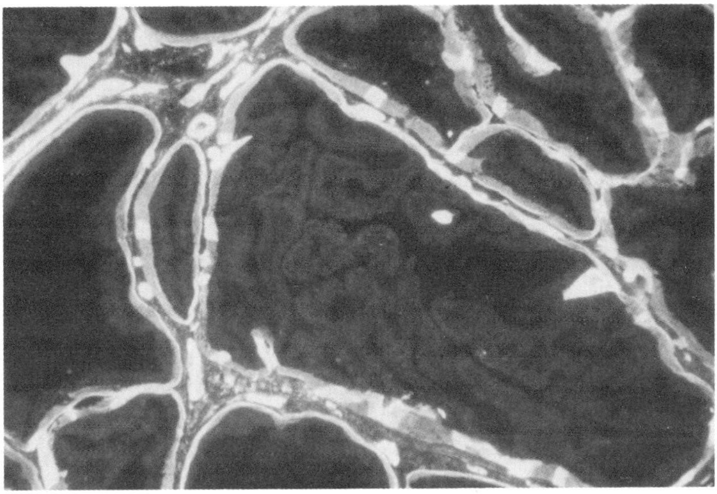

Figure 4. IF staining of laminin in a section of canine prostate. Ribbons of fluorescence surrounding acini represent laminin present in epithelial basement membranes. Basement membranes of smooth muscle and vascular endothelial cells can be seen in the stroma. 130X.

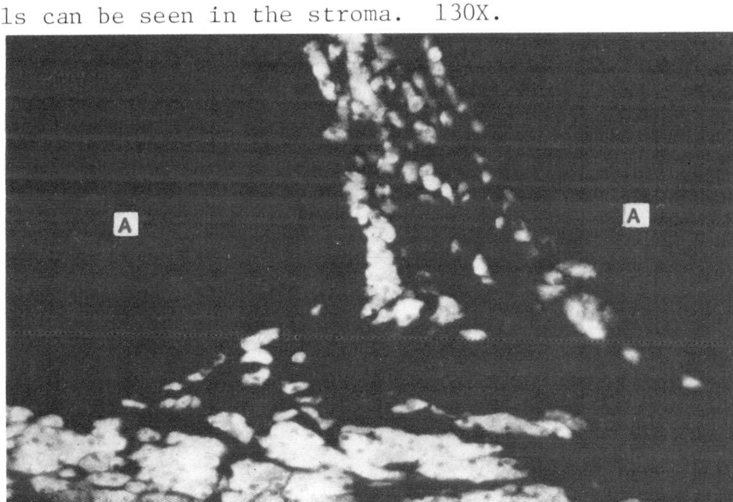

Figure 5. NBD-phallacidin staining of actin in smooth muscle in a section of canine prostate. Acini are denoted by "A". 130X.

Actin: Actin is present as a major component of the cytoplasmic matrix in all cell types, including non-muscle cells, where it is found primarily in the polymerized form in conjunction with myosin and other associated proteins in microfilaments. It is also found, in higher amounts, in the contractile apparatus of muscle cells. Due to the large amount of actin in smooth muscle cells, these cells can be preferentially labelled in prostatic sections using NBD-phallacidin, a fluorescently-tagged mushroom toxin which has a highly specific affinity for F-actin. An example of this staining is shown in Figure 5.

It should be mentioned that no gross alterations were observed in the staining patterns for laminin, fibronectin and actin in BPH glands compared to normal. This might be expected given the fact that overall tissue organization is maintained in BPH.

Keratin: The keratins are a family of highly insoluble proteins of variable molecular weight (40000 - 70000 daltons) which comprise the major intermediate filament component of the cytoplasmic matrix of epithelial cells. Recently it has been demonstrated that different types of epithelium (simple, stratified, or keratinizing) contain different sized keratins as determined by SDS-PAGE (Tseng et al. 1982). Thus, the particular keratins which are present in a given epithelial cell are reflective of the differentiated state of that cell as modulated by its environment.

Immunofluorescent staining of keratin in a section of a normal prostate from a two-year old beagle is shown in Figure 6. Staining can be seen to be restricted to the epithelium. Within the epithelium, the secretory cells stain only faintly, with intense fluorescence seen only in the basal epithelium located along the basement membrane. This intense, basal cell staining is characteristic of young normal glands. Keratin staining of a section of a prostate of a six-year old dog with BPH is shown in Figure 7. Basal cells, although still present, are reduced in number and their presence is somewhat obscured by the increased staining intensity of the secretory epithelium present within the characteristically dilated acini. The reduction of basal-type staining cells is variable in BPH, not only from gland to gland but also within acini of the same gland - in many instances, there is a complete loss of

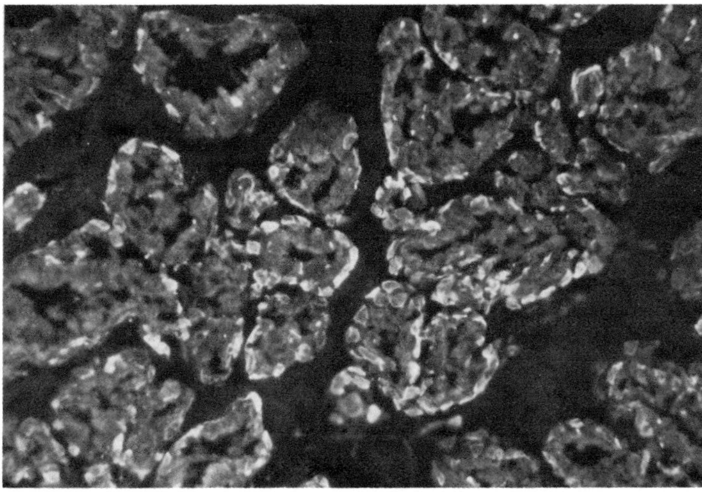

Figure 6. IF staining of keratin in a section of normal canine prostate from a two year old dog. Note prominent staining of the basal epithelium located along the periphery of the acini. Secretory epithelial cells stain only faintly. 130X.

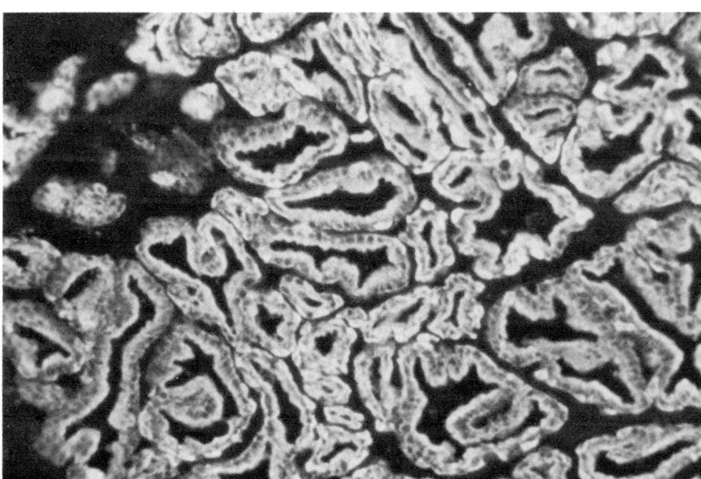

Figure 7. IF staining of keratin in a section of canine prostate from a six year old dog with BPH. Note increased staining of secretory epithelium and marked reduction of basal epithelium when compared to Figure 6. 130X.

distinguishable basal cells. In the cystic acini of complex BPH, the epithelium, often atrophic, invariably stains with uniform intense fluorescence (Figure 8). Whether these changes in the keratin staining patterns in normal versus BPH glands represent alterations in the types of keratins present, or the quantity of keratins present, or both, is not known at present. It is clear, however, that rather dramatic changes occur in a major structural component of prostatic epithelium in BPH.

Canine Prostatic Secretory Protein - A Functional Marker

In order to accurately assess alterations in the prostatic functional capability that may accompany the development of BPH, a specific and sensitive marker of prostatic function is needed. To this end, we have recently identified, isolated and characterized the major secretory protein of the canine prostate (Isaacs, Shaper 1983b). This protein accounts for the majority of the soluble protein in prostates of intact, mature dogs, where its presence is androgen-dependent. It also accounts for over 90% of the total protein found in prostatic fluid. It is composed of two dissimilar subunits (termed H and L), which are linked via disulfide bonds to form the intact protein. A summary of compositional data for the intact secretory protein and its subunits is given in Table L.

In vitro studies of protein synthesis by Dube et al (1983) indicate that this protein is the major protein synthesized by tissue slices from intact animals but, in castrated animals, its synthesis is virtually undetectable. In independent experiments, we have confirmed these observations (Isaacs, Coffey 1983a).

In addition, we have recently identified two functional properties of the secretory protein: 1) it is an enzyme, specifically an arginine esteroprotease. This conclusion is based on the following observations: firstly, secretory protein, purified in its native state, has the ability to covalently bind ^{3}H-diisopropylfluorophosphate, a specific affinity label for the active site serine residue of serine proteases (Figure 9), and secondly, this protein rapidly hydrolyzes esters and amides of arginine derivatives (e.g., benzoyl L-arginine ethyl ester) with little or no activity being demonstrated for the corresponding lysine derivatives (Table 2); 2) the secretory protein specifically binds

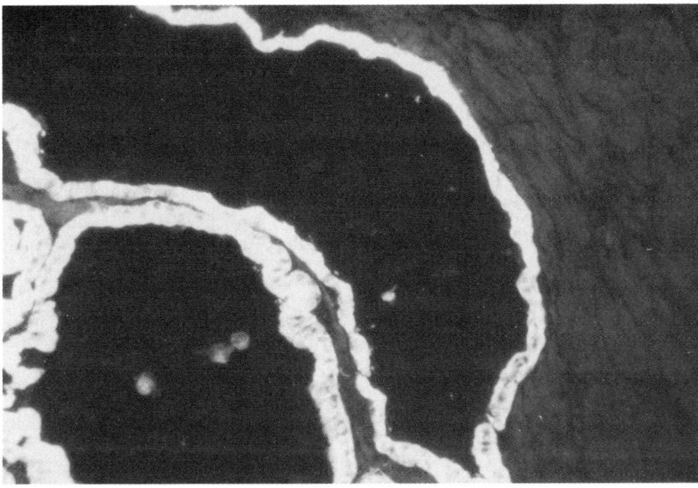

Figure 8.. IF staining of keratin in a section of canine prostate from a six year old dog with BPH. Note intense uniform staining of epithelium lining these cystic acini 130X.

Table 1

Summary of Compositional Data for Canine Prostatic Secretory Protein

	Intact Protein	H Subunits	L Subunits
MW	29,000*	15,000	12,000-14,000
pI	6.5-8.4	8.3-8.6	6.6-7.7
%CHO by weight	3.5	ND	12
Glucosamine (mol/mol protein)	4.5	ND	4.5
NH_2 terminus	Ala and Ileu	Ala	Ileu

ND - not detectable.

*This estimate is based on the mobility of the intact protein on SDS PAGE under nonreducing conditions.

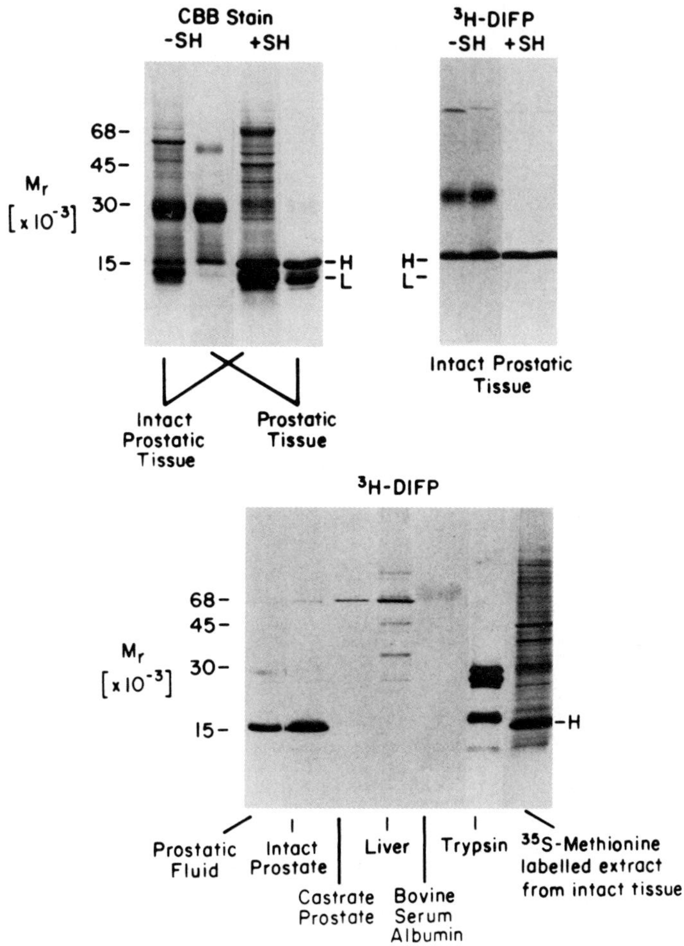

Figure 9. ^{3}H-Diisopropylfluorophosphate (^{3}H-DIFP) labeling of the canine secretory protein. Top left: Coomassie brilliant blue (CBB) staining of SDS gels of reduced (+SH) and nonreduced (-SH) prostatic fluid and intact tissue extracts (H and L denote the subunits of the intact secretory protein). Top right: autoradiograph of reduced and nonreduced samples of ^{3}H-DIFP labeled homogenates of prostatic tissue from an intact animal. Note that over 95% of the total ^{3}H-DIFP is localized in the intact secretory protein and its H subunit. The L subunits do not bind ^{3}H-DIFP. Bottom: Survey of ^{3}H-DIFP binding to various samples and controls. Note absence of binding in castrate prostate.

Table 2
Activity of Canine Prostatic Secretory Protein on Various Synthetic Peptide Substrates

Substrate (specificity)	Activity (nmoles hydrolyzed/min/mg protein)
N-Benzoyl-L-arginine-MCA (arginine amidase)	20.5 ± 3.5
N-Z-L-argining-MCA (arginine amidase)	15.6 ± 2.6
Glutaryl-glycyl-arginine-MCA (urokinase)	10.4 ± 4.4
t-BOC-L-glutamyl-L-lysyl-lysine-MCA (plasmin)	>1.0
t-BOC-L-valyl-L-prolyl-L-arginine-MCA (thrombin)	62.5 ± 14.1
L-Prolyl-phenylalanyl-L-arginine-MCA (glandular kallikrein)	385 ± 86*
N-Z-Glycyl-glycyl-arginine-MCA (plasminogen activators)	19.6 ± 3.1
Methoxysuccinyl-L-alanyl-L-alanyl-L-prolyl-L-valine-MCA (elastase)	>1.0
Glutaryl-L-phenylalanine-MCA (chymotrypsin)	>1.0
L-Leucine-MCA (leucine aminopeptidase)	>1.0

All assays were performed at 22°C in 20 mM NaCl, 50 mM Tris, pH 8.0 and substrate at 0.2 mM. This pH has been determined to be optimum. Using N-benzoyl-L-arginine-MCA as substrate, the following substances were found to affect enzymatic activity: Na^+, K^+ are activators; soy bean trypsin inhibitor, leupeptin, Cu^{++}, Zn^{++} and 2-mercaptoethanol are inhibitors.

Abbreviations: Z, carbobenzoxy; t-BOC, tert-butoxycarbonyl; MCA, 4-methyl-coumarinyl-7-amide.

*This high specific activity of the secretory protein with this substrate prompted us to assay the ability of the secretory protein to cause hypotension in an anesthetized dog (a property of typical glandular kallikrein). The results of this assay were negative.

canine sperm. Using the antiserum described below, the presence of the secretory protein can be demonstrated on the surface of washed, ejaculated sperm, but it is absent from epididymal sperm unless they have been previously exposed to either prostatic fluid or purified secretory protein (Figure 10). Further details of the enzymatic and sperm binding activities of the secretory protein are presented elsewhere (Isaacs, Coffey 1983b, 1984).

As mentioned above, a rabbit antiserum has been prepared against the purified secretory protein (Isaacs, Shaper 1983a). Immunofluorescent staining of sections of normal prostates obtained from intact, mature dogs reveals the strict localization of this protein within the apical portion of the secretory epithelium (Figure 11). It is absent from both basal epithelium and stroma. The androgen dependency of the secretory protein is demonstrated by the absence of staining in prostates obtained from animals which have been castrated or from intact animals which have received exogenous estrogen. The tissue specificity of the secretory protein is indicated by its absence of staining sections of liver, kidney, testes, vas deferens, epididymis, bladder and sartorius muscle.

When BPH prostates are examined for the presence of secretory protein, three types of staining patterns can be observed: 1) normal - intense fluorescence localized to the apical end of the tall, columnar, secretory epithelium. This type of staining is usually found in smaller acini located in the periphery of the gland; 2) diffuse - somewhat less intense staining diffusely localized throughout the cell (Figure 12). This pattern is seen in the larger, hyperplastic acini, lined by hypertrophic epithelium; 3) diminished or absent - little or no fluorescence observable in the attenuated or atrophic epithelium lining the cysts seen in complex hyperplasia (Figure 13).

Prostatic Structure and Function In Vitro

We have been examining the expression of various structural proteins and the secretory protein by prostatic cells *in vitro*, using the immunological probes described above. Using a technique similar to that of Weber (1979) for culturing human prostatic cells, we have

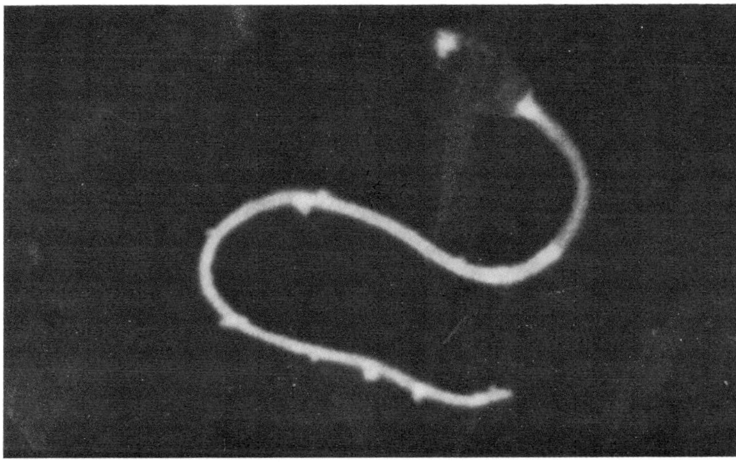

Figure 10. IF staining of secretory protein on the surface of a canine epididymal sperm which had been incubated with purified secretory protein for 1 hour at 37°C and subsequently washed 3 times in Hanks' balanced salt solution. Fluorescence is localized throughout the tail region but is absent from the sperm head. Fluorescence at the tip of the head is thought to be nonspecific. 1200X.

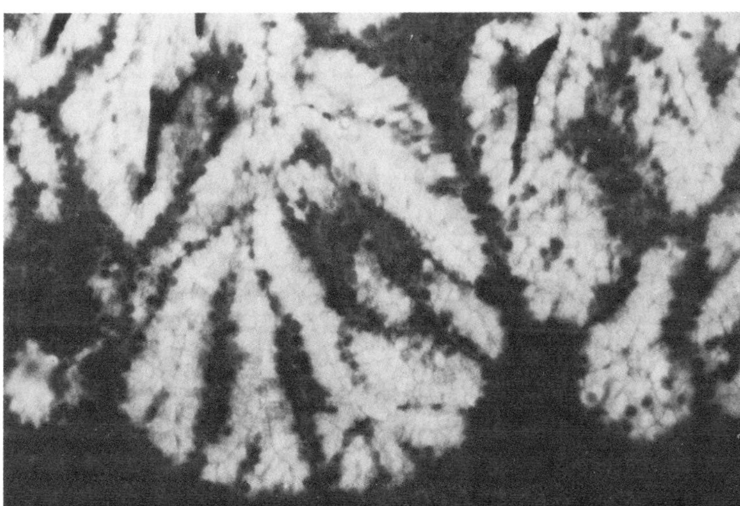

Figure 11. IF staining of secretory protein in a section of normal canine prostate from a two year old dog. Staining is restricted to apical portions of secretory epithelium. 130X.

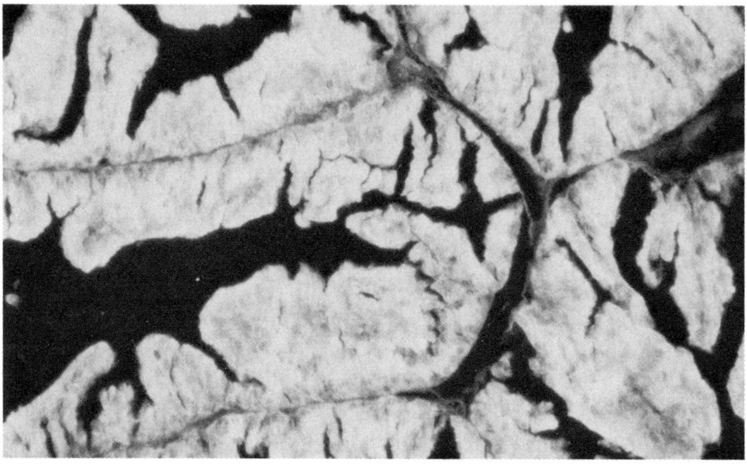

Figure 12. IF staining of secretory protein in a section of canine prostate from a six year old dog with BPH. Note diffuse staining throughout hypertrophic, glandular epithelium. 130X.

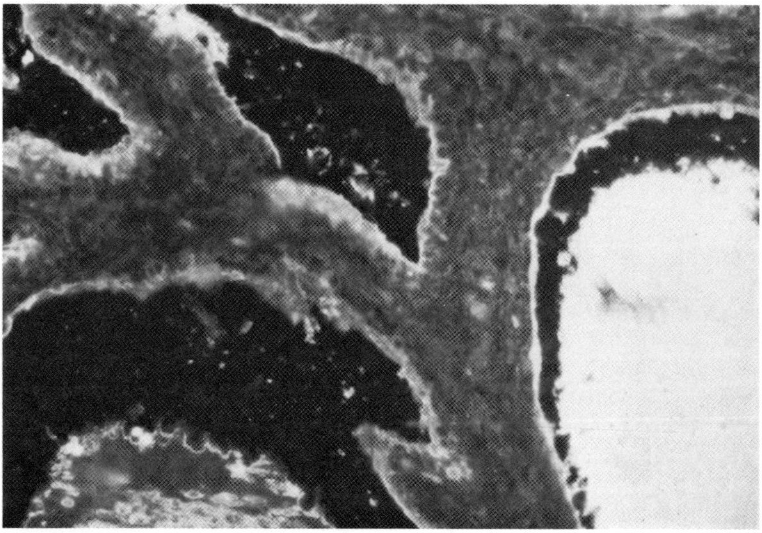

Figure 13. IF staining of secretory protein in a section of canine prostate from a six year old dog with BPH. Note accumulation of staining material within the lumen of the cystic acini. The staining of the atrophic epithelium lining these acini is greatly diminished or absent. 130X.

been able to obtain essentially pure populations of canine prostatic epithelium and fibroblasts.

Fibroblast cultures are characterized by their dense accumulation of fibronectin, stress fibers which can be stained with NBD-phallacidin, and morphology, and their lack of laminin, keratin and secretory protein. Epithelial cell cultures are positively stained for secretory protein (Figure 14), laminin, and keratin (Figure 15), whereas they are stained only faintly for fibronectin and have more irregular and less prominent actin cables.

Several features of the epithelial cell cultures deserve further comment. If one stains the primary cultures of epithelium for secretory protein within one to three days after plating on tissue culture plastic, anywhere from 20% to 60% of the cells are positive. If one examines anti-keratin staining at this time, all the cells are positive (attesting to the lack of fibroblasts) with a variable portion of cells being distinguishable as basal cells by virtue of their more intense fluorescence. After seven to ten days in culture, this distinction in keratin staining is lost, with all cells staining with uniform intensity. In many cases these cells stratify and become squamous as is particularly evident by their characteristic keratin pattern (Figure 16). Concomitant with these alterations in structural protein organization, secretory protein, after seven to ten days of culture can be detected in less than 1% of the cells. Thus, under these conditions of culture, prostatic epithelium quickly lose their secretory phenotype and proceed down a differentiation pathway towards squamous metaplasia. It should be noted that this process occurs in a variety of media and serum and that estrogens do not seem to be essential for its occurrence.

In an effort to maintain the secretory capability of canine prostatic epithelium *in vitro*, we have prepared extracellular matrix from normal canine prostates according to the method of Rojkind et al (1980; Enat et al 1982). Isolated prostatic epithelium attach readily to this material as a culture substrate and maintain a high degree of viability for weeks. In addition, even after one month of culture, a significant amount of secretory protein is detectable within cells attached to this substrate, but not in adjacent cells attached to plastic (Figure 17).

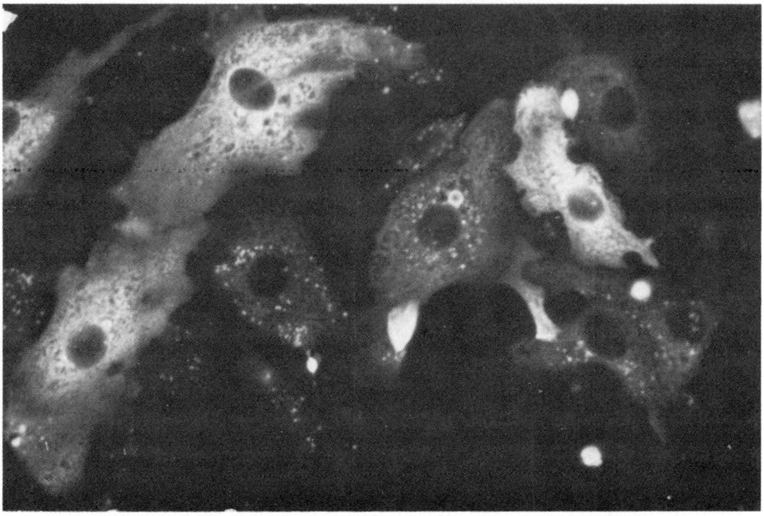

Figure 14. IF staining of secretory protein in a primary culture of canine prostatic epithelial cells two days after plating on plastic. Staining is seen in discrete secretory granules or diffusely distributed throughout the cell.

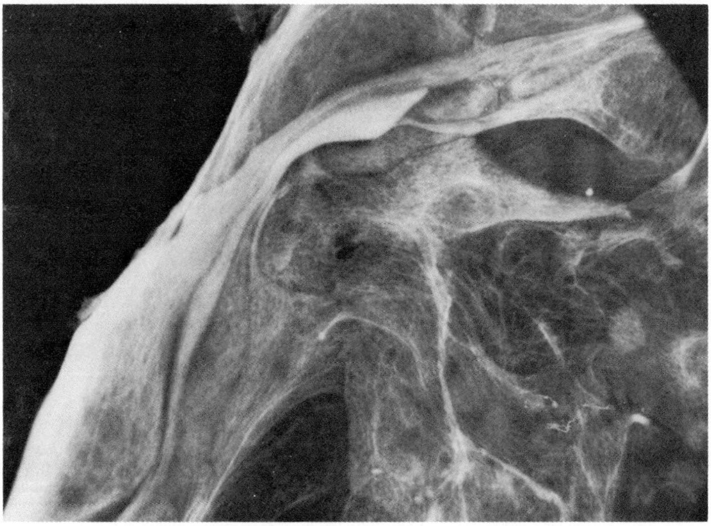

Figure 15. IF staining of keratin in a primary culture of canine prostatic epithelial cells two days after plating on plastic. Keratin can be seen as a profuse network of filaments within the cytoplasm of these cells. 320X.

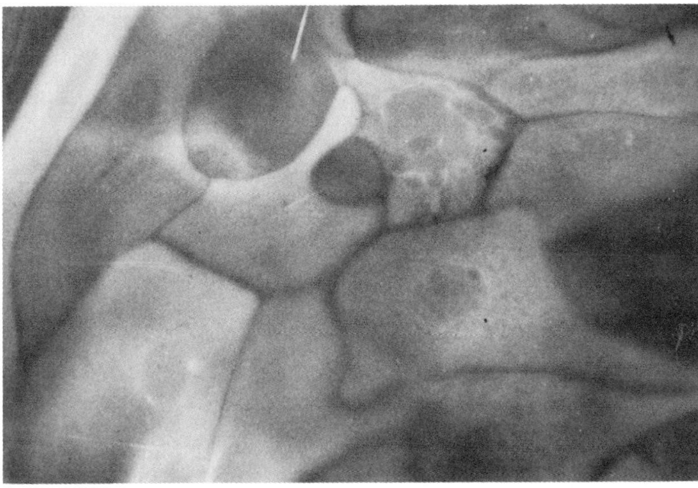

Figure 16. IF staining of keratin in a primary culture of canine prostatic epithelial cells ten days after plating on plastic. The cells have stratified and assumed a squamous morphology. 320X.

Table 3

Summary of Immunohistochemical Study of Canine Prostatic Cell Types *In Vivo* and *In Vitro*

	Cell Type	Secretory Protein	Keratin	Laminin	Fibronectin	Actin
EPITHELIUM	Secretory (normal)	++++	+	+++	+	+
	Basal	-	++++	+++	+	+
	Secretory (BPH)	++++/ ++/- *	+++	+++	+	+
STROMA	Fibroblast	-	-	-	++++	+
	Smooth Muscle	-	-	+	++	++++
	Vascular Endothelium	-	-	+	++	+

*Variable - see text.

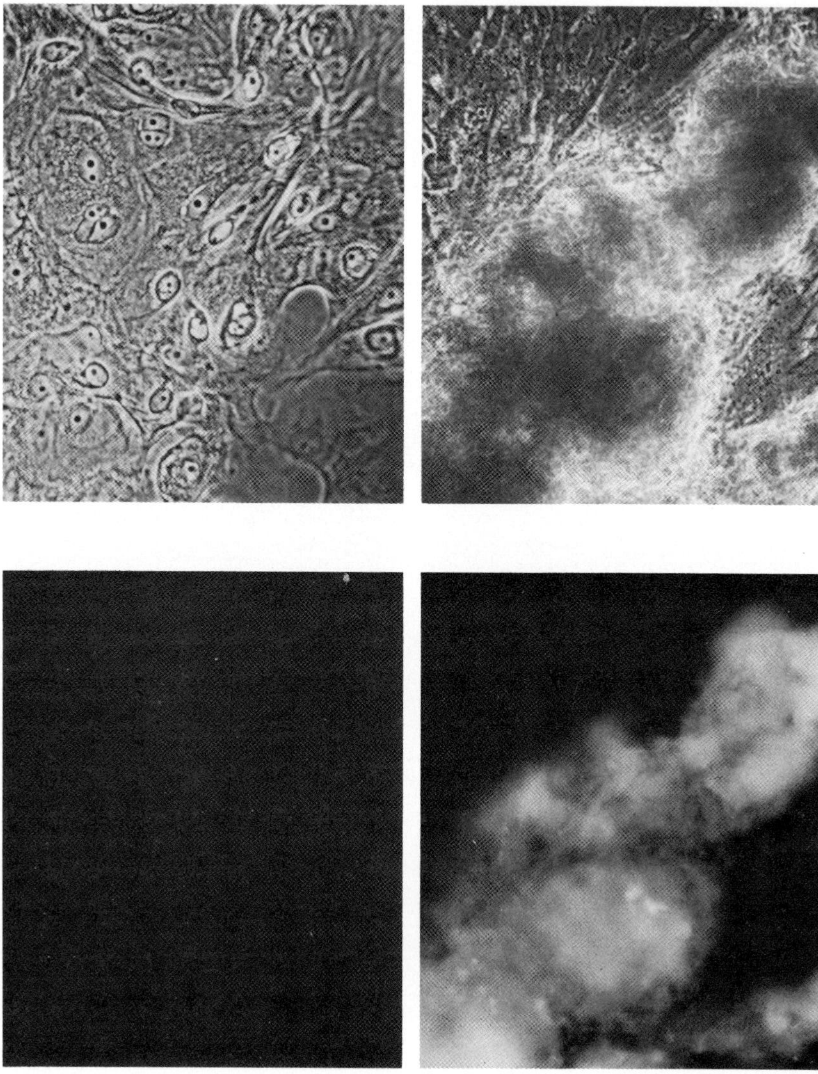

Figure 17. Canine prostatic epithelial cells one month after plating on either plastic (left) or isolated prostatic extracellular matrix (right). Top - phase contrast; Bottom - IF staining for secretory protein. Note that only cells in contact with extracellular matrix are positive for secretory protein. 320X.

Culturing of cells on floating collagen gels results in a similar maintenance of differentiated function, but to a lesser extent.

A summary of the immunohistochemical analysis of the various canine prostatic cells *in vivo* and *in vitro* is presented in Table 3.

Summary - Future Directions

We have presented data on the localization of various structural components of the tissue matrix of the canine prostate. One of these components, the epithelial intermediate filament, keratin, has been shown to undergo dramatic alterations in BPH *versus* normal canine prostates. These alterations can be correlated, to some extent, with changes concomitantly observed in the staining patterns observed for the canine prostatic secretory protein, a specific marker of prostatic function.

Work characterizing the secretory protein has been reviewed. In addition to its usefulness as a highly sensitive marker of androgen action and prostatic function, the secretory protein has been demonstrated to be an arginine esteroprotease which has the capability to specifically bind canine sperm.

In vitro studies have demonstrated that the culture substratum is an important modulator of cell phenotype and state of secretory differentiation. Future work will focus on the possible role of extracellular matrix isolated from BPH prostates in stimulating increased epithelial cell growth when compared to matrix prepared from normal prostates. In any case, further work will be needed to more fully characterize structural changes that occur in BPH, and the possible role that these alterations may play in the etiology of this disease.

Acknowledgments

This work was supported by Grant AM 19300 awarded by NIAMDD and Training Grant CA-09243 from the NIH. The author would like to acknowledge the invaluable advice and encouragement of Drs. D. S. Coffey and J. H. Shaper throughout the course of this work. In addition, the supportive research environment created by Dr. P. C. Walsh within the Brady Urological Institute is gratefully acknowledged. Finally, I would like to thank Ruth Middleton for her excellent editorial assistance in preparing this manuscript.

This work is in partial fulfillment of the requirements for the degree of Doctor of Philosophy from the Johns Hopkins University.

References

Arcardi JA (1954). Role of ground substance in atrophy of normal and malignant prostatic tissue following estrogen administration and orchiectomy. J Clin Endocrinol Metab 14:1113.

Bissell MJ, Hall GH, Parry G (1982). How does the extracellular matrix direct gene expression? J Theor Biol 99:31.

Brendler CB, Berry SJ, Ewing LL, McCullough AR, Cochran RC, Strandberg JD, Zirkin BR, Coffey, DS, Wheaton LG, Hiler ML, Bordy MC, Scott WW, Walsh PC (1983). Spontaneous benign prostatic hyperplasia in the beagle: Age-associated changes in serum hormone levels and the morphology and secretory function of the canine prostate. J Clin Invest 71:1114.

Chung LWK, Cunha GR (1983). Stromal-epithelial interactions. II. Regulation of prostatic growth by urogenital sinus mesenchyme. The Prostate 4:503.

Cunha GR, Chung LWK (1981). Stromal-epithelial interactions. I. Inducation of prostatic phenotype in urethelium of testicular feminized (Tfm/y) mice. J Steroid Biochem 14:1317.

DeKlerk DP, Coffey, DS, Ewing LL, McDermott IR, Reiner WG, Robinson CH, Scott WW, Strandberg JD, Talalay P, Walsh PC, Wheaton LG, Zirkin BR (1979). Comparison of spontaneous and experimentally induced canine prostatic hyperplasia. J Clin Invest 64:842.

Dube JY, Chapdelaine P, Tremblay RR (1983). Effect of testicular hormones on synthesis of soluble proteins by dog prostate slices. Can J Biochem Cell Biol 61:756.

Emerman JT, Enami J, Pitelka DR, Nandi S (1977). Hormonal effects on intracellular and secreted casein in cultures of mouse mammary epithelial cells on floating collagen membranes. Proc Natl Acad Sci USA 74:4466.

Enat R, Ruiz-Oparzo N, Gatmaitan Z, Leinwand L, Reid L (1982). Liver regeneration in vitro: Its dependence on synergies between hormones and extracellular matrix. J Cell Biol 95:131a.

Grahame R (1970). A method for measuring skin elasticity in vivo with observations on the effects of age, sex and pregnancy. Clin Sci 39:223.

Hay ED (1981). IN: Hay ED (Ed.): "The Cell Biology of the Extracellular Matrix", N. Y. Plenum Press, p. 379.

Hay ED (1982). Interaction of embryonic cell surface and cytoskeleton with extracellular matarix. Am J Anat 165:1.

Isaacs JT, Barrack ER, Isaacs, WB, Coffey DS (1981). IN: Murphy GP, Sandberg AA, Karr JP (eds.): "The Prostatic Cell: Structure and Function", N. Y. Alan R. Lliss, p. 1.

Isaacs WB, Coffey DS (1983a). Synthesis of the major canine prostatic secretory protein in normal and hyperplastic prostates. Submitted for publication.

Isaacs WB, Coffey DS (1983b). Characterization of the argininesteroprotease activity of the canine prostate and its secretions. Submitted for publication.

Isaacs WB, Coffey DS (1984). The major canine prostatic secretory protein is an arginine esterase that has the ability to specifically bind canine sperm. Abstract submitted to Am Urol Assn.

Isaacs WB, Shaper JH. (1983a). Immunological characterization of the major androgen dependent secretory glycoprotein of the canine prostate. Submitted for publication.

Isaacs WB, Shaper JH (1983b). Isolation and characterization of the major androgen-dependent glycoprotein of canine prostatic fluid. J Biol Chem 258:6610.

Kleinman HK, Klebe RJ, Martin GR (1981). Role of collagenous matrices in the adhesion and growth of cells. J Cell Biol 88:473.

Lenk R, Ransom L, Kaufmann Y, Penman S (1977). A cytoskeletal structure with associated polyribosomes obtained from HeLa cells. Cell 10:67.

Mao P, Angrist A (1966). The fine structure of the basal cells of human prostate. Lab Invest 15:1768.

Merk FB, Ofner P, Kwan PWL, Leav I, Vena RL (1982). Ultrastructural and biochemical expressions of divergent differentiation in prostates of castrated dogs treated with estrogen and androgen. Lab Invest 47:437.

McNeal JE (1978). Origin and evolution of benign prostatic enlargement. Invest Urol 15:340.

Osborn M, Weber K (1977). The detergent resistant cytoskeleton of tissue culture cells includes the nucleus and the microfilament bundles. Exp Cell Res 106:339.
Pardoll DM, Vogelstein B, Coffey, DS (1980). A fixed site of DNA replication in eucaryotic cells. Cell 19:527.
Robinson SI, Small D, Idzenda R, McKnight GS, Vogelstein B (1983). The association of transcriptionally active genes with the nuclear matrix of chicken oviduct. Nucleic Acids Research 11:5113.
Rojkind M, Gatmaitan Z, Mackensen S, Giambione MD, Ponce P, Reid LM (1980). Connective tissue biomatrix: Its isolation and utilization for long-term cultur of normal rat hepatocytes. J Cell Biol 87:255.
Terranova VP, Rohrback DH, Murray JC, Martin GR, Yuspa SH (1980). The role of laminin in epidermal cell attachment to basement membrane collagen. IN: "Cold Spring Harbor Symposium on the Biology of the Vascular Cell", Cold Spring Harbor, N.Y.: Cold Spring Harbor Press.
Tseng SCG, Jarvinen MJ, Nelson WG, Huang JW, Woodcock-Mitchell J, Sun TT (1982). Correlation of specific keratins with different types of epithelial differentiation: Monoclonal antibody studies. Cell 30:361.
Walsh PC. Human benign prostatic hyperplasia: Etiological considerations. (This volume.)
Weber MM (1979). Normal and benign human prostatic epithelium in culture. I. Isolation. In Vitro 15:967.
Yamada KM, Olden K (1978). Fibronectins: Adhesive glycoproteins of cell surface and blood. Nature (London) 275:179.

Discussion

Chung: What is the culture medium for the epithelium. Are there hormones in it? What kinds?

W. Isaacs: It's not a defined medium. I haven't been able to get the extracellular matrix to support the function of epithelial cells without having serum present. We are currently working on a defined medium in which we could look specifically at what hormones are involved.

McNeal: Are the keratin filaments in the normal dog prostatic epithelium mainly concentrated in the basal cells?

W. Isaacs: It's hard to get an idea when looking at just staining. There certainly appears to be more stain concentrated in the basal cells, however there are keratin filaments present in the secretory epithelium also. As you could see, the intensity is much less in the secretory epithelium but any time you're dealing with changes in intensity, you have to be very careful. So, I'm not absolutely sure what the answer to that question is.

McNeal: There was a change in the dog hyperplasia. There appeared to be very few basal cells with stained keratin filaments and more filaments stained in the secretory cells.

W. Isaacs: That's correct.

McNeal: How about older dogs without BPH?

Isaacs: I haven't done any systematic study of older dogs without BPH. We've been concentrating mainly on what we see in BPH. We don't have any dogs that have normal histology over six years of age.

McNeal: What happens after castration?

W. Isaacs: There appears to be an overall decrease in the amount of staining of keratins after castration. You also lose any distinction between a basal or a secretory epithelium. They all look like the same type of cell.

New Approaches to the Study
of Benign Prostatic Hyperplasia, pages 333–344

PROSTATIC WEIGHT AND ZINC CONCENTRATION

Lars E Tisell[1] and Karl H Leissner

[1]Associate Professor of Surgery

Sahlgren's hospital, Göteborg, Sweden

The weight of the normal prostatic gland in the adult man has usually been reported to be about 20 g (Haugen, Harbitz 1972; Liavåg 1967; Simmonds 1918; van Teem 1936). In these previous reports no information was given concerning the way the prostatic gland was delimited from periurethral and surrounding tissues. As the prostatic gland is dependent on androgens for its growth (Price, Williams-Ashman 1961), the prostatic weight reflects the hormonal status of the subject. For a correct interpretation of this relationship it is important to include only true prostatic tissue when weighing the prostate. By using the anatomical dissection technique described by Tisell & Salander (1975) we have studied the weight of the human prostate and its lobes in an autopsy series including more than 200 individuals.

Fig. 1 shows that in newborn boys the prostatic weight is only about half a g. Before puberty the prostatic weight is about one g. The multifold increase in prostatic weight associated with puberty emphasizes the importance of androgens for prostatic growth. The prostate reaches adult size in the third decade of life and did not change further with increasing age. The mean prostatic weight for the adult men who had died without previous disease was 11.3 g with a range of 7 to 16 g.

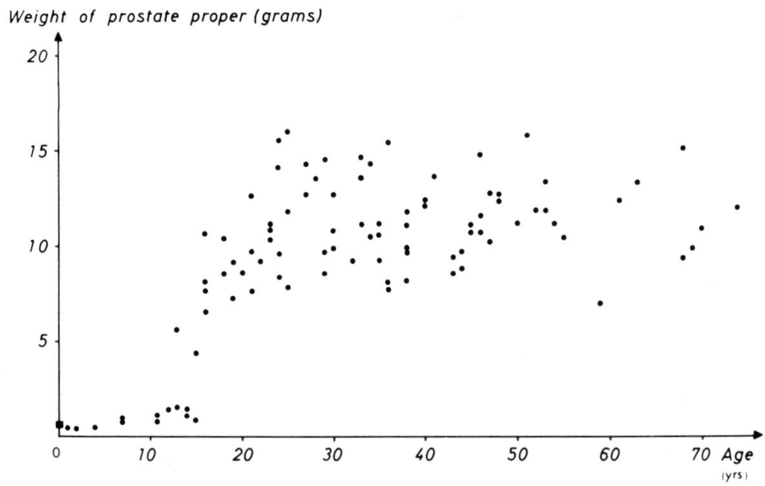

Fig. 1. Scatter diagram of age-weight relationship concerning 99 prostatic glands obtained from individuals who had died suddenly and who had no periurethral adenomas.
■ denotes mean prostatic weight of five newborn infants.

Subjects with chronic debilitating diseases have reduced testis weight (Harbitz 1973a) and Leydig cell mass (Harbitz 1973b) and also low plasma testosterone concentrations (Young, Kent 1968). To investigate whether androgen deficiency could influence on the prostatic weight in the adult man we compared the prostatic weights in patients who had died from debilitating disease with those of men who had an acute death.

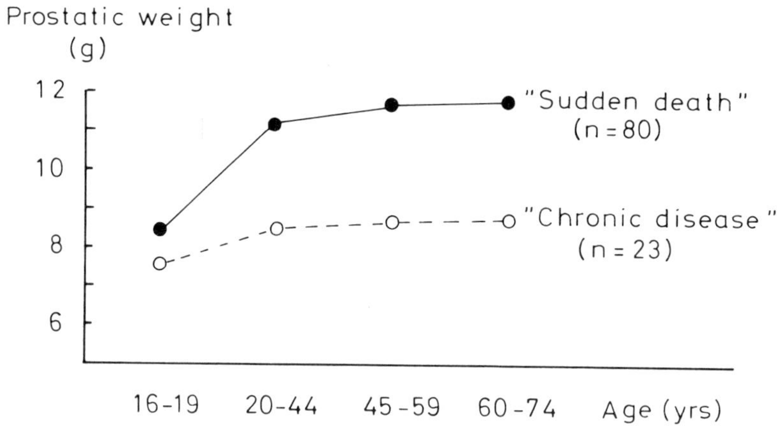

Fig. 2. Prostatic weight related to cause of death

As seen in Fig. 2 we found a more than 20 per cent reduction of the prostatic weight in subjects with chronic disease. In unselected autopsy series the majority of the older subjects probably died from prolonged wasting disease. This can explain why in such series lower prostatic weights were found at advanced age in subjects without periurethral adenomas (Liavåg 1967; Simmonds 1918; Swyer 1944).

Our method of dissection made it possible to define the prostate proper even in cases with periurethral adenomas. Contrary to the opinion that the so-called "surgical capsule" after adenomectomy consists of compressed atrophic prostatic glandular tissue (Semple 1963) we found higher weights of the prostate proper in cases with periurethral adenomas (13.9 $\pm$ 2.5 g) than in subjects of the same age without adenomas (11.7 $\pm$ 1.9 g). These findings indicate that the factors promoting the growth of periurethral adenomas also stimulate the growth of the prostate proper. Our observations concerning the weight of the prostate proper in adult men can be summarized as follows: 1. Mean weight 11 g (range 7 - 16). 2. No weight change with age 3. Debilitating disease -

lower prostatic weight. 4. Occurrence of periurethral adenomas - higher weights of prostate proper (Leissner, Tisell 1979a).

When we studied the weight of the separate prostatic lobes we found that in all age-groups the medial lobes made up the largest part of the prostate (Fig. 3). The preponderance of the medial lobes was most marked in children in whom it formed about 50 % of the prostatic gland compared to 38 % in adult men. In subjects who had suffered from prolonged disease all the prostatic lobes decreased in weight to about the same extent (Leissner, Tisell 1979b).

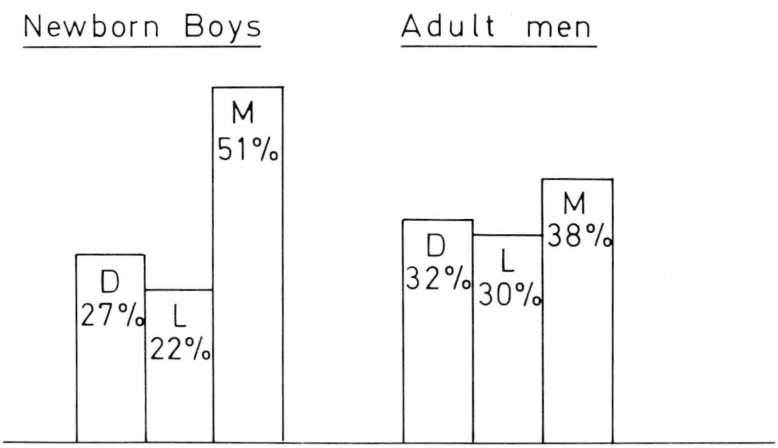

Fig. 3. The percental share of the prostate for the dorsal, lateral and medial lobes.

It has been known for a long time that the prostatic gland is exceptionally rich in zinc (Bertrand, Vladesco 1921). Previous studies of prostatic zinc in man have concerned only a few cases. Only a few investigators have reported the age and previous state of health of the men whose prostatic zinc concentrations were studied. In most previous studies values from pieces or slices of the prostate have been used to represent those of the whole glands (Boström, Andersson 1971; Habib, Hammond, Lee, Dawson, Mason, Smith, Stitch 1976; Hoare, Delory, Penner 1956; Mawson, Fischer 1952, Schrodt, Hall, Whitmore 1964).

We have studied the zinc content and concentration in about a hundred prostatic glands and have related the results to age and clinical data (Leissner, Fjelkegård, Tisell 1980; Tisell, Fjelkegård, Leissner 1982). In an unselected series of 42 men more than 29 years old we found that the prostatic zinc concentration ranged from 2 to 29 µmole/g of dry weight. In some patients zinc concentration was as low as in the extraprostatic tissue. When we separated the subjects into two groups according to the situation before death we found that the subjects who had died acute without previous disease had three times higher zinc concentration in their prostatic glands than those who had died from chronic disease. Subjects with periurethral adenomas are excluded from this comparison (Fig. 4).

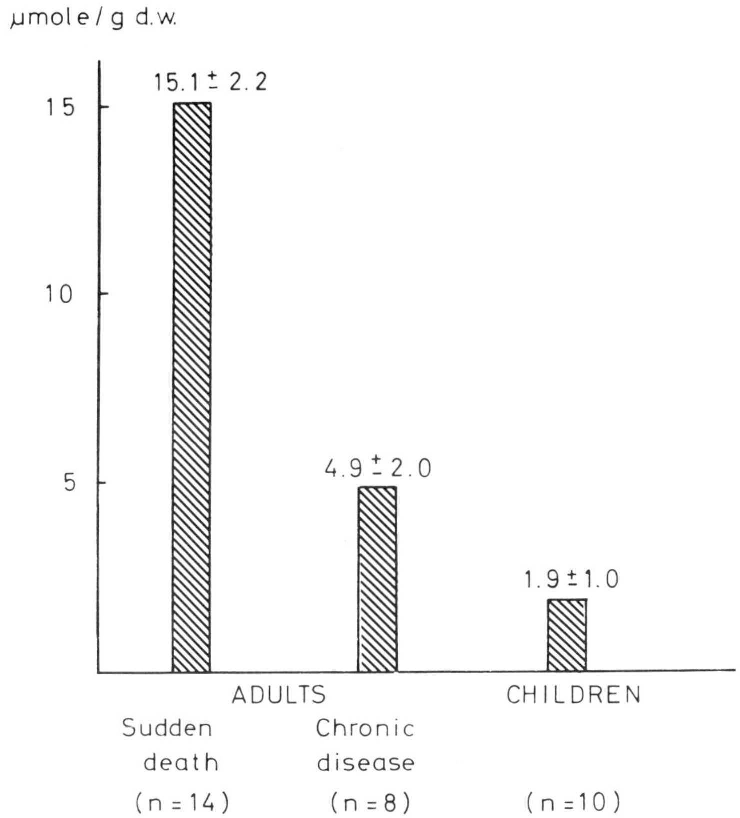

Fig. 4. Zinc concentration of prostate proper (mean ± SD)

On the other hand the zinc concentration of non-prostatic tissue adhering to the prostate was not dependent on whether the subject had died from an acute or a chronic wasting disease. Similarly McBean et al. (1972) found no difference in zinc concentrations of bone, muscle, liver, pancreas and kidney when subjects with sudden accidental death were compared with those who had died from various diseases. These observations indicate that the low prostatic zinc concentration in subjects with chronic disease was not attributable to general effects of the disease. Fig. 4 also demonstrates that the prostatic zinc concentration in children is very low. The age of the children whose prostatic zinc concentration is presented in Fig. 4 was 5 years or less.

In adult men who had died suddenly the zinc concentration was lower before the age of thirty (10 µmole/g.d.w.) than after (15 µmole/g.d.w.) in spite of similar prostatic weights. After the age of thirty the zinc concentration of the prostate did not change with age.

The fact that the zinc concentration increases with puberty and decreases in connection with wasting disease warrants the conclusion that male sex hormones are the major factors controlling the accumulation and maintenance of zinc in the prostate.

Other investigators have observed great intraprostatic variations in zinc concentration. They could not correlate their findings to the anatomy of the prostate as it was intrepreted in those days (Györkey, Min, Huff, Györkey 1967; Kerr, Keresteci, Mayoh 1960). As the anatomy of the prostate now has been defined (Tisell, Salander 1975) we thought it convenient to investigate whether the observed variations in prostatic zinc concentration could be related to the anatomically defined prostatic lobes.

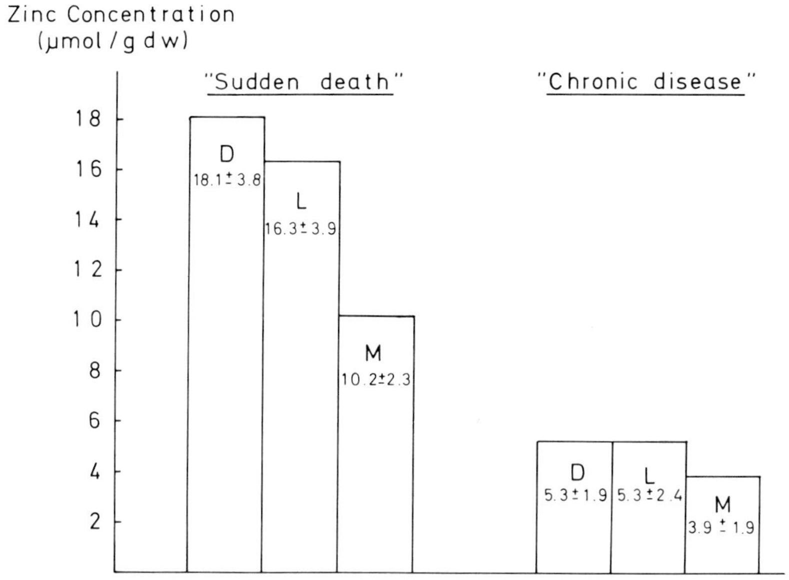

Fig. 5. Zinc concentration of the prostatic lobes related to cause of death.

As seen in fig. 5 the prostatic lobes in adult men, aged from 30 to 69 years, who had died suddenly without previous disease differ concerning their zinc concentrations (n=21). The dorsal lobes have the highest, the medial lobes the lowest and the lateral lobes intermediate zinc concentrations. Thus our findings demonstrate that the previously observed variations in zinc distribution can be related to the anatomically defined prostatic lobes. Our findings also facilitate the interpretation of some earlier observations on intraprostatic zinc distribution. Kerr et al. (1960) noted that the concentration of zinc in the prostate increases from the region near the bladder towards the apex of the gland. These findings fit very well with our observations as the medial lobes are situated near the bladder and the dorsal lobes form the apex of the prostate (Tisell, Salander 1975).It has previously been demonstrated that the prostatic lobes in man can be anatomically separated by dissection (Tisell, Salander 1975) and that each lobe has its own histological characteristics (Salander, Johansson, Tisell 1981). The observation that the zinc concentrations differ between the lobes adds biochemical confirmation of the concept that the human prostate is composed of three paired lobes. The histological and chemical differences between the lobes indicate that they are functionally different.

Subjects who had died after chronic debilitating disease had very low zinc concentrations in the prostatic lobes and the differences in zinc concentration between the lobes were leveled (Fig. 5). This indicates that the differences in zinc concentrations between the lobes is not maintained in androgen deficient states. However, subjects who had died from chronic disease and had adenomas in the periurethral tissue had preserved zinc levels in their prostatic lobes.

The zinc concentration of periurethral adenomas in twelve subjects who had an acute death was 24.1 ± 16.2 µmole/g.d.w. This zinc concentration was twice that of the medial lobes from which the periurethral adenomas had been dissected free and it also differed significantly from that of the total prostate proper ($p < 0.01$). The great difference in zinc concentration between the periurethral adenomas and the medial lobes which are located so close to each other emphasizes the importance of an anatomical dissection.

Our findings in these studies concerning weight and zinc concentration of the prostate and its lobes may have wider implications in prostatic research. They demonstrate the importance of considering the health of the subject whose prostate is studied. They also show the importance of considering the lobar anatomy of the prostate when sampling tissue for analyses.

Bertrand G, Vladesco R (1921). Intervention probable du zinc dans les phénomènes de fécondation ches lez animaux vertébrates. C R Acad Sci 173:176.

Boström K, Andersson L (1971). Creatinine phosphokinase relative to acid phosphatase, lactate dehydrogenase, zinc and fructose in human semen with special reference to chronic prostatitis. Scand J Urol Nephrol 5:123.

Györkey F, Min KW, Huff JA, Györkey P (1967). Zinc and magnesium in human prostate gland: normal, hyperplastic and neoplastic. Cancer Res 27:1348.

Habib FK, Hammond GL, Lee IR, Dawson JB, Mason MK, Smith PK Stitch SR (1976). Metal-androgen interrelationships in carcinoma and hyperplasia of the human prostate. J Endocrinol 71:133.

Harbitz TB (1973a). Testis weight and the histology of the prostate in elderly men. An analysis in an autopsy series. Acta Pathol Microbiol Scand A 81:148.

Harbitz TB (1973b). Morphometric studies of the Leydig cells in elderly men with special reference to the histology of the prostate. An analysis in an autopsy series. Acta Pathol Microbiol Scand A 81:301.

Haugen OA, Harbitz TB (1972). Prostatic weight in elderly men. Acta Pathol Microbiol Scand A 80:769.

Hoare R, Delory GE, Penner DW (1956). Zinc and acid phosphatase in the human prostate. Cancer 9:721.

Kerr WK, Keresteci AG, Mayoh H (1960). The distribution of zinc within the human prostate. Cancer 13:550.

Leissner KH, Tisell LE (1979a). The weight of the human prostate. Scand J Urol Nephrol 13:137.

Leissner KH, Tisell LE (1979b). The weight of the dorsal, lateral and medial prostatic lobes in man. Scand J Urol Nephrol 13:223.

Leissner KH, Fjelkegård B, Tisell LE (1980). Concentration and content of zinc in the human prostate. Invest Urol 18:32.

Liavåg I (1967). Carcinoma of the prostate. Diss Scand University Books, Oslo.

Mawson CA, Fischer MI (1952). The occurrence of zinc in the human prostate gland. Can J Med Sci 30:336.

McBean LD, Dove JT, Halsted JA, Smith JC (1972). Zinc concentration in human tissues. Am J Clin Nutr 25:672.

Price D, Williams-Ashman HG (1961). The accessory reproductive glands of mammals. In Sex and Internal Secretions (ed. W.C. Young) 3rd ed. Williams & Wilkins, Baltimore, vol. 1, pp. 366–448.

Salander H, Johansson S, Tisell LE (1981). The histology of the dorsal, lateral and medial prostatic lobes in man. Invest Urol 18:479.

Schrodt GR, Hall T., Whitmore WF (1964). The concentration of zinc in diseased human prostate gland. Cancer 17:1555.
Semple JE (1963). Surgical capsule of benign enlargement of the prostate. Br Med J 1:1640.
Simmonds M (1918). Über Prostatahypertrophie. Frankf Pathol 21:178.
Swyer GIM (1944). Post-natal growth changes in the human prostate. J Anat 78:130.
Teem van M (1936). Size and weight of the normal and of the pathologic prostate gland. Arch Pathol 22:817.
Tisell LE, Salander H (1975). The lobes of the human prostate. Scand J Urol Nephrol 9:185.
Tisell LE, Fjelkegård B, Leissner KH (1982). Zinc concentration and content of the dorsal, lateral and medial prostatic lobes and of periurethral adenomas in man. J Urol 128:403.
Young HH, Kent JR (1968). Plasma testosterone levels in patients with prostatic carcinoma before and after treatment. J Urol 99:788.

The authors wish to acknowledge the editor of Scand J Urol Nephrol for permission to publish figure 1.

Discussion

Schwende: What is known about the microscopic distribution of zinc? Is it associated with epithelial cells or glandular cells?

Tissel: We have not done such studies by ourselves, but other studies have shown that it is located mostly in the epithelial cells.

McNeal First, Dr. Tissel, I'd like to comment on your findings about the weights of the prostate. I did 75 prostates in the same way that you did, dissecting out the periurethral tissues and measuring the true prostate weights. My findings were just about identical to your findings. I think its very interesting that the prostate weight doesn't decline in men in their 60's and 70's, I wonder if you attach any significance to that?

Tissel: I don't know if I understood you.

McNeal: The prostate weight in men in their 70's is not reduced from the prostate weight in the 30 year old's. Yet the androgen levels are supposed to be lower at that age. How do you interpret that?

Tissel: I have no answer, but perhaps it can be due to a relative increase in estrogens. Because in the cases with periurethral adenomas the prostate proper was increased in weight and a change in the estrogen-androgen ratio has often been implicated in the genesis of prostatic hyperplasia. These are only speculations. Have you the answer?

McNeal: Epithelial activity is high in many men in their 70's. Either there is some altered hormonal status that is stimulating the epithelium more than the original testosterone level did, or the epithelium is becoming partially independent of androgen stimulation. These are two speculations that would occur to me.

Another question about the zinc concentrations. Are the zinc concentrations different statistically in the dorsal lobe versus the lateral lobe?

Tissel: Yes, that was done with nonparametric tests. You saw that the standard deviation was rather high. The zinc concentration was higher in the dorsal lobe in almost every case. The difference in zinc concentration between the dorsal and lateral lobe was significant ($p < 0.01$).

McNeal: The concentration of zinc in the periurethral adenomas was about 30% higher than in the dorsal and lateral lobes. If the zinc concentration is entirely in the epithelium and if Dr. Bartsch's comment is correct that the periurethral adenomas represent almost entirely an increase in stroma, then this would represent a fantastic increase in the concentration of zinc per epithelial cell, wouldn't you suspect?

Tissel: Yes, perhaps zinc is in the secretion also.

Ofner: Two questions: There is a report that zinc might be bound to a low molecular weight species, namely citrate, and citrate, of course is a constitutent of the prostate. Have you or anyone any evidence on prostate citrate content?

My second question is, I'm intrigued about the low level of zinc in chronic diseased prostates. You felt that it may not have anything to do with the hormonal background. What do you propose that the low zinc content in these patients is due to?

Tissel: I can answer the last question. I believe that the low zinc levels in chronic disease is due to lower androgen levels. I think it's interesting that both the weight and the zinc content is maintained in old men.

Ofner: Is the ability of prostatic epithelial cells to concentrate zinc a feature of a fully mature prostatic epithelial cell, or does it also occur in the fetal prostate?

Tissel: I don't know if there is any zinc in the fetal prostate. We have not investigated it.

New Approaches to the Study
of Benign Prostatic Hyperplasia, pages 345–361

PROGESTERONE RECEPTORS IN THE PROSTATE

John A. Belis, M.D.
Eli F. Lizza, M.D.
William F. Tarry, M.D.

Department of Urology
West Virginia University School of Medicine
Morgantown, West Virginia 26506

Studies of the mechanism of action of sex steroid hormones in normal human prostate and benign prostatic hyperplasia (BPH) have concentrated on the dihydrotestosterone (DHT) receptor in cytosol and nucleus (Wilson 1980). In the course of these studies a specific cytosol receptor in BPH with the characteristics of a progesterone receptor has been identified (Asselin 1976, Cowan 1977, Menon 1978, Gustafsson 1978, Ekman 1982). The cytosol progesterone receptor has all of the characteristics of a classical receptor demonstrating high specificity, high affinity, low capacity, and sensitivity to heat denaturation (Ekman 1982). The progesterone receptor in BPH cytosol has a dissociation constant of approximately 1.0nM.

In order to avoid ligand binding to plasma sex hormone binding globulin, the synthetic ligand, methyltrienolone (MT) has been used for androgen receptor studies in the prostate (Asselin 1976). Progestational agents were more effective competitors than androgens for ^{3}H-MT binding by BPH cytosol while androgens were more effective competitors for ^{3}H-MT binding by BPH nuclear extract (Asselin 1976, Menon 1978). In comparison, androgens were more effective competitors than progestins for ^{3}H-MT binding in the rat ventral prostate, (Menon 1978) and progestins were more effective competitors for ^{3}H-MT binding in human myometrium (Asselin 1976).

Because MT binds to both androgen receptors and

progesterone receptors, other investigators have measured specific cytosol progesterone binding using the synthetic ligand R5020 (Gustafsson 1978, Tilley 1980). Binding of ^{3}H-R5020 to BPH cytosol had a K_d of approximately 1nM. DHT and cortisol were poor competitors for BPH cytosol ^{3}H-R5020 binding (Gustafsson 1978). Using R5020, quantification of the progesterone receptor varied from 1 to 40 fmol/mg cytosol protein, with a greater number of binding sites usually detected in open surgical specimens than those obtained by transurethral resection (Gustafsson 1978).

Competition of unlabelled steroids for ^{3}H-R5020 binding by BPH cytosol again showed the progestational agents to be more effective competitors than androgens (Gustafsson 1978). The progesterone receptor-like binding sites have been reported in BPH tissue which was almost completely fibromuscular as well as those with mixed glandular and stromal elements (Gustafsson 1978). Investigators who attempted to separate the epithelial and stromal elements of BPH reported that the cytosol progesterone binding sites were found predominantly in the fibromuscular stroma (Cowan 1977).

Further efforts to eliminate the progesterone receptor from interference with characterization of the cytosol BPH androgen receptor led to the addition of unlabelled triamcinolone acetonide (TA) to the receptor assays to block binding of ^{3}H-MT to the progesterone receptor (Zava 1979).

Recently TA has been used in combination with ^{3}H-MT to simultaneously estimate the quantities of androgen receptor and progesterone receptor in BPH cytosol (Ekman 1982). Incubation of BPH cytosol with ^{3}H-MT in the presence of TA produced relative binding affinities that were typical of an androgen receptor. Subtracting the binding of ^{3}H-MT in the presence of a 500-fold excess of TA plus increasing concentrations of each competitor, from the binding of ^{3}H-MT at each corresponding concentration of competitor, produced relative binding affinity values with a pattern of steroid specificity of a progesterone receptor (Ekman 1982). The progesterone receptor level obtained with this method was similar to those obtained with ^{3}H-progesterone, ^{3}H-R5020, and ^{3}H-medroxyprogesterone acetate.

In order to better understand the cytosol progesterone receptor in BPH, animal studies have been performed in the dog and rat. The dog prostate, which spontaneously develops a form of BPH, and in which experimental BPH has been induced (Walsh 1976, DeKlerk 1979), has a measurable level of cytosol progesterone receptor which can be significantly increased by estradiol injections (Dube 1979, Frenette 1982). The unenhanced level of cytosol progesterone receptor in dog BPH is similar to those noted in human BPH (Dube 1979, Frenette 1982).

The rat ventral prostate has been shown to be lacking in cytosol progesterone receptors (Asselin 1976, Dube 1976, Menon 1978, Zava 1979) but it has previously been demonstrated that the rat lateral prostate increases in weight in castrate animals treated with a high dosage of progesterone (Price 1955).

With the ultimate goal of resolving the functional significance of the cytosol progesterone receptor in the prostate, the present study attempted to define the effects of progesterone on the prostate, and to determine those which are distinct from the action of androgen acting on an androgen receptor. Because the castrate rat lateral prostate has been reported to grow in response to progesterone, this organ was selected as one where progesterone action may be independent from androgen action, and may be correlated with specific cytosol receptors for progesterone. Estrogen-progesterone interaction was also studied in the rat lateral prostate since this organ has been reported to be sensitive to estrogen (Tisell 1971, Belis 1983), and progesterone activity is known to often be dependent on prior estrogen stimulation (Leavitt 1977).

METHODS

Sexually mature Wistar rats, 300 grams average body weight at the beginning of each experiment were used throughout the study. The animals were housed in the medical center animal quarters for one week before treatment and were provided water and standard laboratory diet.

Hormone therapy

Bilateral orchiectomy was performed using ether anesthesia. Animals treated with hormones received daily subcutaneous injections of drugs suspended in peanut oil, or oil alone beginning the morning after surgery in the regression experiments, and beginning 14 days after surgery in the restoration experiments. Injections were performed daily for 14 days, and the animals were sacrificed by cervical dislocation on day 15. The ventral prostate, lateral prostate, and seminal vesicles were excised, blotted and weighed.

In order to determine the optimum effects of estradiol and progesterone on weight of the sex accessory organs, dose-response studies were performed with each hormone. Dosages ranged from 0.5 to 4.0 mg/kg/day for progesterone and 0.001 to 0.1 mg/kg/day for estradiol.

Quantification of cytosol ^{3}H-R-5020 binding

Cytosols for competitive binding studies were prepared at 4 degrees centigrade according to methods previously described (Robinette 1978b). Aliquots of cytosols that contained 3-5 mg of total protein were incubated at 4°C for 4 hours with various concentrations of ^{3}H-R-5020 and non-radioactive competitors. A 100-fold excess of unlabelled steroid was used in competition studies. A 4 hour period of incubation was sufficient to obtain an equilibrium of protein-bound and free steroid, and the protein contents utilized were on the linear portion of the protein-hormone binding relationship. To terminate the incubation procedure and to separate the free and bound steroid fractions, samples received additions of dextran-coated charcoal. Cytosol protein content was determined by a standard method (Bradford 1976). Column chromatography was used to repurify radioactive steroids (Butcher 1974). The purity of radioactive steroids after this procedure was confirmed using Silica Gel G chromatography.

Scatchard plot analysis

Scatchard plot analysis of ^{3}H-R-5020 binding in the male sex accessory organ cytosols was performed as described previously (Robinette 1978b). A 4 hour incubation period was chosen for the binding assay as this interval was sufficient to achieve equilibrium of the binding reaction. When the assays were performed as described, the reaction exhibited a linear protein dependency. A 10-fold excess of unlabelled DHT was added to each assay to block binding of ^{3}H-R5020 to the androgen receptor. Only non-specific binding of ^{3}H-R-5020 was detected in samples of rat plasma.

Although low concentrations of ^{3}H-R-5020 were used to emphasize specific binding, non-specific interactions accounted for approximately 50% of the hormone bound in the lateral prostate. Correction for the contributions of non-specific binding to the Scatchard plots was performed as previously described (Robinette 1978b). Statisical analysis was performed using the students T-test, with significant difference at $p \leq 0.05$.

All radioactive materials were obtained from New England Nuclear, organic solvents from Burdick and Jackson, and steroids and other dry chemicals from Sigma Chemical Company.

DNA and RNA

DNA was measured by the method of Schneider (Schneider 1957). RNA was measured by the method of Hutchinson and Munro (Hutchinson 1961).

RESULTS

Hormone Therapy

DHT restored the weights of the lateral prostate and ventral prostate to pre-castrate levels in both the regression (Table 1) and restoration experiments (not shown). Flutamide at a maximum effective dose of 20 mg/kg/day completely blocked the effects of DHT.

Progesterone at a maximum effective dose of 4 mg/kg/day produced a small but not significant increase in weight of the lateral prostate and no change in the weight of the ventral prostate. Estradiol at a dosage of 0.01 mg/kg/day had no effect on the sex accessory organs after a 14 day regression but did partially inhibit regression in the lateral prostate and seminal vesicles when administered

TABLE 1

Effects of Progesterone and Estradiol on Regression of Castrate Adult Male Rat Sex Accessory Organ Weight[a]

Treatment	Lateral Prostate	Ventral Prostate	Seminal Vesicles
Castrate	23 ± 4[b]	20 ± 2	43 ± 5
Castrate + DHT (5.0mg/kg/day)	248 ± 19*	313 ± 25*	348 ± 34*
Castrate + DHT + flutamide (20mg/kg/day)	30 ± 4	25 ± 3	49 ± 4
Castrate + E_2 (0.01mg/kg/day)	47 ± 5*	22 ± 2	65 ± 7*
Castrate + P (4.0mg/kg/day)	31 ± 5	21 ± 2	52 ± 4
Castrate + E_2 + P	95 ± 8*	23 ± 3	59 ± 3*
Castrate + E_2 + P + flutamide	93 ± 6*	19 ± 2	61 ± 5*

a=animals received treatment for 14 days beginning 24 hours after castration.
b=mg tissue wet weight, mean $\pm$ s.e.m., n>6.
*=significantly increased from control, $p \leq 0.01$.

immediately after castration.

The combination of estradiol (0.01 mg/kg/day) and progesterone (4.0 mg/kg/day) produced a statistically significant increase in the weight of the lateral prostate but had no effect on the ventral prostate in both the regression (Table 1) and restoration studies. Flutamide had no effect on the weight changes in the lateral prostate produced by the combination of estradiol and progesterone. In order to determine the most effective dosage for estradiol and progesterone in these studies, dose-response studies were performed. A dosage of 0.01 mg/kg/day for estradiol and 4.0 mg/kg/day for progesterone was then selected for use throughout the remainder of the studies.

In order to exclude the possibility of estradiol-progesterone effects ultimately being mediated through a common pathway with androgens in the lateral prostate, the anti-androgenic effect of flutamide was examined in the estrogen-progesterone treated animals. A dosage of flutamide of 20.0 mg/kg/day was used throughout the experiment as this level produced a maximum regression in male sex accessory organ weights in castrate rats which were treated with DHT in dosages ranging from 2.0 mg/kg/day to 10.0 mg/kg/day. Although flutamide reduced male sex accessory organ weight to near castrate levels in the DHT treated animals it had no significant effect on the changes produced by estradiol-progesterone (Table 1).

DNA and RNA

Animals receiving only oil after castration had low DNA and RNA content in the lateral prostate after 14 days of treatment (Table 2). Animals treated with estradiol and progesterone had significantly greater DNA and RNA content than animals receiving oil, but less than animals receiving DHT. Similar results were noted when hormonal therapy was initiated 14 days after castration (not shown).

Cytosol Progestin Binding

A low level of specific cytosol ^{3}H-R5020 binding (7 ± 3 fmol/mg cytosol protein, K_d = 0.8 nM) was detected in the lateral prostate of control rats. Treatment with estradiol (0.01 mg/kg/day) for 2 weeks did not alter the binding affinity but caused an approximately 3-fold increase in the number of cytosol ^{3}H-R5020 binding sites (24 ± 5 fmol/mg cytosol protein). Specific ^{3}H-R5020 cytosol binding sites could not be demonstrated in measurable quantities in the castrate rat ventral prostate in either the control group or the estradiol-treated group.

Analysis of the steroid specificity of cytosol ^{3}H-R5020 binding in lateral prostate demonstrated preferential

TABLE 2

DNA and RNA Content in Castrate Rat Lateral Prostate

Treatment[a]	DNA (μg/organ)	RNA (μg/organ)
Oil	159±13	94±7
Estradiol (0.01 mg/kg/day)+ progesterone (4.0 mg/kg/day)	384±21*	323±26*
DHT (5.0 mg/kg/day)	794±82*	1040±148*

a=animals received treatment for 14 days beginning 24 hours after castration
*=significantly increased from control, $p \leq 0.01$, mean ± s.e.m., n>6.

affinity for progestins. R-5020 and progesterone were very effective while DHT was a weak competitor and estradiol and cortisol had no effect.

DISCUSSION

Cytosol Progesterone Binding in Rat Prostate

The physiologic function of the progesterone receptor in human BPH cytosol remains unknown, but may be of importance in the regulation of prostatic growth and function. The influence of estradiol on the development of BPH in the dog (Walsh 1976, DeKlerk 1979), evidence that estradiol levels in men increase with age (Rubens 1974), and the possibility that estradiol may regulate cytosol progesterone receptor levels in BPH as it does in many other tissues (Leavitt 1977) suggest the need for further investigation of the physiology of progesterone receptors in the prostate. Studies of cytosol progestin binding in the prostate in animals have focused on the dog and rat.

The present investigation has demonstrated that the castrate rat lateral prostate has a low level of specific cytosol progesterone binding which can be increased by injections of estradiol. Under conditions of increased cytosol progesterone receptors levels in the lateral prostate of the castrate adult rat, administration of progesterone produced an increase in weight and DNA which was limited to the lateral prostate and appeared to be independent of the potential androgenic activity of progesterone mediated by the androgen receptor. This observation did not occur in the ventral prostate of the same animals and may be explained by a low level of specific cytosol estradiol binding in this organ (Bouton 1981, Blondeau 1982) which is undetectable 3 days after castration (Ginsburg 1980, Bouton 1981), along with very low or absent specific cytosol progestin binding (Asselin 1976, Dube 1976).

Price and co-workers described some of the effects of progesterone on male rat sex accessory organs (Price 1955). Castrated male rats, 8-10 weeks of age were treated with 25mg progesterone subcutaneously for 20 days beginning 6 weeks after castration. Although fructose and citric acid production, acinar size and epithelial height were increased in all sex accessory tissues, a significant increase in wet weight was noted only in the lateral prostate. This study used a dosage of progesterone which was similar to 5 micrograms of testosterone propionate per day. The authors concluded that the observation was a weak androgenic action of progesterone. The present investigation examined a smaller dosage of progesterone (4mg/kg/day) given subcutaneously daily for two weeks beginning 24 hours after castration or beginning two weeks after castration, and no significant change in wet weight or DNA was noted in any of the sex accessory organs.

It seems unlikely that biotransformation of progesterone to C_{19} steroids is responsible for the week androgenic activity of progesterone as flutamide does not block the progesterone effect. Progesterone also is not metabolized to DHT in the rat prostate (Mowszowicz 1974).

When the effects of progestins were measured in the ventral prostates of castrate rats, progesterone and its derivatives had only minimal androgenic effects, while compounds structurally related to 19-nor-testosterone had greater androgenic effects (Edgren 1967). Synthetic progestins with androgenic activity appeared to produce this activity by binding to androgen receptors (Mowszowicz

1974). Potent synthetic progestins at high dosage also exhibited anti-androgenic activity by interaction with the androgen receptor.

In contrast, synandrogenic activity of potent synthetic progestational anti-androgens at low dosage was related to progestational rather than androgenic activity (Mowszowicz 1974). Non-progestational anti-androgens did not demonstrate synandrogenic activity (Mowszowicz 1974). Synandrogenic activity occurred in mouse kidney but not in mouse prostate (Mowszowicz 1974). This observation may be related to the presence or absence of cytosol progesterone binding in these tissues.

Although the presence or absence of a cytosol progesterone receptor could explain the difference in synandrogenic response to low dosage synthetic progestins, it is also possible that progestational anti-androgens are synandrogenic by binding to another binding site on an allosteric androgen receptor (Mowszowicz 1974). Metabolism of progestins to androgens also does not explain how one steroid may be both synandrogenic and anti-androgenic (Mowszowicz 1974). Therefore, the mechanism for synandrogenic activity of potent synthetic progestins remains to be determined.

Cytosol binding of ^{3}H-pregnenolone and ^{3}H-progesterone to unspecified lobes of the non-castrate adult rat prostate has been reported using sucrose density gradients following a 4 hour incubation of the cytosol with the ligand at 37 degrees C. (Karznia 1969). However, more recent reports examining binding of ^{3}H-MT to rat ventral prostate cytosol failed to detect specific cytosol progesterone binding as DHT was a very good competitor for ^{3}H-MT binding while unlabelled R5020 and progesterone were poor competitors (Dube 1976). Other investigators have confirmed that androgens are more effective competitors than progesterone for cytosol ^{3}H-MT binding by rat ventral prostate (Menon 1978, Zava 1979). Use of ^{3}H-R5020 as a ligand in rat ventral prostate cytosol also failed to reveal significant binding (Asselin 1976).

In the present investigation estradiol injections were initiated within 24 hours of castration and increased cytosol progestin binding in the rat lateral prostate. When injections of estradiol were initiated three weeks after castration, a similar increase in cytosol progestin binding was noted and was possibly mediated once again through the binding of estradiol to the cytosol estrogen receptor which has been reported to return to normal levels in the rat ventral prostate by 14 days after castration (Ginsburg 1980).

R5020 has been reported to bind to glucocorticoid receptors that are present in most mammalian tissues but were not found in juvenile rat prostate (Ballard 1974) or in human prostate (Ekman 1982). In the present study, neither the affinity nor capacity of ^{3}H-R5020 binding in rat lateral prostate cytosol was changed by addition of a constant ratio of 10-fold unlabelled cortisol.

Cytosol Progesterone Binding in Dog Prostate

Several investigators have studied the cytosol progesterone receptor in the dog prostate. BPH occurs spontaneously in the dog prostate, and prostatic hypertrophy has been experimentally induced in the castrate dog (Walsh 1976, DeKlerk 1979). Estradiol was necessary for the experimental induction of prostatic hypertrophy in the dog (Walsh 1976, DeKlerk 1979), the dog prostate was rich in specific cytosol estradiol receptors (Robinette 1978a), and estradiol regulated cytosol DHT binding (Moore 1979).

The presence of progesterone receptors in dog prostate cytosol has been demonstrated by sucrose density gradient analysis using ^{3}H-R5020 or ^{3}H-MT.[18] Normal and hyperplastic dog prostate had a similar cytosol progesterone receptor level (30$\pm$1 fmol/mg cytosol protein) (Dube 1979). However, 5 days after a single injection of estradiol valerate, cytosol progesterone binding was increased by a magnitude of 10 (Dube 1979). Relative affinity of competitor steroids for cytosol progesterone binding sites showed that the unlabelled synthetic progestins and progesterone were highly competitive while DHT and cortisol were poor competitors (Dube 1979).

In addition to assay of cytosol progesterone binding with ^{3}H-R5020 the authors measured specific cytosol progesterone binding in the dog prostate by incubating the cytosol with ^{3}H-MT with and without unlabelled DHT (Dube 1979). Because of the relatively low affinity of dog prostate cytosol for ^{3}H-R5020, higher concentrations were needed to obtain saturation. Non-specific binding was high and could completely obscure low levels of specific binding. MT was bound with a higher affinity than ^{3}H-progesterone or ^{3}H-R5020 and had very low non-specific binding (Dube 1979). In dog prostate cytosol this appeared to be a more accurate method to determine low concentration of specific cytosol progesterone binding (Dube 1979).

Further studies of the effects of estradiol treatment on specific cytosol estradiol, androgen and progesterone binding in the dog prostate showed that repeated injections of estradiol enhanced the cytosol levels of all three receptors with the largest increase occurring in progesterone receptors (Frenette 1982). The ability of estradiol to enhance cytosol ^{3}H-DHT binding in the dog prostate may be an important mechanism by which estradiol and androgens together contribute to experimental BPH in the dog (Moore 1979), while the significance of cytosol progestin binding in the dog prostate remains to be determined.

Cytosol Progesterone Binding in BPH

The relevance of the observations in the rat lateral prostate for those noted in hyperplastic dog prostate and human prostate are unknown. Both circulatory and prostatic progesterone levels have been reported to be low in men (Hammond 1978, Lukkarinen 1980), and progesterone is not considered to be a major trophic hormone for male sex accessory organs (Menon 1978). Other agonists for the cytosol progesterone receptor, possibly androgens, must be considered.

The progesterone receptor was not detected in the nuclear fraction of BPH homogenates, but this does not exclude a physiologic role for the progesterone receptor in BPH cytosol (Menon 1978, Ekman 1982). It has been postulated that the abscence of an intranuclear progesterone receptor in BPH may be due to low levels of circulating progesterone or the possibility that the receptor may act in an extranuclear compartment (Liang 1977).

No difference has been noted in the quantity of progesterone receptor in BPH cytosol compared to normal prostate cytosol obtained from the peripheral area of the prostate gland (Nozumi 1981, Ekman 1982), but it has been reported that the incidence of a detectable cytosol progesterone receptor in human BPH increases with age (Tilly 1980).

If the cytosol progesterone receptor in human BPH is regulated by estradiol in a manner similar to that noted in rat lateral prostate and dog prostate , both estradiol and the cytosol progesterone receptor may be factors in the development of BPH. Circulating estradiol has been reported to increase with age (Rubens 1974) and may enhance the formation of cytosol progesterone receptor in the prostate which in turn may mediate some of the hormonal events which contribute to prostatic hyperplasia.

SUMMARY

The lateral prostate of the castrate rat has low levels of specific cytosol progesterone binding which can be increased by treatment of the animals with estradiol. Although progesterone alone is a relatively ineffective agonist in either the ventral prostate or the lateral prostate, treatment of animals with a combination of progesterone and estradiol caused selective growth of the lateral prostate. This response did not occur in the ventral prostate which had a very low or undectectable level of specific cytosol progesterone binding which did not respond to treatment with estradiol.

The effects of progesterone in the lateral prostate were not mediated via the androgen receptor suggesting that the cytosol progesterone receptor is capable of mediating a growth response to an agonist in the lateral prostate. An endogenous agonist for the cytosol progesterone receptor in the prostate remains to be identified, and its relevance to BPH remains to be defined.

REFERENCES

Asselin J, Labrie F, Gourdeau Y, Bonne C, Raynaud JP (1976). Binding of ^{3}H-Methyltrienolone (R 1881) in rat prostate and human benign prostatic hypertrophy (BPH). Steroids 28:449.

Ballard PL, Baxter JD, Higgins SJ, Rousseau GG, Tomkins GM

(1974). General presence of glucocorticoid receptors in mammalian tissues. Endocr 94:998.

Belis JA, Adlestein LB, Tarry WF (1983). Influence of estradiol on accessory reproductive organs in the castrated male rat. J Androl 4:144.

Blondeau JP, Baulieu EE, Robel P (1982). Androgen-dependent regulation of androgen nuclear receptor in the rat ventral prostate. Endocr 110:1926.

Bouton MN, Pornin C, Brandadam JA (1981). Estrogen regulation of rat prostate androgen receptor. J Steroid Biochem 15:403.

Bradford MM (1976). A rapid and sensitive method for the quantitation of microgram quantities of protein utilizing the principle of protein-dye binding. Anal Biochem 72: 248.

Butcher RL, Collins WE, Fugo NW (1974). Plasma concentration of LH, FSH, prolactin, progesterone and estradiol-17-beta throughout the four day estrous cycle of the rat. Endocr 94:1704.

Cowan RA, Cowan SK, Grant JK (1977). Binding of methyltrienolone (R 1881) to a progestrone receptor-like component of human prostatic cytosols. J Endocr 74:281.

DeKlerk DP, Coffey DS, Ewing LL, McDermott IR, Reiner WG, Robinson CH, Scott WW, Strandberg JD, Talalay P, Walsh TC, Wheaton LG, Zirkin BR (1979). Comparison of spontaneous and experimentally induced canine prostatic hyperplasia. J Clin Invest 64:842.

Dube JY, Chapdelaine P, Tremblay RR, Bonne C, Raynaud JP (1976). Comparative bindings specificity of methyltrienolone in human and rat prostate. Horm Res 7:341.

Dube JY, Lesage R, Tremblay RR (1979). Estradiol and progesterone receptors in dog prostate cytosol. J Steroid Biochem 10:459.

Edgren RA, Jones RC, Peterson DL (1967). A biological classification of progestational agents. Fertil Steril 18:238.

Ekman P, Barrack ER, Walsh PC (1982). Simultaneous measurement of progesterone and androgen receptors in human prostate: A microassay. J Clin Endocr Metab 55: 1089.

Frenette G, Dube JY, Tremblay RR (1982). Effect of hormone injection on levels of cytosolic receptors for estrogen, androgen and progesterone in dog prostate. J Steroid Biochem 17:271.

Ginsburg M, Jung-Testas I, Baulieu EE (1980). Specific high-affinity oestradiol binding in rat ventral prostate.

J Endocr 87:285.
Gustafsson JA, Ekman P, Pousette A, Snochowski M, Hogberg B (1978). Demonstration of a progestin receptor in human benign prostatic hyperplasia and prostatic carcinoma. Invest Urol 15:361.
Hammond GL (1978). Endogenous steroid levels in the human prostate from birth to old age: A comparison of normal and diseased tissues. J Endocr 78:7.
Hutchinson WC, Munro HN (1961). The determination of nucleic acids in biological materials. Analyst 86:768.
Karsznia R, Wyss RH, Heinrichs WL, Herrmann WL (1969). Binding of pregnenolone and progesterone by prostatic receptor proteins. Endocr 84:1238.
Leavitt WW, Chen TJ, Allen TC (1977). Regulation of progesterone receptor formation by estrogen action. Ann NY Acad Sci 286:210.
Liang T, Castaneda E, Liao S (1977). Androgen and initiation of protein synthesis in the prostate. J Biol Chem 252:5692.
Lukkarinen O, Hammond GL, Kontturi M, Vihko R (1980). Peripheral and prostatic vein steroid concentrations in benign prostatic hypertrophy patients before and after removal of the adenoma. Scand J Urol Nephrol 14:225.
Menon M, Tananis CE, Hicks LL, Hawkins EF, McLoughlin MG, Walsh PC (1978). Characterization of the binding of a potent synthetic androgen, methyltrienolone, to human tissues. J Clin Invest 61:150.
Moore RJ, Gazak JM, Wilson JD (1979). Regulation of cytoplasmic dihydrotestosterone binding in dog prostate by 17 β-estradiol. J Clin Invest 63:351.
Mowszowicz I, Bieber DE, Chung KW, Bullock LP, Bardin CW (1974). Synandrogenic and antiandrogenic effect of progestins: Comparison with nonprogestational antiandrogens. Endocr 95:1589.
Nozumi K, Sato R, Ito H, Maruoka M, Shimazaki J (1981). Binding of dihydrotestosterone, R 1881 and R5020 in cytosols from normal, benign hypertrophic and cancerous human prostates. Urol Int 36:79.
Price D, Mann T, Lutwak-Mann C (1955). The stimulating effect of female hormones on the metabolic activity and histological structure of male rat accessory reproductive glands. Anat Rec 122:363.
Robinette CL, Blume CD, Mawhinney MG (1978a). Androphilic and estrophilic molecules in canine prostate glands. Invest Urol 15:425.
Robinette CL, McGraw RG, Cricco RP, Mawhinney MG (1978b).

Localization, metabolism and binding of estrogens in the male rat. Arch Biochem Biophys 191:234.
Rubens R, Dhont MD, Vermeulen A (1974). Further studies on leydig cell function in old age. J Clin Endocr Metab 39:40.
Schneider WC (1957). Determination of nucleic acids in tissues by pentose analysis. In: Methods in Enzymology, SP Coldwick and NO Kaplan eds New York: Academic Press 3:680.
Tilley WD, Keightley DD, Marshall VR (1980). Oestrogen and progesterone receptors in benign prostatic hyperplasia in humans. J Steroid Biochem 13:395.
Tisell LE (1971). The growth of the ventral prostate, the dorsolateral prostate, the coagulating glands and the seminal vesicles in castrated adrenalectomized rats injected with oestradiol and/or cortisone. Acta Endocr 68:485.
Walsh PC, Wilson JD (1976). The induction of prostatic hypertrophy in the dog with androstanediol. J Clin Invest 57:1093.
Wilson JD (1980). The pathogenesis of benign prostatic hyperplasia. Am J Med 68:745.
Zava DT, Landrum B, Horwitz KB, McGuire WL (1979). Androgen receptor assay with ^{3}H-methyltrienolone (R1881) in the presence of progesterone receptors. Endocr 104:1007.

Discussion

Chung: Was the lateral prostate that you induced to grow by progesterone treatment predominantly stroma or epithelium or both?

Belis: That is a very good point. We haven't looked at the histology but I think it would be important to determine if it is stromal or epithelial growth.

Chung: When you used progesterone as a ligand compared with methyltrienalone in the presence of cortisol there seems to be a change in the Kd. Why does it change the Kd?

Belis: That was Ekman's work (Ekman et al, 1982) and not something that I did. I don't have an explanation why the Kd was different using progesterone as a ligand. As you are aware, binding of progesterone to transcortin makes it a difficult ligand to use. Perhaps Dr. Walsh may comment in this regard.

Chung: The V_{max} is not changing?

Belis: The V_{max} was not changed. If anything, probably a good point in our assay would be to look at methyltrienealone in combination with triamcinolone acetonide as perhaps a better ligand system than R5020.

Mawhinney: John, would you comment on the importance of prolactin.

Belis: I didn't really compare it in this particular study, but we have looked at the effect of prolactin on the lateral prostate previously. The work of Jack Grayhack shows a fairly specific effect of prolactin on lateral prostate. Prolactin acts much like estrogen, that is, it inhibits regression. It doesn't actually produce growth after regression has occurred. We have looked at DNA and RNA content following treatment with prolactin using autotranspanted pituitaries to raise prolactin levels. We find there is a permanent change in RNA, not DNA content, suggesting perhaps a secretory effect or a cytoplasmic effect, and not a nuclear effect.

Mawhinney: Do you have any evidence that prolactin is involved in this synergistic response with progesterone?

Belis: We haven't done any combinations of prolactin in this model. Perhaps that is worth doing.

Walsh: I can comment on Ekman's prostatic paper. The Kd for progesterone binding to the human prostatic progesterone receptor was found for an animal (man) where the synthetic progestational agents had higher affinity than progesterone. That is why synthetic progestins are preferable for assay purposes.

Reference:
Ekman P, Barrack ER, Walsh PC (1982). Simultaneous measurements of progesterone and androgen receptors in human prostate: A microassay.

New Approaches to the Study
of Benign Prostatic Hyperplasia, pages 363–380

ANDROGEN METABOLISM IN CULTURED PROSTATIC CELLS

Peter Ofner, Ph.D.*, Louis Terracio, Ph.D.+ and
Richard L. Vena, B.A.*
*Department of Urology, Tufts University School of Medicine, Boston, MA 02111 and +Department of Anatomy, University of South Carolina School of Medicine, Columbia, S.C. 29208

The essential nature of mesenchymal-epithelial interaction in the morphogenesis, cytodifferentiation and hormonal responsiveness of the prostate is becoming well documented as a result of work with tissue recombinants (Cunha, Lung 1979; Cunha et al 1983a,b; Lasnitzki, Mizuno 1980). The possibility that the inductive potential of the mesenchyme may resurface in the adult in the form of stromal-epithelial interactions and that such interactions may play a significant role in prostatic disease is an interesting hypothesis.

We have reported the isolation of highly-enriched epithelial cells and fibroblasts of rat ventral prostate (Douglas et al 1980; Ofner et al 1982) and canine prostate (Terracio et al 1982; Ofner et al 1982) by means of a collagenase-digestion differential-attachment procedure. We shall describe here the application of this procedure to the isolation of enriched epithelial and fibroblast cell populations from human BPH specimens removed during open prostatectomy (a more detailed account of an earlier version has been submitted for publication). A procedure utilizing collagenase digestion and low-speed centrifugation for the separation of cells from human BPH tissue was described by Webber (1979). The present paper provides a survey of our preliminary studies of comparative C_{19}-radiosteroid metabolism in primary monolayer cultures of epithelial cells and fibroblasts from rat ventral and canine prostate and human BPH tissue.

Epithelial cells and fibroblasts from human BPH specimens were established as follows: BPH nodules were minced into 1-3 mm^3 pieces and the tissue fragments were washed with F12K tissue culture medium and digested on a reciprocating shaker at 37°C with F12K containing 700 U/ml collagenase (Worthington type I) plus 1% fetal bovine serum (FBS). After 30 min of digestion, the tissue fragments were allowed to settle and the enzyme solution containing small cellular aggregates and single cells was removed, diluted with F12K-10% FBS, centrifuged (50 x g for 5 min), suspended in F12K-10% FBS and stored on ice. The collagenase solution was again added to the tissue fragments and the procedure was repeated until the tissue was totally digested (~5-6 cycles). The cellular aggregates were pooled and washed 3 times with F12K-10% FBS by gentle centrifugation (50 x g for 3 min). The washed aggregates were plated into 100 mm culture dishes containing 10 ml of F12K-10% FBS (5 dishes/BPH specimen). The cultures were maintained for 8-12 h in an incubator at 37°C with a gas phase of 5% v/v CO_2 in air. After 8-12 h *in vitro* the medium and unattached cellular aggregates were removed from the 100 mm dishes and centrifuged at 50 x g for 5 min. The aggregates were suspended in F12K-10% FBS and evenly distributed into new culture vessels.

Within 48 h the aggregates attached and spread out to yield a semiconfluent monolayer of distinctly epithelial cells (Fig. 1a). The human cultures contained less than 10% fibroblasts at day 14 as determined by morphometric analysis (Terracio, Douglas 1982a). These excess fibroblasts could be removed by gentle trypsin-EDTA treatment (Owens et al 1974). The original culture dishes were washed and re-fed with F12K-10% FBS. These dishes contained attached single cells that are predominantly fibroblasts (>99%). These cultures grow rapidly and could be easily passaged.

Both cell types have been characterized by light microscopy (LM), electron microscopy (EM) and histochemistry (HC). The epithelial cell cultures possessed features characteristic of prostatic epithelial cells. Even when tightly packed, the epithelial cells retained their polygonal morphology (Fig. 1a). By EM the cells were shown to be attached to one another by tight junctions and desmosomes to form "lumen-like" structures and to possess tonofilaments and possible secretory granules (Fig. 2a). HC for prostatic acid phosphatase (PAP) (Fig. 3a) indicated that the cultured epithelial cells possess immunoreactive PAP.

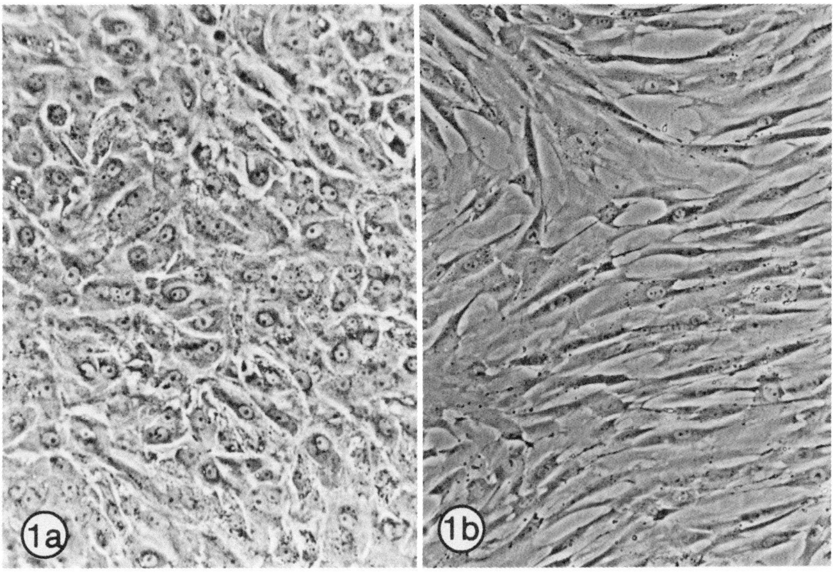

Figure 1 a) is a phase contrast micrograph of a seven day culture of human prostatic epithelial cells. Note the polygonal shape of the epithelial cells even when tightly packed together. 155 x. b) is a phase contrast micrograph of human prostate fibroblasts in culture. These cells have the characteristic elongated spindle shape of fibroblasts *in vitro*. 130 x.

The fibroblasts in culture contained the following characteristic features: they had an elongated spindle shape (Fig. 1b) and would multilayer in culture. EM revealed that the fibroblasts were not attached by cell junctions, and had characteristic dilated profiles of RER (Fig. 2b). HC revealed that the fibroblasts did not contain immunoreactive PAP (Fig. 3b) but did produce detectable amounts of collagen (data not shown).

C_{19}-Radiosteroids were incubated in primary monolayer cultures of prostatic epithelial cells and fibroblasts and metabolic patterns obtained as described previously (Ofner et al 1982). Tables 1 and 2 provide a comparative survey of data from our preliminary studies in which two preparations of morphologically-characterized epithelial cells and fibroblasts of rat ventral prostate and canine prostate were isolated with little cross-contamination. These cultures were exposed in duplicate 24 h incubations at 37°C to each of four C_{19}-radiosteroids at 300 nM and 3 nM substrate concentrations in serum-free F12K medium.

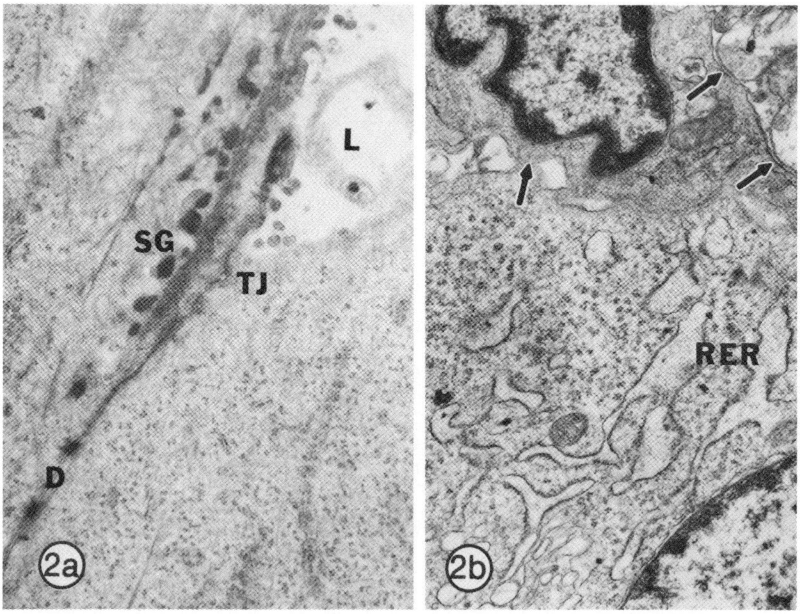

Figure 2 a) is an EM micrograph of human prostatic epithelial cells in primary culture. The adjacent cells are attached by tight junctions (TJ) and desmosomes (D) to form lumen-like structure (L). The cells possess possible secretory granules (SG) near the surface of the cell. 11,050 x. b) is an EM micrograph of human prostate fibroblasts. Note that even when the cells are in close proximity they do not form junctions between the adjacent cells (→). These cells possess characteristic dilated rough endoplasmic reticulum (RER). 16,200 x.

Recoveries as unchanged radiosubstrates from control incubations in the absence of cells were never less than 93% of the added radioactivity. In the presence of cells, recovered substrate and metabolites accounted for at least 90% of the added radioactivity. Separate extraction of the cells recovered in each case amounted to <1.5% of the added radioactivity and yielded patterns that were qualitatively similar to those derived by extracting the media. The proviso needs to be emphasized that several of our

24 h incubations, including those with human prostate cells, resulted in >90% metabolism of radiosubstrate at 0.15-0.85 mg cell protein. Studies with shorter incubation times and low cell protein are in progress.

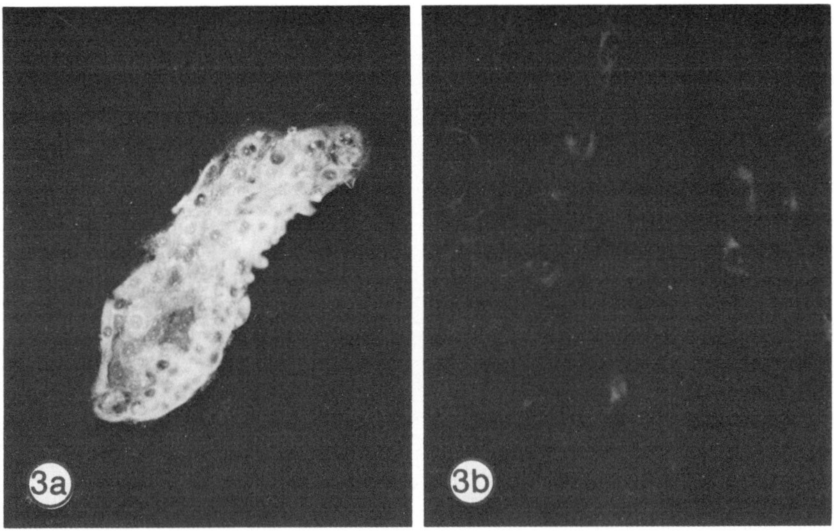

Figures 3a and 3b are fluorescence micrographs of epithelial cells and fibroblasts reacted with an anti-PAP antibody in an indirect immunofluorescence procedure. The epithelial cells (a) are highly immunofluorescent indicating the presence of PAP, while the fibroblasts (b) do not possess immunoreactive PAP and are only visible due to autofluorescence. 225 x and 265 x.

A summary of our findings as reported (Ofner et al 1982) and condensed in Tables 1 and 2 follows:

1. Levels of testosterone 5α-reduction were very low in rat ventral and canine prostate fibroblasts compared with their epithelial counterparts. 5α-Dihydrotestosterone was the principal epithelial radiotestosterone metabolite

2. 3α-Hydroxysteroid dehydrogenation was substantially greater than testosterone 5α-reduction in epithelial cells and fibroblasts of both species and thus 3α-androstanediol (5α-androstane-3α,17β-diol) was a more effective precursor of 5α-dihydrotestosterone than testosterone.

Table 1. C_{19}-Radiosteroid Metabolism in Primary Cultures of Prostatic Epithelial Cells and Fibroblasts

Source	Rat Ventral Prostate				Canine Prostate			
Cell Type	E		F		E		F	
^{3}H-Steroids+	2400 pmoles substrate, 300 nM							
Testosterone	79	140	12	19	>48*	120	27	38
Dihydrotestosterone	47	110	29	49	>47*	150	42	66
3α-Androstanediol		>610*		53		380		230
3β-Androstanediol	150	170	160	75	>46*	320	260	240
	24 pmoles substrate, 3 nM							
Testosterone	1.7	2.9	0.21	0.33	>0.48*	2.6	0.35	0.69
Dihydrotestosterone	0.77	1.5	0.33	0.58	>0.48*	2.3	0.49	1.2
3α-Androstanediol		>6.2*		1.9		>4.0*		3.2
3β-Androstanediol	1.6	4.3	>2.3*	2.0	>0.46*	>4.1*	3.4	4.3

E = Epithelial F = Fibroblast

+pmoles metabolized/mg protein/h. For comparison normalized data were derived from results obtained with 24 h -incubations of the cited radiosubstrate at single cell-protein concentrations in 8 ml serum-free F12K at 37°C, as published in J. Androl. (1982)3:269.

*Radiosubstrate transformation exceeded 90%.

Table 2. Enzymatic Contributions to C_{19}-Radiosteroid Metabolism by Epithelial Cells and Fibroblasts

Source	Rat Ventral Prostate				Canine Prostate			
Cell Type	E		F		E		F	
C_{19}-Steroid Metabolism[+]	2400 pmoles substrate, 300 nM							
5α-Reduction	65	110	8	9	>25*	35	4.7	10
17β-OH Dehydrog.	8	22	3	7	>30*	120	23	38
3α-OH Dehydrog.		>550*		19		230		130
3β-OH Hydroxyl.	6	20	130	50	>44*	230	220	130
	24 pmoles substrate, 3 nM							
5α-Reduction	1.4	2.5	0.13	0.19	>0.24*	2.1	0.09	0.28
17β-OH Dehydrog.	0.2	0.4	0.05	0.11	>0.23*	1.7	0.30	0.50
3α-OH Dehydrog.		>4.0*		1.0		>1.5*		0.67
3β-OH Hydroxyl.	1.1	2.1	2.2	1.6	>0.44*	>3.6*	>3.0*	3.3

E = Epithelial F = Fibroblast

+pmoles metabolites formed by specified reactions/mg protein/h. Normalized data were derived from published results (see Table 1).

*Radiosubstrate transformation exceeded 90%.

Table 3. Metabolism of Radiotestosterone by Primary Epithelial-Cell and Fibroblast Cultures of Human Prostate with Benign Hyperplasia

Prostate Specimen	I				II	
Cell Type	E	F	E	F	E	F
Protein (mg)	0.85	0.75	0.85	0.75	0.30	0.57
Substrate Molarity (nM)	300	300	3	3	3	3
% Substrate Recovered	3	5	1	5	17	3
% as Metabolites						
Δ^4A	18	61	2	49	24	60
A	7	4	10	4	21	5
Androsterone	53	20	54	25	21	18
DHT	2	5	3	1	3	2
$C_{19}O_3$-steroids	11	2	20	3	5	3
5α-$C_{19}O_2$-steroids	68	32	77	43	54	34
17-oxo-$C_{19}O_2$-steroids	82	89	72	88	72	92

The cells derived from open prostatectomy specimens were incubated with the labeled steroid for 24 h at 37°C in 8 ml serum-free F12K medium.

E = Epithelial F = Fibroblast

Δ^4A, 4-androstene-3,17-dione; A, 5α-androstane-3,17-dione

3. High levels of 3β-androstanediol (5α-androstane-3β, 17β-diol) hydroxylation and low levels of competing 3β-hydroxysteroid dehydrogenation were characteristic features of rat ventral and canine prostate epithelial cells and fibroblasts. For rat prostatic fibroblasts this pathway appears to be a differentiated function, since rat-lung fibroblasts actively converted 3β-androstanediol to 5α-dihydrotestosterone and 3α-androstanediol.

4. 17β-Hydroxysteroid dehydrogenation by canine prostate cells greatly exceeded the level in rat prostate cells.

It is instructive to relate these findings to patterns of radiolabeled testosterone disposition by rat ventral and canine prostate in serum-free organ cultures which retain the morphological integrity of the explants (Ofner et al 1979, 1983). We established that the terminal $C_{19}O_3$-radiometabolites which accumulate in the culture medium with increasing incubation time have the 3β-hydroxy 5α-androstane configuration. These metabolites proved inactive in bioassays for androgenic activity (Isaacs et al 1979a; Sunde et al 1982; Cellotti et al 1983). Thus androgen inactivation and egress is effected mainly by the coupled 3-oxo-5α-C_{19}-steroid reductase/3β-hydroxysteroid hydroxylase reactions. Since in low-protein epithelial cell and fibroblast cultures 5α-dihydrotestosterone metabolism was scant but 3β-androstanediol hydroxylation extensive, we surmise that the reductase link of the coupled enzyme system is a limiting factor in the disposition of the active hormone and that it therefore has a major role in regulating the concentration of intracellular androgens. How coupling of the enzymes occurs, and how the stromal-epithelial components interact to facilitate it, remain to be investigated.

Results of our preliminary studies of radiotestosterone metabolism in 24 h primary cultures of human BPH epithelial cells and fibroblasts are given in Table 3. They differ in several aspects from the metabolite patterns obtained with cells isolated from normal rat ventral and canine prostate.

Thus, based on experience with cells isolated from two surgical specimens, levels of 5α-reduction by BPH fibroblasts were considerably higher than those obtained with rat ventral and canine prostate, although still substantially lower than levels found in BPH epithelial cell cultures. The latter conclusion is evident from comparison of the metabolite ratios 5α-reduced $C_{19}O_2$-steroids/4-androstene-3,17-dione, again with the proviso that 0.30-0.85 mg cell protein metabolized 83-99% of 300 nM and 3 nM radiosubstrate in 24 h. Use of this pathway ratio underestimates epithelial vs fibroblast 5α-reduction, as the $C_{19}O_3$-products are almost certainly 5α-reduced 3β-hydroxysteroids, although not yet identified in this series of experiments.

The major 5α-reduction products generated in 24 h by both BPH cell types were 5α-androstane-3,17-dione and, predominantly, androsterone, rather than 5α-dihydrotestosterone. Their formation demonstrates the presence of high dehydrogenase levels of 17β-hydroxysteroid oxidoreductase and reductase levels of 3α-hydroxysteroid oxidoreductase.

This result agrees with findings of Schweikert et al (1982). Their report compared radiotestosterone metabolism, by fibroblasts only, from human BPH, prostatic adenocarcinoma, and nongenital and genital skin. The fibroblasts were passaged and used between passages 5 and 15. Fibroblast cell strains isolated from three BPH specimens obtained at open prostatectomy converted the substrate more extensively to identified 5α-reduced $C_{19}O_2$-radiosteroids than fibroblasts from genital skin which in turn were substantially more active than fibroblasts from adenocarcinoma and much more so than those from nongenital skin. However, here the preponderant enzymatic reaction of BPH fibroblasts was also 17-oxosteroid formation which, together with considerable conversion to 3α-hydroxysteroid radiometabolites, distinguished these cells from one cell strain of genital skin and two cell strains of prostatic adenocarcinoma. Extensive radiotestosterone metabolism to androsterone in our 24 h primary cultures of BPH epithelial cells contrasts with predominant 5α-dihydrotestosterone formation in 24 h monolayer cultures of low-passage and high-passage-number MA 160 cells incubated with radiotestosterone in F10 medium (Ofner et al 1977). This permanent cell line originated from human BPH (Fraley et al 1970).

We have seen that hydroxylated 5α-3β-hydroxysteroids are terminal metabolites of radiotestosterone in organ cultures of rat ventral and canine prostate (Ofner et al 1983), while these metabolites could be generated in primary cell cultures only at high epithelial cell-protein concentrations (Ofner et al 1982). However, in studies with human BPH explants under the same radiotestosterone-incubation conditions, release of labeled 5α-dihydrotestosterone into the organ-culture medium consistently exceeded that of the 5α-$C_{19}O_3$-radiosteroids (6α-,7β- and predominantly 7α-hydroxylated 3β-hydroxysteroids). Concomitantly labeled 5α-dihydrotestosterone, and to a smaller extent 3α-androstanediol and androsterone, accumulated in the explants (Ofner et al 1983, and additional unpublished data). The ability of explants from the same prostatectomy specimens to transform 3β-androstanediol extensively to 6α-, 7β- and predominantly 7α-hydroxylated metabolites was clearly established in parallel organ cultures (submitted for publication). These results suggest deficient formation of 3β-androstanediol and isoandrosterone as an explanation for the abnormally high 5α-dihydrotestosterone content of BPH tissue (Siiteri, Wilson 1970; Geller et al 1976); additional comparative studies with normal and hyperplastic canine (Ofner et al 1983) and human prostate are needed.

In our differential-attachment procedure cellular aggregates on plastic substrate are the source of cells with the described differentiated epithelial characteristics and function. Canine prostate cells displaying exclusively epithelial morphology have been isolated by spillage from deep parallel tissue incisions, expression of cells into the medium by gentle compression, and cell growth in monolayer cultures on type I collagen substrate (Eaton, Pierrepoint 1982). The work of these authors supports the findings of Chevalier et al (1980) who separated secretory and nonsecretory epithelial cells of canine prostate which were then studied in primary culture.

The aggregates isolated by our collagenase-digestion differential-attachment procedure do not possess nonsecretory epithelial cells. We confirm that, when grown on three-dimensional collagen sponge matrix (Gelfoam Upjohn Co),prostatic secretory epithelial cells derived from the collagenase-isolated aggregates maintained a histological organization similar to the prostatic acinus. They retained their columnar orientation and possessed an increased number of secretory granules compared with our control monolayer culture on plastic substrate (Terracio, Douglas 1982b).

A controversial issue in prostatic C_{19}-steroid metabolism has been the location of 4-en-3-oxosteroid 5α-reductase, specifically of testosterone 5α-reduction to 5α-dihydrotestosterone, in the epithelial-stromal compartments. Relying upon mechanical separation procedures, several groups have concluded that 5α-reductase is mainly located in the stroma (Cowan et al 1977, 1979; Bruchovsky et al 1980) and that human BPH stroma has substantially higher activity than its normal counterpart (Wilkin et al 1980; Krieg et al 1981). A serious problem with such procedures is that any time physical separation methods are used, loss of cellular viability occurs although cell markers indicative of cell viability can still be found. Epithelial cells incur greater damage due to their more rigid cytoskeleton and their constituents may be dislodged and become bound to stromal elements. Our preliminary data point to a higher level of testosterone 5α-reduction in BPH epithelium than in fibroblasts associated with acini. It remains to be seen whether fibroblasts from periurethral areas devoid of epithelium have a different 5α-reductase content. Isolation and morphological and steroid-biochemical characterization of smooth muscle cells from BPH tissue are under investigation.

Although much information has become available in recent years which bears on androgen, estrogen, prolactin and aging effects and target-organ androgen metabolism in relation to BPH (reviewed recently by Hamilton, Ofner 1982; Leav, Ofner 1982), little is known of the action and interaction of these factors in the stromal and epithelial compartments of the human prostate. The action of these hormones in primary and passaged cell cultures is obviously a promising area for future research.

In closing I give two examples of possible regulatory mechanisms in which epithelium and stroma may play interactive roles in androgen disposition. Stromal cells, here demonstrated in the case of fibroblasts, may exert control over the extent of epithelial 5α-reduction of testosterone to 5α-dihydrotestosterone through competitive inhibition by the predominantly stromal testosterone metabolite 4-androstene-3,17-dione. Estradiol-17β is an inhibitor of the 5α-reductase (Thouvenot, Morfin 1980) and of the terminal 5α-3β-hydroxysteroid hydroxylases (Isaacs et al 1979b; Ofner et al 1979). Thus estrogen effects on metabolic androgen disposition will be determined by the extent of differential uptake of the hormone into prostatic stroma and epithelium. Study of their sex steroid content, metabolism and binding-site characteristics will be necessary to understand prostatic androgen and estrogen homeostasis and significant abnormalities in proliferative diseases of the target organ.

ACKNOWLEDGEMENTS

This work was supported by USPHS grant 29513 from the National Cancer Institute and by appropriations from the Commonwealth of Massachusetts, Item No. 4532-0001-01.

Bruchovsky N, Rennie PS, Wilkin RP (1980). New aspects of androgen action in prostatic cells: stromal localization of 5α-reductase, nuclear abundance of androstanolone and binding of receptor to linker deoxyribonucleic acid. In Schröder FH, de Voogt HJ (eds): "Steroid Receptors, Metabolism and Prostate Cancer," Amsterdam-Oxford-Princeton, p. 57.

Celotti F, Avosadri N, Ferraboschi P, Motta M, Nesri-Cesi P, Santaniello E (1983). Effects of 6- and 7-hydroxy metabolites of 3β,17β-dihydroxy-5α-androstane on gonadotrophin and prolactin secretion and on sex accessories weight of male rats. J Steroid Biochem 18:397.

Chevalier S, Bleau G, Roberts KD, Chapdelaine A (1980) Characterization of canine prostatic cells from normal and hyperplastic glands. Mol Cell Endocrinol 20:59.

Cowan RA, Cowan SK, Grant JK, Elder HY (1977). Biochemical investigations of separated epithelium and stroma from benign hyperplastic prostatic tissue. J Endocr 74:111.

Cowan RA, Cook B, Cowan SK, Grant JK, Sirett DAN, Wallace AM (1979). Testosterone 5α-reductase and the accumulation of dihydrotestosterone in benign prostatic hyperplasia. J Steroid Biochem 11:609.

Cunha GR, Lung B (1979). The importance of stroma in morphogenesis and functional activity of urogenital epithelium. In Vitro 15:50.

Cunha GR, Fujii H, Neubauer BL, Sannon JM, Sawyer L, Reese BA (1983a). Epithelial-mesenchymal interactions in prostatic development I. Morphological observations or prostatic induction by urogenital sinus mesenchyme in epithelium of the adult rodent urinary bladder. J Cell Biol 96:1662.

Cunha GR, Shannon JM, Taguchi O, Fujii H, Meloy B (1983b). Epithelial-mesenchymal interactions in hormone-induced development. In Sawyer RH, Fallon JF (eds): "Epithelial-Mesenchymal Interactions in Development," New York: Praegar Publishers, p. 51.

Douglas WHJ, Terracio L, Glass H (1980). Isolation, culture and characterization of epithelial cells derived from rat ventral prostate. Anat Rec 197:239.

Eaton CL, Pierrepoint CG (1982). Epithelial and fibroblastoid cell lines derived from the normal canine prostate I. Separation and characterization of epithelial and stromal components. The Prostate 3:277.

Fraley EE, Ecker S, Vincent MM (1970). Spontaneous *in vitro* neoplastic transformation of adult human prostatic epithelium. Science 170:540.

Geller J, Albert J, Lopez D, Geller S, Niwayama G (1976). Comparison of androgen metabolites in benign prostatic hypertrophy (BPH) and normal prostate. J Clin Endocrinol Metab 43:686.

Hamilton DW, Ofner P (1982). Androgen action and target-organ androgen metabolism. In Hamilton D, Naftolin F (eds): "Basic Reproductive Medicine Vol. 2 Reproductive Function in Man," Cambridge MA: MIT Press, p. 142.

Isaacs JT, McDermott IR, Coffey DS (1979a). The identification and characterization of a new $C_{19}O_3$-steroid metabolite in the rat ventral prostate: 5α-androstane-3β, 6α,17β-triol. Steroids 33:639.

Isaacs JT, McDermott IR, Coffey DS (1979b). Characterization of two new enzymatic activities of the rat ventral prostate: 5α-androstane-3β,17β-diol 6α-hydroxylase and 5α-androstane-3β,17β-diol 7α-hydroxylase. Steroids 33:675.

Krieg M, Klotzl G, Kaufmann J, Voigt KD (1981). Stroma of human benign prostatic hyperplasia: preferential tissue for androgen metabolism and oestrogen binding. Acta Endocrinologica 96:422.

Lasnitzki I, Mizuno T (1980). Prostatic induction: interaction of epithelium and mesenchyme from normal wild-type mice and androgen-insensitive mice with testicular feminization. J Endocr 85:423.

Leav I, Ofner P (1982). Proliferative diseases of the prostate: anatomy, pathology and hormone effects. In Hamilton D, Naftolin F (eds): "Basic Reproductive Medicine Vol. 2 Reproductive Function in Man," Cambridge MA: MIT Press, p. 223.

Ofner P, Vena RL, Barowsky NJ, Singer RM, Tashjian AH Jr (1977). Comparative C_{19}-radiosteroid metabolism by MA 160 and HeLa cell lines. In Vitro 13:378.

Ofner P, Vena RL, Leav I, Hamilton DW (1979). Metabolism of C_{19}-radiosteroids by explants of canine prostate and epididymis with disposition as hydroxylated products: a possible mechanism for androgen inactivation. J Steroid Biochem 11:1367.

Ofner P, Vena RL, Terracio L, Douglas WHJ (1982). Comparative C_{19}-radiosteroid metabolism in primary monolayer cultures of epithelial cells and fibroblasts from rat ventral prostate, canine prostate, and rat lung. J Androl 3:269.

Ofner P, Sousa RL, Vena RL, Krinsky-Feibush P, LeQuesne PW (1983). Metabolism of radiotestosterone to 3β,6α- and 3β,7α-dihydroxy 5α-steroids by rat ventral, canine and human prostate in organ culture. J Steroid Biochem 18:415.

Owens RB, Smith HS, Hackett AJ (1974). Epithelial cell cultures from normal glandular tissue of mice. J Natl Cancer Inst 53:261.

Schweikert HU, Hein HJ, Romijn JC, Schröder FH (1982). Testosterone metabolism of fibroblasts grown from prostatic carcinoma, benign prostatic hyperplasia and skin fibroblasts. J Urol 127:361.

Siiteri PK, Wilson JD (1970). I. Formation and content of dihydrotestosterone in the hypertrophic prostate of man. J Clin Invest 49:1737.

Sunde A, Aareskjold K, Haug E, Eik-Nes KB (1982). Synthesis and androgen effects of 7α,17β-dihydroxy-5α-androstan-3-one, 5α-androstan-3α,7α,17β-triol and 5α-androstane-3β,7α,17β-triol. J Steroid Biochem 16:483.

Terracio L, Douglas WHJ (1982a). Densitometric and morphometric evaluation of growth in primary cultures of rat ventral prostate epithelial cells. The Prostate 3:183.

Terracio L, Douglas WHJ (1982b). Characterization of prostatic epithelial cells in organotypic culture. Proc Elec Microsc Soc Amer 40:256.

Terracio L, Douglas WHJ, Pennachio D, Vena RL, Ofner P (1982). Primary epithelial cell cultures derived from canine prostate: isolation, culture and characterization. Amer J Anat 164:311.

Thouvenot D, Mortin RF (1980). Interferences of zearalenone, zearalanol or estradiol-17β with the steroid metabolizing enzymes of the human prostate gland. J Steroid Biochem 13:1337.

Webber MM (1979). Normal and benign human prostatic epithelium in culture. I. Isolation. In Vitro 15:967.

Wilkin RP, Bruchovsky N, Shnitka TK, Rennie PS, Comeau TL (1980). Stromal 5α-reductase activity is elevated in benign prostatic hyperplasia. Acta Endocrinologica 94:284.

Discussion

Katzenellenbogen: Could you say a little more about your sponge cultures?

Ofner: We use Gelfoam® (The Upjohn Company) as a substrate for the epithelial cells. The epithelial cells are innoculated directly onto the Gelfoam. The interesting thing then is that the epithelial cells sit directly on that substrate. It forms a sort of biomembrane. We've shown the viability of the epithelial cells in this system. There is apprently some reaggregation and acini and lumen formation. It reconstitutes the acinus and that is what we're really interested in. We're not really all that interested in epithelial cells per se, we're much more interested in the epithelial acinus. I think perhaps a comparison of organ culture, explant culture, organotypic culture and cell culture will answer different questions.

Chung: I have one comment and two questions. The comment is, we reported 5-alpha reductase activity in isolated rat ventral prostatic epithelium and in stroma in 1981. We agree with your talk today that most of the 5-apha reductase activity is in the epithelium. There's very little in the stroma based on the metabolites that we assayed by HPLC.

I'm not sure about the $C_{19}O_3$-radiometabolite that you described. What is that metabolized to? I'm curious about the production of the 6-alpha and 7-alpha diols. Do they belong to your $C_{19}O_3$-products? It is 17-hydroxylated plus the triols. Is it all combined?

Ofner: All the $C_{19}O_3$ steroids are classical androgens up to the diol stage. The 3-beta diol gets hydroxylated with an extra hydroxyl function. Work done both in our lab and Dr. John Isaac's lab, showed that the 3-beta androstanediol, together with isoandrostene, that's the ketone analog of 3-beta androstanediol, are specific substrates for 6- and 7-hydroxylation. These are water soluble, they come out into the medium, they're not androgenically active, they're not bound, and they are terminal metabolites.

Chung: As you indicated, these are microsomal P450 reactions. Which of the metabolites or metabolite are the predominant metabolite produced by the stroma?

Ofner: There's no difference between stroma and epithelium. It is species-specific. In other words, it's mainly 6-alpha in the rat and in the dog, it's mainly 7-alpha. We've done both rat ventral prostate fibroblasts and epithelial cells and found them. Do you agree, Dr. Isaacs?

J. Isaacs: Yes.

Ofner: It does look, even in the canine, that there is some 7-beta hydroxylation. There's not too much difference between the human and dog, but certainly in the human and the dog 7-hydroxylation predominates. When you use smooth muscle, e.g., diaphragmatic muscle, you go from dihydrotestosterone to the 3-alpha diol. In other words, it is not in the prostate that 3-alpha androstanediol is mainly in the oxided form, the dehydrogenation mode goes to dihydrotestosterone and the 3-alpha diol is not hydroxylated. It is the 3-beta diol which is specifically hydroxylated.

Chung: Do you want to speculate on the biological function of 3-beta diol in organ cultures?

Ofner: First, I wanted to say that I believe that the reductase is the limiting factor. I believe that this particular enzyme reaction determines the overall disposition of dihydrotesterone and it may be that when that particular enzyme reaction is deficient, dihydrotestosterone accumulation occurs. We've seen that it doesn't accumulate in content but 3-alpha diol, together with estrogen, produced massive hyperplasias in the canine prostate. That is because 3-alpha diol is such a very good precursor for dihydrotestosterone.

Regarding the question of 3-beta androstanediol function, the interesting thing is that 3-beta androstanediol is in about six different tissues. We have done work in the prostate and shown that 3-beta androstanediol binds to the cytoplasmic estrogen receptor at a moderate affinity (paper in press). We have not yet found 3-beta androstanediol in the nucleus but we can dissociate estrogen off its cytoplasmic receptor with 3-beta androstanediol. This is true in the prostate and uterus. Also, 3-beta androstanediol has recently been shown by Adams to be estrogenic. In other words, you get 3-beta androstanediol and you can restore uterine activity in the castrate. Whether 3-beta androstene has an additional function of promoting secretion is not known. We know now that it is binding to the estrogen receptor. What it's real molecular action *per se* is, whether it mediates secretion, perhaps by nongenetic, epigenetic mechanisms, or level of translation, we don't know. It's an unresolved problem which we are hoping to address.

Index

PROGRESS IN CLINICAL AND BIOLOGICAL RESEARCH

Vol 1: **Erythrocyte Structure and Function,** George J. Brewer, *Editor*

Vol 2: **Preventability of Perinatal Injury,** Karlis Adamsons, Howard A. Fox, *Editors*

Vol 3: **Infections of the Fetus and the Newborn Infant,** Saul Krugman, Anne A. Gershon, *Editors*

Vol 4: **Conflicts in Childhood Cancer: An Evaluation of Current Management,** Lucius F. Sinks, John O. Godden, *Editors*

Vol 5: **Trace Components of Plasma: Isolation and Clinical Significance,** G.A. Jamieson, T.J. Greenwalt, *Editors*

Vol 6: **Prostatic Disease,** H. Marberger, H. Haschek, H.K.A. Schirmer, J.A.C. Colston, E. Witkin, *Editors*

Vol 7: **Blood Pressure, Edema and Proteinuria in Pregnancy,** Emanuel A. Friedman, *Editor*

Vol 8: **Cell Surface Receptors,** Garth L. Nicolson, Michael A. Raftery, Martin Rodbell, C. Fred Fox, *Editors*

Vol 9: **Membranes and Neoplasia: New Approaches and Strategies,** Vincent T. Marchesi, *Editor*

Vol 10: **Diabetes and Other Endocrine Disorders During Pregnancy and in the Newborn,** Maria I. New, Robert H. Fiser, *Editors*

Vol 11: **Clinical Uses of Frozen-Thawed Red Blood Cells,** John A. Griep, *Editor*

Vol 12: **Breast Cancer,** Albert C.W. Montague, Geary L. Stonesifer, Jr., Edward F. Lewison, *Editors*

Vol 13: **The Granulocyte: Function and Clinical Utilization,** Tibor J. Greenwalt, G.A. Jamieson, *Editors*

Vol 14: **Zinc Metabolism: Current Aspects in Health and Disease,** George J. Brewer, Ananda S. Prasad, *Editors*

Vol 15: **Cellular Neurobiology,** Zach Hall, Regis Kelly, C. Fred Fox, *Editors*

Vol 16: **HLA and Malignancy,** Gerald P. Murphy, *Editor*

Vol 17: **Cell Shape and Surface Architecture,** Jean Paul Revel, Ulf Henning, C. Fred Fox, *Editors*

Vol 18: **Tay-Sachs Disease: Screening and Prevention,** Michael M. Kaback, *Editor*

Vol 19: **Blood Substitutes and Plasma Expanders,** G.A. Jamieson, T.J. Greenwalt, *Editors*

Vol 20: **Erythrocyte Membranes: Recent Clinical and Experimental Advances,** Walter C. Kruckeberg, John W. Eaton, George J. Brewer, *Editors*

Vol 21: **The Red Cell,** George J. Brewer, *Editor*

Vol 22: **Molecular Aspects of Membrane Transport,** Dale Oxender, C. Fred Fox, *Editors*

Vol 23: **Cell Surface Carbohydrates and Biological Recognition,** Vincent T. Marchesi, Victor Ginsburg, Phillips W. Robbins, C. Fred Fox, *Editors*

Vol 24: **Twin Research, Proceedings of the Second International Congress on Twin Studies,** Walter E. Nance, *Editor* Published in 3 volumes: Part A: **Psychology and Methodology** Part B: **Biology and Epidemiology** Part C: **Clinical Studies**

Vol 25: **Recent Advances in Clinical Oncology,** Tapan A. Hazra, Michael C. Beachley, *Editors*

Vol 26: **Origin and Natural History of Cell Lines,** Claudio Barigozzi, *Editor*

Vol 27: **Membrane Mechanisms of Drugs of Abuse,** Charles W. Sharp, Leo G. Abood, *Editors*

Vol 28: **The Blood Platelet in Transfusion Therapy,** G.A. Jamieson, Tibor J. Greenwalt, *Editors*

Vol 29: **Biomedical Applications of the Horseshoe Crab (Limulidae),** Elias Cohen, *Editor-in-Chief*

Vol 30: **Normal and Abnormal Red Cell Membranes,** Samuel E. Lux, Vincent T. Marchesi, C. Fred Fox, *Editors*

Vol 31: **Transmembrane Signaling,** Mark Bitensky, R. John Collier, Donald F. Steiner, C. Fred Fox, *Editors*

Vol 32: **Genetic Analysis of Common Diseases: Applications to Predictive Factors in Coronary Disease,** Charles F. Sing, Mark Skolnick, *Editors*

Vol 33: **Prostate Cancer and Hormone Receptors,** Gerald P. Murphy, Avery A. Sandberg, *Editors*

Vol 34: **The Management of Genetic Disorders,** Constantine J. Papadatos, Christos S. Bartsocas, *Editors*

Vol 35: **Antibiotics and Hospitals,** Carlo Grassi, Giuseppe Ostino, *Editors*

Vol 36: **Drug and Chemical Risks to the Fetus and Newborn,** Richard H. Schwarz, Sumner J. Yaffe, *Editors*

Vol 37: **Models for Prostate Cancer,** Gerald P. Murphy, *Editor*

Vol 38: **Ethics, Humanism, and Medicine,** Marc D. Basson, *Editor*

Vol 39: **Neurochemistry and Clinical Neurology,** Leontino Battistin, George Hashim, Abel Lajtha, *Editors*

Vol 40: **Biological Recognition and Assembly,** David S. Eisenberg, James A. Lake, C. Fred Fox, *Editors*

Vol 41: **Tumor Cell Surfaces and Malignancy,** Richard O. Hynes, C. Fred Fox, *Editors*

Vol 42: **Membranes, Receptors, and the Immune Response: 80 Years After Ehrlich's Side Chain Theory,** Edward P. Cohen, Heinz Köhler, *Editors*

Vol 43: **Immunobiology of the Erythrocyte,** S. Gerald Sandler, Jacob Nusbacher, Moses S. Schanfield, *Editors*

Vol 44: **Perinatal Medicine Today,** Bruce K. Young, *Editor*

Vol 45: **Mammalian Genetics and Cancer: The Jackson Laboratory Fiftieth Anniversary Symposium,** Elizabeth S. Russell, *Editor*

Vol 46: **Etiology of Cleft Lip and Cleft Palate,** Michael Melnick, David Bixler, Edward D. Shields, *Editors*

Vol 47: **New Developments With Human and Veterinary Vaccines,** A. Mizrahi, I. Hertman, M.A. Klingberg, A. Kohn, *Editors*

Vol 48: **Cloning of Human Tumor Stem Cells,** Sidney E. Salmon, *Editor*

Vol 49: **Myelin: Chemistry and Biology,** George A. Hashim, *Editor*

Vol 50: **Rights and Responsibilities in Modern Medicine: The Second Volume in a Series on Ethics, Humanism, and Medicine,** Marc D. Basson, *Editor*

Vol 51: **The Function of Red Blood Cells: Erythrocyte Pathobiology,** Donald F. H. Wallach, *Editor*

Vol 52: **Conduction Velocity Distributions: A Population Approach to Electrophysiology of Nerve,** Leslie J. Dorfman, Kenneth L. Cummins, Lary J. Leifer, *Editors*

Vol 53: **Cancer Among Black Populations,** Curtis Mettlin, Gerald P. Murphy, *Editors*

Vol 54: **Connective Tissue Research: Chemistry, Biology, and Physiology,** Zdenek Deyl, Milan Adam, *Editors*

Vol 55: **The Red Cell: Fifth Ann Arbor Conference,** George J. Brewer, *Editor*

Vol 56: **Erythrocyte Membranes 2: Recent Clinical and Experimental Advances,** Walter C. Kruckeberg, John W. Eaton, George J. Brewer, *Editors*

Vol 57: **Progress in Cancer Control,** Curtis Mettlin, Gerald P. Murphy, *Editors*

Vol 58: **The Lymphocyte,** Kenneth W. Sell, William V. Miller, *Editors*

Vol 59: **Eleventh International Congress of Anatomy,** Enrique Acosta Vidrio, *Editor-in-Chief.* Published in 3 volumes: Part A: **Glial and Neuronal Cell Biology,** Sergey Fedoroff, *Editor* Part B: **Advances in the Morphology of Cells and Tissues,** Miguel A. Galina, *Editor* Part C: **Biological Rhythms in Structure and Function,** Heinz von Mayersbach, Lawrence E. Scheving, John E. Pauly, *Editors*

Vol 60: **Advances in Hemoglobin Analysis,** Samir M. Hanash, George J. Brewer, *Editors*

Vol 61: **Nutrition and Child Health: Perspectives for the 1980s,** Reginald C. Tsang, Buford Lee Nichols, Jr., *Editors*

Vol 62: **Pathophysiological Effects of Endotoxins at the Cellular Level,** Jeannine A. Majde, Robert J. Person, *Editors*

Vol 63: **Membrane Transport and Neuroreceptors,** Dale Oxender, Arthur Blume, Ivan Diamond, C. Fred Fox, *Editors*

Vol 64: **Bacteriophage Assembly,** Michael S. DuBow, *Editor*

Vol 65: **Apheresis: Development, Applications, and Collection Procedures,** C. Harold Mielke, Jr., *Editor*

Vol 66: **Control of Cellular Division and Development,** Dennis Cunningham, Eugene Goldwasser, James Watson, C. Fred Fox, *Editors.* Published in 2 volumes.

Vol 67: **Nutrition in the 1980s: Contraints on Our Knowledge,** Nancy Selvey, Philip L. White, *Editors*

Vol 68: **The Role of Peptides and Amino Acids as Neurotransmitters,** J. Barry Lombardini, Alexander D. Kenny, *Editors*

Vol 69: **Twin Research 3, Proceedings of the Third International Congress on Twin Studies,** Ligi Gedda, Paolo Parisi, Walter E. Nance, *Editors.* Published in 3 volumes: Part A: **Twin Biology and Multiple Pregnancy** Part B: **Intelligence, Personality, and Development** Part C: **Epidemiological and Clinical Studies**

Vol 70: **Reproductive Immunology,** Norbert Gleicher, *Editor*

Vol 71: **Psychopharmacology of Clonidine,** Harbans Lal, Stuart Fielding, *Editors*

Vol 72: **Hemophilia and Hemostasis,** Doris Ménaché, D. MacN. Surgenor, Harlan D. Anderson, *Editors*

Vol 73: **Membrane Biophysics: Structure and Function in Epithelia,** Mumtaz A. Dinno, Arthur B. Callahan, *Editors*

Vol 74: **Physiopathology of Endocrine Diseases and Mechanisms of Hormone Action,** Roberto J. Soto, Alejandro De Nicola, Jorge Blaquier, *Editors*

Vol 75: **The Prostatic Cell: Structure and Function,** Gerald P. Murphy, Avery A. Sandberg, James P. Karr, *Editors.* Published in 2 volumes: Part A: **Morphologic, Secretory, and Biochemical Aspects** Part B: **Prolactin, Carcinogenesis, and Clinical Aspects**

Vol 76: **Troubling Problems in Medical Ethics: The Third Volume in a Series on Ethics, Humanism, and Medicine,** Marc D. Basson, Rachel E. Lipson, Doreen L. Ganos, *Editors*

Vol 77: **Nutrition in Health and Disease and International Development: Symposia From the XII International Congress of Nutrition,** Alfred E. Harper, George K. Davis *Editors*

Vol 78: **Female Incontinence,** Norman R. Zinner, Arthur M. Sterling, *Editors*

Vol 79: **Proteins in the Nervous System: Structure and Function,** Bernard Haber, Jose Regino Perez-Polo, Joe Dan Coulter, *Editors*

Vol 80: **Mechanism and Control of Ciliary Movement,** Charles J. Brokaw, Pedro Verdugo, *Editors*

Vol 81: **Physiology and Biology of Horseshoe Crabs: Studies on Normal and Environmentally Stressed Animals,** Joseph Bonaventura, Celia Bonaventura, Shirley Tesh, *Editors*

Vol 82: **Clinical, Structural, and Biochemical Advances in Hereditary Eye Disorders,** Donna L. Daentl, *Editor*

Vol 83: **Issues in Cancer Screening and Communications,** Curtis Mettlin, Gerald P. Murphy, *Editors*

Vol 84: **Progress in Dermatoglyphic Research,** Christos S. Bartsocas, *Editor*

Vol 85: **Embryonic Development,** Max M. Burger, Rudolf Weber, *Editors.* Published in 2 volumes: Part A: **Genetic Aspects** Part B: **Cellular Aspects**

Vol 86: **The Interaction of Acoustical and Electromagnetic Fields With Biological Systems,** Shiro Takashima, Elliot Postow, *Editors*

Vol 87: **Physiopathology of Hypophysial Disturbances and Diseases of Reproduction,** Alejandro De Nicola, Jorge Blaquier, Roberto J. Soto, *Editors*

Vol 88: **Cytapheresis and Plasma Exchange: Clinical Indications,** W.R. Vogler, *Editor*

Vol 89: **Interaction of Platelets and Tumor Cells,** G.A. Jamieson, *Editor*

Vol 90: **Beta-Carbolines and Tetrahydroisoquinolines,** Floyd Bloom, Jack Barchas, Merton Sandler, Earl Usdin, *Organizers*

Vol 91: **Membranes in Growth and Development,** Joseph F. Hoffman, Gerhard H. Giebisch, Liana Bolis, *Editors*

Vol 92: **The Pineal and Its Hormones,** Russel J. Reiter, *Editor*

Vol 93: **Endotoxins and Their Detection With the Limulus Amebocyte Lysate Test,** Stanley W. Watson, Jack Levin, Thomas J. Novitsky, *Editors*

Vol 94: **Animal Models of Inherited Metabolic Diseases,** Robert J. Desnick, Donald F. Patterson, Dante G. Scarpelli, *Editors*

Vol 95: **Gaucher Disease: A Century of Delineation and Research,** Robert J. Desnick, Shimon Gatt, Gregory A. Grabowski, *Editors*

Vol 96: **Mechanisms of Speciation,** Claudio Barigozzi, *Editor*